DIFFERENTIATING NURSING PRACTICE

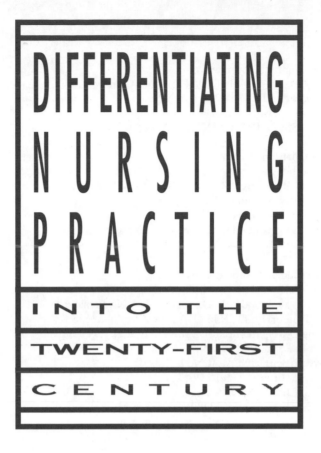

DIFFERENTIATING NURSING PRACTICE

INTO THE
TWENTY-FIRST
CENTURY

SELECTED PAPERS
FROM THE
18TH ANNUAL MEETING AND 1990 CONFERENCE
OF THE AMERICAN ACADEMY OF NURSING

OCTOBER 14-15, 1990
CHARLESTON, SOUTH CAROLINA

EDITED BY
IRMA E. GOERTZEN, M.S., R.N., F.A.A.N.

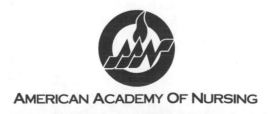

AMERICAN ACADEMY OF NURSING

Conference Planning Committee
Irma E. Goertzen, M.S., R.N., F.A.A.N., Chairperson
Nola J. Pender, Ph.D., R.N., F.A.A.N.
Laura Skeggs, M.S., R.N.
Gloria R. Smith, Ph.D., R.N., F.A.A.N.

AAN Staff to Planning Committee
Office of the American Academy of Nursing:
Lyndall D. Eddy, M.P.A., R.N., CAE, Administrator
Dorothy A. Young, Staff Specialist
Gloria Diaz Garver, Staff Assistant
ANA Staff Consultant to Planning Committee:
Sharon R. Lunn, M.S., R.N.

**American Academy of Nursing Governing
Council (1989-90)**
Nancy Fugate Woods, Ph.D., R.N., F.A.A.N., President
Nola J. Pender, Ph.D., R.N., F.A.A.N., President-Elect
Suzanne Lee Feetham, Ph.D., R.N., F.A.A.N., Secretary
Patricia R. Forni, Ph.D., R.N., F.A.A.N., Treasurer
Beverly A. Benfer, M.A., R.N., F.A.A.N.
Dorothy A. Brooten, Ph.D., R.N., F.A.A.N.
Peggy L. Chinn, Ph.D., R.N., F.A.A.N.
Constance R. Curran, Ed.D., R.N., F.A.A.N.
Joanne C. McCloskey, Ph.D., R.N., F.A.A.N.
Grayce M. Sills, Ph.D., R.N., F.A.A.N.

The American Academy of Nursing was established in 1973 under the aegis of the American Nurses Association.

ISBN 1-55810-065-2

Published by
American Academy of Nursing
2420 Pershing Road
Kansas City, Missouri 64108

G-182   2.5M   10/91

The 1990 Conference
on

Differentiating Nursing Practice: Into the Twenty-First Century

was sponsored by

American Academy of Nursing
and
American Nurses Association
in collaboration with
American Organization of Nurse Executives

Statement of Purpose

To examine differentiated nursing practice within the context of future projections for health care and nursing as the basis for designing cost-effective nursing systems.

Contents

Preface

"A nurse is a nurse is a nurse." This phrase has been quoted for a number of years, but we all now know that it is true.

During the last three decades, the professional organizations, the specialty nursing organizations, the educational institutions, and the practice settings all have sought to define not only professional nursing, but also the roles of the various nursing practitioners in today's health care environment. Consequently, it was timely and appropriate for the American Academy of Nursing and the American Nurses Association, in conjunction with the American Organization of Nurse Executives, to sponsor an October 1990 conference titled "Differentiating Nursing Practice: Into the Twenty-First Century." The conference's stated purpose was "to examine differentiated nursing practice within the context of future projections for health care and nursing as the basis for designing cost-effective nursing systems."

The content of the conference was devised to give nursing leaders information about current models of differentiated practice, as well as educational approaches that would help prepare them for differing practitioner roles. Strategies for evaluation and documentation of the models were also presented.

This book, dedicated to the proceedings from the conference, examines models of differentiated practice currently being developed or already in operation. Several papers address the evolution and outcome of differentiated nursing practice. Nursing theories and their application to practice are herein made available to the nurse leader for the development of organizational practice models.

Many thanks are due to the conference presenters for their time and unflagging energy. The information they provided stimulated active dialogues, discussions, questions, and creative problem-solving throughout the meetings. Participants left not only with new ideas, but also with specific challenges to pursue, such as the question of how nursing will contribute to the public welfare during the next century.

It is equally important to recognize the members of the planning committee: Nola Pender, PhD, RN, FAAN; Laura Skaggs, MS, RN; and Gloria Smith, PhD, RN, FAAN, who took differentiated practice — a concept not widely understood or accepted — and transformed it into a successful conference topic.

The support of the American Nurses Association (ANA) and the American Organization of Nurse Executives (AONE) as conference co-sponsors is greatly appreciated, with special thanks going to Sharon Lunn, MS, RN, ANA senior staff specialist, educational services, and Carol Boston, MS, RN, AONE executive director. The active support of the American Academy of Nursing staff — Lyndall D. Eddy, MPA, RN, CAE, administrator; Dorothy A. Young, staff specialist; and Gloria Diaz Garver, staff assistant — is gratefully acknowledged. Mollie A. Robinson, ANA publications manager, also merits special recognition and appreciation.

IRMA E. GOERTZEN M.S., R.N., F.A.A.N.
Chairperson, Planning Committee

Introduction

Margaret L. McClure, Ed.D., R.N., F.A.A.N.

T he concept of differentiated nursing practice has become increasingly visible in both our literature and our thinking. The term means different things to different people, yet it is a natural concern for a profession whose work is carried out by such a widely diverse group of individuals — diverse in terms of educational preparation, knowledge, and skill.

On an informal basis, differentiated practice among registered nurses exists in every setting. Nurses, physicians, and patients have always differentiated nurses by their demonstrated competence. The concept is effected each time a head nurse plans a staffing schedule so that there is an appropriate mix of individuals on any given tour of duty at any point in time (Koerner, 1990). Similarly, physicians and patients develop a sixth sense about the abilities of the nurses with whom they interact, which greatly affects their actions and responses.

Differentiated practice had its formal origins in World War II, when a shortage of nurses in civilian hospitals led to the creation of assistive roles — namely, practical nurses and nursing assistants. Once the war was over, and the need for nurses did not abate, these position titles were institutionalized. It was clear that they represented more than a temporary solution to a short-term problem. Throughout the remainder of the twentieth century, the education and utilization of these two distinct assistive levels has gradually become more formal and codified.

Of course, the current discussion of differentiated practice presented herein surpasses any concern for these assistive roles. The

1

roots of our dialogue and debates today are, instead, deeply embed-
ded in the "entry into practice" issue. This paper, therefore, will be
confined to an examination of the concepts and considerations of
differentiated practice as they relate to current and future individuals practicing as registered and/or professional nurses.

Before embarking on a discussion of differentiated practice, it is
appropriate to examine the role and functions of the nurse in some
detail. These topics can then form the context for our discussion.

For several years, I have been developing theories about the
nurse's two-fold role. In one role, the nurse is a caregiver; in the
other, an integrator. The caregiver is the role most of us consider to
be basic to nursing practice. It includes a number of functions
designed to meet the following patient needs:

- Dependency (hygiene, nutrition, safety, etc.).
- Comfort (both physical and psychological).
- Education (including coping mechanisms).
- Therapeutic (medications and other treatments). [Tech-
  nology is introduced within this category. This factor
  requires substantial attention, for its complexity is increasing at a staggering pace and has come to represent a clear
  and present danger to patients in all settings. For this
  reason, technology is often a critical and objective variable
  in determining both patient acuity and the level of staff
  expertise required to render care.]
- Monitoring (collecting, interpreting, and acting on
  patient data).

The foregoing categories are somewhat hierarchical in terms of
the knowledge and skill levels required. Thus, assistive and/or less
expert personnel are better able to meet dependency and comfort
needs than therapeutic and monitoring needs. Further, the categories are not mutually exclusive.

In many respects, the true measure of the nurse's expertise is
taken within the area of monitoring, which requires the most knowledge and judgement. The functions within this category require the
ability to interpret a patient's signs and symptoms that indicate
whether he/she is following the normal trajectory for recovery or
whether he/she is deviating from the norm. Obviously, much of the
data collection is part of the tasks and activities performed within
the other four categories. Thus, a task as mundane as a bath can
provide an opportunity to observe important changes in a patient's

2

condition that might otherwise go undetected. The more expert the nurse, the better able he/she is to identify the subtle, often insidious signs and symptoms of problems that require further medical attention.

The monitoring function is not a passive one; rather, it entails the responsibility to act — or to see that others act — appropriately in response to the data presented. This implies that the nurse has the requisite knowledge to determine what interventions are needed and to see that such interventions are provided in a timely fashion. The responsibility for one's own actions is understood; the responsibility to oversee the actions of others is less well understood and is certainly, in many situations, more difficult to achieve. It is, however, a logical and essential component of the monitoring function (Benner, 1984).

In many respects, it is the monitoring function that links the caregiver role to the integrator role. The term *integrator*, in this context, has been coined by Lawrence and Lorsch (1967), two organizational theorists who have studied complex organizations extensively. By definition, such organizations consist of a large number of highly specialized departments — each of which becomes a sort of subculture, capable of developing its own values and norms — somewhat divorced from the larger organization and its goals. Lawrence and Lorsch have labeled this process *differentiation*. They have observed that complex organizations must develop a complementary process, which they call *integration*, in order for the work or output of the differentiated departments to come together and create a product. They further indicate that in each organization responsibility for this integration falls to one particular position which, by nature of its placement in the structure, has the knowledge to perform as the integrator. Lawrence and Lorsch perceive this role to be an extremely powerful one.

It is clear that, regardless of the setting, nurses have always played the integrator role. What Lawrence and Lorsch have defined is not a new function, but rather a new description of a responsibility nurses have assumed since Nightingale's time. By virtue of the moment-to-moment knowledge requirement, the nurse is the only person able to carry out this responsibility. In a hospital, this means integrating each department's contribution — interacting with individuals of varying skill, from the maintenance worker to the physician — and doing so on a routine as well as emergency basis. It also

3

involves a concern for integrating services that is well beyond the bounds of the institution.

It is my belief that we have long undervalued the integrator responsibility, viewing it more as an interruption or unnecessary nuisance than as a vitally important component of the nursing function. It is impossible to conceive of nursing practice that does not include integration activity; therefore, we need to better understand and appreciate its centrality to our care of patients. Excellent nursing practice must involve expertise in both the integrator and caregiver subsets.

Differentiated practice has been defined as "a philosophy that focuses on the structuring of roles and functions of nurses according to education, experience, and competence" (Boston, 1990). In keeping with this, Koerner (1990) would add that such a philosophy embodies differentiated sets of values, beliefs, attitudes, and behaviors.

Beyond the definition, it is important to consider the various rationales for such an approach. First, differentiated practice, if carried out properly, can serve to improve patient care and contribute to patient safety. Second, there is the benefit to be gained from a structure that enables the most effective and efficient utilization of scarce resources — a significant goal, considering the state of the economy and the continuing shortage of professional nurses. Third, there is the opportunity to provide increased satisfaction for nurses themselves as they are better able to optimize their practice. Encompassed within both notions of the effective utilization of resources and increased satisfaction for practitioners is the final rationale — namely, the opportunity to compensate nurses fairly based on their expertise, contribution, and productivity.

While the definition and rationales for differentiated practice can be presented somewhat simply, several rather complex issues remain that need to be addressed and clarified. The first centers around the key variables upon which practice should be differentiated. There are two major approaches suggested in the literature.

The most common view is that educational preparation should be the differentiating factor (Hawken, 1990; Joel, 1990; Koerner, 1990; Primm, 1990). Taking this approach, the MAIN project, headed by Peggy Primm, has done extensive and impressive work in this area. Beginning with accepted ADN and BSN competencies, the project has developed job specifications which are being tested in several practice settings (Primm, 1990).

4

The second major differentiating variable that has been described is demonstrated clinical competence. Although it was not the specific intent of her research, the seminal contribution to the conceptual basis for this approach was made by Benner (1984) in her important study, *From Novice to Expert*. In it, she defines five levels of practitioner — novice, advanced beginner, competent, proficient, and expert. In doing so, she makes a case for these empirically derived stages of growth and levels of practice. Many others have taken a more applied approach to this idea and conceived and implemented clinical ladders designed specifically to differentiate and reward varying levels of clinical practice (Deckert et al., 1984, Durio et al., 1986; Hesterly and Sebilia, 1986; Kneedler et al., 1987; Murphy and DeBack, 1990; Sanford, 1987).

On closer examination, it becomes clear that these two methods of differentiating variables (i.e., education versus demonstrated competence) are a function of a far deeper difference. According to Primm (1990), "Differentiated nursing practice is a philosophical construct addressing the multiple levels of educational preparation for and the *resulting* multilevel conceptual framework of nursing as a practice."

Clearly, Primm's point of view is that practice levels should be designed to reflect educational levels. But is that as it should be? Is it not more appropriate for education to be defined by practice? It would seem that a practice model can only succeed if it uses patient needs as its basis and is congruent with the role and functions that fulfill those needs. Thus, while educators need to play a role of visionary leadership in the development of nursing practice, the basis for direction must come from the substance of that practice. It may well be that many of the problems concerning the definition of differentiated practice have stemmed from the failure to connect patient needs with practice models.

Aside from the question of differentiating variables, there is another important conceptual issue to be examined — namely, the way in which the several differentiated practices fit together to form the whole. Interestingly enough, this question arises only if one uses basic education as the differentiating variable. The early developmental years of the technical/professional practice approach fostered many differences of opinion concerning this matter and, while much of that controversy has died down, some issues remain unresolved.

I have found Venn diagrams to be most useful in describing the concept in question. The two points of view under consideration stipulate that, on one hand, the practice role of the ADN-level nurse is distinct from that of the BSN-level nurse. The possibility for advancement from novice to expert is possible within each level (Koerner, 1990). This is called the collegial model (Figure 1-a). The other point of view is that ADN practice is a subset of the larger BSN role (Joel, 1990; McClure, 1976; Primm, 1990), and can be labeled as the delegated model (Figure 1-b). Most of the nurse leaders working in this area have agreed on the delegated model, but we must be absolutely clear about this concept, as it seriously affects differentiated practice. The first view creates two independent practices; the second maintains a single scope of practice.

The foregoing leads me to conclude that a differentiated practice model should be built on levels of demonstrated competence — i.e., the clinical ladder approach. This idea is actually more compatible with the ADN/BSN practice levels than it might appear at first. Given the fact that all types of education in nursing today are competency-based (Primm, 1987), differentiation according to educational preparation would appear to occur *de facto* in the practice arena, based on the levels of competency demonstrated by various graduates.

Clearly, this has been the experience in the South Dakota experiment, the single most important trial that has attempted to approximate the education-based model (Koerner, 1990). Moreover, the competency-based approach is one that allows for and, more importantly, encourages and rewards the professional growth of the individual nurse. In light of the fact that large numbers of A.D.N. and diploma nurses continue their education, their continued development can reflect their work situation as they demonstrate new competencies. The model, therefore, is designed to match practice progress with educational progress, and can be conceptualized as a series of increasingly large concentric circles (Figure 2).

It also is interesting to consider initiating the competency-based model in such a way that it extends beyond the direct caregiver levels into the management realm. Benner (1984) has pointed out that, "Providing patient care involves risks for both nurse and patient." I believe that, in most settings, we have the potential to provide a safety net for the less expert nurses and their patients through the supervisory structure that is already in place. Unfortunately, in too many agencies, first line and middle managers are chosen for their administrative abilities rather than their clinical expertise. Moreover, once appointed, many of these supervisors are so bogged down by administrative responsibilities that whatever clinical skills they have are not fully utilized to the benefit of their staff and patients. We must reverse this trend and insist that the primary responsibility of these managers is to demonstrate effective leadership in nursing practice.

Of course, the clinical ladder itself needs to be structured for the direct caregivers in such a way that oversight and mentoring of juniors by seniors becomes an expectation and even a criterion for promotion. At New York University Medical Center, a clinical ladder has been in place for the past 23 years. Part of our success in delivering high-quality care to patients is due to the fact that nurses are promoted not only for their clinical skills, but also for their willingness and ability to share their knowledge with less expert nurses and with students.

Widespread implementation of differentiated practice will not be easy to achieve. We need to consider the social, political, and economic forces that we must confront if we are committed to making the concept a reality.

Undoubtedly, the most important issue is that of supply and demand. It is probably safe to say that the shortage of professional nurses in the United States today is well understood by almost every citizen. Depending on the strategy used, this single factor of supply and demand could make or break our efforts. The rationale that has proved most successful in selling the concept of clinical ladders over the years is its effect on nurse satisfaction and retention of staff in agencies and institutions. This fact has been demonstrated in several studies (McClure et al., 1983; McKibbin, 1990). One hospital recently reported that following the introduction of differentiated practice on two pilot units, turnover rates were greatly reduced (on one unit the rate fell from 68% to 32%). Recruitment dramatically improved and the use of supplemental staffing decreased by more than 50% (Malloch, Milton, and Jobes, 1990).

In considering supply and demand, we also need to give careful attention to the data regarding credentialing. It has been reported that 76% of the RNs currently delivering care in clinical settings hold associate degrees or are diploma-prepared (Joel, 1990). Add to that statistic the fact that baccalaureate graduates are not evenly distributed in all geographic areas and it becomes evident that some settings will experience more difficulty than others in implementing differentiated practice.

In the end, each institution or agency needs to evaluate their own circumstances as they develop the criteria and job descriptions for their various differentiated levels. To do otherwise would result in models that would be, at best, unrealistic.

A second highly important factor to be addressed is that of economics. The introduction of differentiated practice levels in most health care settings in this country will come with a very high price tag amounting to millions of dollars for the average agency. We will need to make a strong cost/benefit argument if we are to succeed. Obviously, one positive factor will be the savings in recruitment and retention mentioned earlier. Productivity needs to be emphasized as well, especially when almost all industries are developing pay-for-performance approaches (French, 1988).

Another economic factor is that health care has become so highly regulated in recent years that in some parts of the country individual institutions are virtually unable to change salaries without permission. On the positive side, however, one hospital in Denver reported that the creation of a competency-based clinical ladder actually caused their rate-setting commission to approve a salary increase for nurses — the selling point being that the increases would not be given to all practitioners automatically (Kneedler et al., 1987).

The management implications for differentiated practice also require our attention. In each agency, the standards for promotions, job descriptions, and titles will need to gain wide acceptance both within and outside of nursing — creating an opportunity for strong participative management. Staff members are generally enthusiastic about the notion of a clinical advancement opportunity and will contribute immeasurably to the development of a plan that will best fit the setting. Further, the model must be clear and logical enough to gain acceptance from the non-nurse influentials important to its success.

A differentiated practice initiative will only be successful if it is accompanied by a carefully conceived staff development program designed to foster the growth of individual practitioners from their earliest novice days. One very important benefit to a clinical ladder is that it allows beginning nurses to start out with realistic expectations — a benefit that can support them in their earliest, and perhaps most important, developmental phase.

Obviously, those institutions with collective bargaining units in place will have the most difficulty implementing competency-based differentiated practice. Traditionally, unions have rejected any compensation programs based on management and/or peer assessment, preferring instead to have all rewards determined by seniority. Unfortunately, units comprised of registered nurses, even those represented by the professional associations, have proven to be no different. In those settings, it will require dedicated time, effort, and close work with the unions to make differentiated practice a reality.

In discussing the social, political, and economic issues, I have purposefully avoided the suggestion that we study the impact of differentiated practice on the quality of patient care. This should not be construed to mean that such an impact will not occur, but rather that such a claim is extraordinarily difficult to prove. Just as we were unable to prove our educational ideas related to the quality outcome issue, we will have equal difficulty proving that differentiated practice will have a positive clinical effect. Substantiating our convictions regarding improved quality of care could easily divert us from accomplishing our more important goal.

In the final analysis, differentiated practice has been slow in coming to nursing and is long overdue. Practice in recent decades has been marked by dramatically increased responsibilities related to an explosion of phenomenal knowledge in all areas of health care. One can only predict that this pace will continue, making the advancement from novice to expert increasingly difficult. Concomitantly, clinical expertise will be of greater value to both patients and health care institutions. It will take real commitment and a great deal of perseverance to make differentiated practice a reality, but I believe that it is a cause worthy of our best and most creative efforts.

❏ ❏ ❏

Figure 1
Education-Based Differentiated Practice

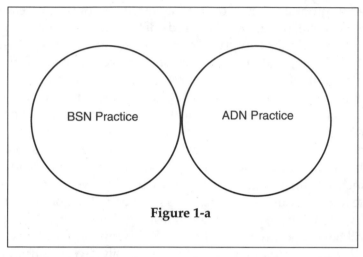

BSN Practice   ADN Practice

Figure 1-a

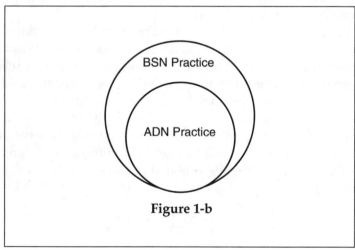

BSN Practice

ADN Practice

Figure 1-b

Figure 2
Competency-Based Differentiated Practice

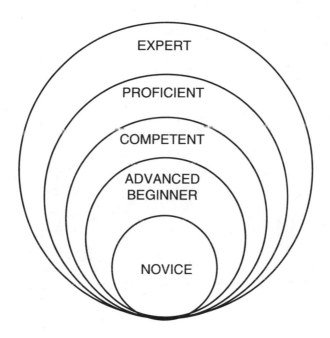

PART I

Differentiated Practice
and the
Health Care Crisis Today

The Crisis of the Health Care Nonsystem

Pamela H. Mitchell, M.S., A.R.N.P., F.A.A.N.
Janelle C. Krueger, Ph.D., R.N., F.A.A.N.
Linda E. Moody, Ph.D., R.N.,C., F.A.A.N.

Although American policymakers agree about little else, they concur that a crisis exists in the provision of health care in the United States. Costs are rising exponentially, indicators of the national health (such as infant mortality and life expectancy) are not changing in relation to these expenditures, and 37 million Americans are without health insurance. Proposals to deal with these problems range from providing state-subsidized insurance to select uninsured citizens, to completely nationalizing the provision of health care.

The basic problem is not simply that providers charge too much, or that health care consumers are not discriminating enough, or that access is differentially distributed among economic and social classes. More fundamentally, the system by which health care is provided in the United States is not a system at all. It is a patchwork of categorical approaches to providing health care (and limited personal medical care) to certain segments of the public, and personal curative and palliative medical care to others. Health care is more than medical treatment of disease, but our current approach to the "health care crisis" emphasizes curative therapy, promotes a disintegration of true health care services, and exacerbates the symptoms

The authors are members of Workgroup I, American Academy of Nursing. They are indebted to Gloria Smith, Patricia Benner, and Sheila Ryan for review and critique of this paper.

of what is truly a systemic crisis. In this paper, we will explore the symptoms of the crisis, analyze the likely impact of currently proposed solutions, and discuss the critical importance of an active nursing presence in the national dialogue.

The Crisis of Health Care in a Fragmenting Society

T. H. Huxley said that the most tragic event in science is the slaying of a beautiful theory by an ugly fact (Dossey, 1982). The theory is that ours is the best medical care system in the world. Yet a number of undeniable societal facts bring us to the realization that our health care system is in disarray, and that a transformation must occur. Among those facts facing the United States are the following:

- Our natural environment, upon which human and plant life are dependent for air, water and food, has been seriously damaged by overpopulation and industrial technology.
- Nutritional and infectious diseases, as well as the disorders of civilization in the form of cancer, alcoholism, and suicide, are increasing.
- Lack of attention to the problems of the chronically mentally ill has become a national scandal.
- Social disintegration — manifested by violent crime, alcoholism, drug abuse, accidents, and suicides — is increasing, along with the numbers of children with learning disabilities and behavioral disorders.
- The United States spends nearly three times as much per person for health care as does our nearest neighbor, Canada — yet has higher death and infant mortality rates.
- The economy is destabilized from ever-increasing inflation, variable employment opportunities, and uneven distribution of income and resources (including access to health care).

More disturbing facts specifically symptomatic of the crisis in the provision of sickness care can be categorized in terms of cost, access, and quality.

Costs

The costs of both institutional and outpatient medical care have risen in all industrialized countries since the end of World War II, but the United States has the dubious distinction of spending a larger share of its gross national product (GNP) on such care than any other nation (Schrieber and Pouillier, 1987). In 1989, we spent $600 billion on health care, or 11.5% of the GNP. At the current rate of increase (10.4% per year), it is estimated that health care spending will reach 15% of the GNP by the turn of the century (Kimball, 1990; Division of National Cost Estimates, 1987). While cost-containment efforts have reduced the rate of increase for hospital expenditures, outpatient and other noninstitutional spending continues to rise at a rate of 15% per year (National Center for Health Statistics, 1985), with the rate of increase doubling for private health insurance costs (Health Insurance Premiums to Soar in '89, 1988).

Providers and insured consumers have largely been insulated from these rising costs because increases in the price of care were passed on to willing payers by insurance companies and the federal government. However, the payers are becoming increasingly alarmed at the size of their bills and have instituted a variety of measures of cost containment, such as prospective payment, coinsurance, higher deductibles, etc. Further, insurers have markedly increased the premiums for private insurance. Business and industry, who have faced increases in premiums of 30-40% over the past year, are concerned about their ability to continue to provide the health care benefits that workers have come to expect (Can You Afford to Get Sick?, 1989).

Access

Despite the considerable private and public expenditures for health care in the United States, significant portions of the population have limited access to such care. A variety of factors, such as geographic, financial, and attitudinal barriers, may affect accessibility.

Geographic Barriers. Geographic barriers exist when a population is located far from a source of health care, as in many rural areas. Cost can exacerbate geographic barriers through market factors. As the movement to contain costs of hospital care gains momentum, small hospitals providing illness care to rural areas become less and less financially secure. That lack of viability is reflected in the high rate of hospital closures in small, often rural, hospitals (Murphy and McNeil, 1986).

Financial Barriers. Financial barriers to accessible health care occur when people lack funds to pay for personal, acute, and chronic care. The number of United States residents with adequate public or private medical insurance coverage is decreasing. Although the number of people covered by private hospital insurance rose rapidly from the 1940s through the 1970s, it peaked in 1980 with a high of 83%. This trend has reversed during the past decade, with only 75.7% of the population covered in 1987, and an estimated 37 million having no insurance at all (Health Insurance Association of America, 1989; U.S. Bureau of the Census, 1989).

It is likely that this trend toward decreasing private insurance coverage will continue due to changes in the job market. Part-time and service industry jobs, which provide little or no health insurance, are increasing while the manufacturing and transportation jobs that traditionally provided full insurance coverage are decreasing (Hudson Institute, 1987).

Private insurance is not the sole source of financial access to medical care. An additional 9.3% of the U.S. population is covered by Medicaid, federally funded and administered through cost sharing with individual states. While Medicaid was instituted to improve access to health care for the poor, recent federal budget cuts have drastically reduced the number of indigent persons actually served by this program of federally funded "insurance." While the number of persons living below the federally-established poverty level has grown by nearly one-third since 1978, the number of Medicaid recipients has remained stable. This stabilization is largely due to tighter eligibility requirements, so that individuals or families must be much "poorer" in relation to the poverty level than ever before (Curtis, 1986; Darling, 1986; Oberg and Polich, 1988).

In addition to Medicaid, the federal government administers three other forms of medical care payments: 1) CHAMPUS (Civilian Health and Medical Program of the Uniformed Services) for dependents of military personnel, 2) Medicare for those over 65 and other selected groups (for example, those with terminal renal disease), and 3) Veterans Administration benefits. Taken together, these private and public forms of coverage provide at least some aspects of care for approximately 86% of Americans (Health Insurance Association of America, 1989).

Those with combined forms of public and private coverage differ in respect to the services covered. Thus, they may have selective financial barriers to services many consider to be basic health care. For example, prenatal care and well-child care are often excluded from "basic" insurance packages (Alan Guttmacher Institute, 1987; Hughes et al., 1989).

Lacking any kind of health insurance is the most obvious financial barrier to access to health care. The percentage of those without insurance has been steadily increasing since 1970, with as many as 37 million currently estimated to have no insurance. Twelve million of these are children (Anderson et al., 1987; Sloan, Blumstein, and Perrin, 1988; Health Insurance Association of America, 1989; Hughes et al., 1989). Only 18% of the uninsured are unemployed workers or their dependents. The remainder are part-time or full-time workers and their dependents (34% and 48%, respectively), whose employers do not offer health insurance. Estimates of the "underinsured" (those with some insurance but who would face severe financial hardship or even ruin with a major illness) range from 8-26% of the insured. These uninsured and underinsured are less likely than the adequately insured to seek preventive care or early attention to existing health problems. Together, these two groups are estimated to account for approximately 27% of the U.S. population, or nearly 56 million people (Senate Special Committee on Aging, 1985; Farley, 1984).

In the past, the costs of care for the uninsured medically indigent were borne by providers through the practice of cross-subsidization — increasing the price for the insured to create a "fund" available for uncompensated care. Such practices are nearly impossible in a truly competitive environment employing cost-containment measures such as prospective payment. Thus, the costs of uncompensated care are borne directly by the providers, and can threaten the economic viability of providers who either have traditionally provided large amounts of "charity care" or who are geographically located so as to attract large numbers of the medically indigent. Economic failure of these providers and institutions threatens to further reduce access to care for the medically indigent (Bazzoli, 1986; Onek, 1988).

Attitudinal Barriers. Attitudinal barriers to accessible health care have traditionally linked beliefs and attitudes about the efficacy of health care, or cultural differences between provider and client that are barriers to communication. This analysis will set aside this traditional view. Instead, it will focus on political attitudes and beliefs about what constitutes health care as significant barriers to integrating the patchwork system and providing true *health* — as opposed to sickness — care.

Although we call it health care insurance, the majority of public and private plans that compensate individuals for the costs of care do so for episodes of disease, sickness, or health care visits that can be forced into a category of disease. A true health care system would encompass the promotion of health as well as prevention, treatment, and rehabilitation from disease. As Milio (1983, 1989) has eloquently pointed out, a true health care system would use a "health-promoting, public policy strategy" and would integrate social factors, such as adequate housing and nutrition, that affect the development of disease, with the long-term support and personal services required by chronic illness. Attitudes that reify diagnostic and curative technology for acute disease serve to perpetuate a patchwork system and act as a strong barrier to integrating health and sickness care. Further, the common tendency to define health promotion in terms of prevention or early detection of specific diseases perpetuates the medicalization of health care. It identifies health-promoting activities as marketplace commodities, and relegates the promotion of community and societal health to outside the "health care system."

Quality

The third symptom of the crisis in our patchwork nonsystem is widespread dissatisfaction with health quality indicators, despite huge expenditures for sickness care. *Quality* is used here to mean indices of health (or sickness) outcome, rather than indices of delivery system structures, processes, or effective outcome (such as satisfaction with care).

There is no question that the poorest overall health status exists among those with the least financial access to care — namely, the poor and the near poor. Infant mortality rates in the U.S. are among the worst in the world, "rivaling those of the Third World" (National Commission to Prevent Infant Mortality, 1990). While the overall infant mortality rate has fallen since 1950, the decline has been much slower for blacks, and is still double the rate for whites. Further, the rates for nonwhites who also are less likely to have adequate access to prenatal care began to rise in the 1980s (Hughes et al., 1989). Infant mortality is related to very low birth weight, for which late or no prenatal care is the strongest predictor. Financial and geographic barriers to access are the primary factors contributing to late or no prenatal care in the United States (Institute of Medicine, 1985; 1988).

Low-income and uninsured Americans perceive their overall state of health to be worse than those with higher incomes, and have a higher prevalence of chronic disease such as hypertension, hearing impairment, heart disease, and stroke. Days of disability in bed also are higher for racial minorities and low- income families (Bayer, Caplan, and Daniels, 1983; Kaspar, 1986). Finally, our overall death rate and infant mortality rates exceed those of our Canadian neighbors, who have an equally diverse population but an integrated health care system. These facts have resulted in a situation in which nine out of 10 Americans polled want fundamental changes in the health care system, with seven times as many Americans as Canadians perceiving that financial barriers prevent them from receiving needed medical care (Blendon and Taylor, 1988).

What Are the Solutions?

Taken together, these serious problems of cost, access, and quality have led many observers to agree with Himmelstein and Woolhandler (1989): "Our health care system is failing. It denies access to many in need and is expensive, inefficient, and increasingly bureaucratic."

Although the problems of cost and access to health care have become increasingly severe in recent years, they have been concerns for the better part of this century, with some form of national or universal health insurance recurrently proposed. A similar sense of crisis led to the passage of the Social Security Act of 1935, which came close to including national health insurance. Since 1935, numerous bills have been introduced into nearly every Congressional session, but only Medicare (enacted in 1965) has become law, providing an entitlement for the aged.

The strongest support for a national system came in the 1970s, when a crisis in medical care costs and access was once again declared. The human rights movement sparked the claim for health care as a basic right. Proponents recognized that satisfying that claim required a structural reform if costs were to be controlled (Starr, 1982). These proposals included expansion of Medicare to additional groups, as well as a nationally operated health system similar to Great Britain's. However, interest faded as organized medicine and the insurance industry formed opposition to any kind of nationalized health system. The proposal, which failed, was changed from advocating universal health care to categorical insurance coverage for all workers (Starr, 1982; Koch, 1988).

Regarding this latest crisis, Relman (1989) published two distinct proposals, declaring that the time has finally arrived for universal health insurance. The Enthoven-Kronick plan is market-oriented, based on controlling costs through private competitive managed-care plans. Universal access would be created by a sliding scale subsidy of premiums through employers and governments (Enthoven and Kronick, 1989). The second proposal is representative of social justice-based plans similar to the Canadian system that provide universal insurance administered locally and funded by the federal government (Himmelstein, Woolhandler, and the Writing Committee, 1989).

These plans, as well as numerous others, are surfacing at the state and federal level, and serve to stimulate and focus dialogue regarding the future of financing health care. However, the more they focus on providing insurance for sickness care, the more they divert attention from the real problem: lack of integration in components of a true health care system. Providing hospital insurance to cover the hundreds of thousands of dollars required to care for a 1200-gram infant will not help create a system that provides adequate preventive prenatal care to women who cannot find providers. Nor does the answer lie in setting up large market-oriented clinics providing three to five minutes of time per client. Insuring the costs of after-the-fact sickness does nothing to provide preventive care. Current proposals are couched in what Milio calls "health services, illness-control policy." According to Milio (1983), what is needed is a "health-promoting, public policy strategy."

Nursing's Opportunity to Lead a Transformation of Health Care

Our current pattern of care distinguishes health care from personal sickness care. This distinction was deliberately made to maintain control over personal services by practitioners of medicine. It has resulted in our being the only country in the world in which public health is considered to be a separate entity from "health care" (i.e., curative and palliative medical care). Nursing bridges both kinds of care, but to the public it is a force relatively indistinguishable from medicine.

The United States, a democratic country committed to free enterprise, has invested heavily in a physician-controlled system of disease care that depends on technology and a hard-science model of medicine. With 12% of our gross national product being spent for health care, the health of our people does not seem to be improving — possibly because the model has become outmoded, expensive, and ineffective.

Why Now?

A number of authors view these facts as globally interdependent aspects of the same crisis — trying to apply concepts of an outdated mechanistic world view based on Cartesian-Newtonian science to a reality that no longer supports these concepts (Capra, 1982; Dossey, 1982; Ferguson, 1987; Harman, 1977). Toynbee (1972) notes that the genesis of civilizations follows a pattern of "challenged response." After reaching a peak of vitality, civilizations tend to lose their cultural flexibility and decline. A challenge from the physical or social environment can provoke a society to reverse such a decline.

Capra (1982) believes that we are at the confluence of three transitions — the decline of patriarchy, the decline of fossil fuel, and a shift to a belief that the "scientific method" as the only valid approach to knowledge needs radical revision. Of the three, the "most profound transition is due to the slow and reluctant but inevitable decline of patriarchy" (Capra, 1982). We are now at that turning point.

Why Nursing?

At least since the time of Florence Nightingale's contributions in the 1860s, if not before, nursing has espoused a holistic approach to care that integrates the person, the nurse as caregiver (rather than curer), society/environment, and health. [See Meleis, 1985, for an historical overview of these themes.] Outside the realm of nursing, others have proposed radical changes in the technological paradigm. Ferguson (1980) states that, "We have oversold the benefits of technology and external manipulations; we have undersold the importance of human relationships and the complexity of nature." She contrasts the assumptions of the old paradigm of medicine with the new paradigm of health. The latter describes a "holistic" or qualitatively different approach that "respects the interaction of mind, body, and environment." Others, educated within the traditional

23

biomedical approach, are suggesting the need for considerable departure from the existing model. The new view of health is socially defined, emphasizing care more than curative features (Dossey, 1982; Callahan, 1990). Nursing's century-old message is being spread and revivified.

The resurgence of interest in universal health insurance presents an opportunity to restructure health care, not merely to provide insurance. It provides a window of opportunity for nursing to be an active player in redesigning the patchwork nonsystem into a true *health* care system, spanning the spectrum from health promotion to acute and long-term sickness care. While individual efforts to transform the organizations in which nurses work can and should continue, our only real hope lies in transforming the system of which nursing is a part.

Components of a Transformed Health Care System

A transformed, *true* health care system would incorporate:

- A policy that recognizes the pivotal nature of housing, nutrition, education, and the environment in promoting healthy environments and practices.
- A universal *access* system, incorporating separate arenas of public health — acute and chronic sickness care and long-term care.
- An overall goal to decrease institutionalization in both acute and long-term illness and to promote both self-care and community care.

Such a system calls for new coalitions of providers with outcome-oriented financial accountability. It would require a combination of centralized funding with local control in order to create the mechanisms for integration and prioritizing. As Maraldo (1989) has pointed out, such a cost-effective, cost-conscious system would make efficient use of a variety of health workers, with nurses working in all parts of the spectrum — ranging from primary care in health promotion and maintenance, to highly skilled technological care in tertiary institutions.

A variety of public and political strategies are necessary for nursing's voice to be heard in this effort to transform the nation's health care system. Publicly, we need to make clear to policymakers why nursing is a knowledgeable and forceful means for gaining equity and access in health care (and not simply a subset of medicine):

- More than any other type of provider, nurses are providing services at every level of health care: health promotion, and primary, secondary, and tertiary prevention. Numerous studies comparing nurses with other providers indicate that these services are cost-effective and of high quality (Maraldo, 1989).
- Historically, nursing has represented the moral and ethical values underlying equality of access. While we stand to gain in terms of self-interest from a greater voice and presence in a unified system, our own pocketbooks are not a motivating force, since we are generally absent from the fee-for-service areas that are publicly viewed as greedy.
- Finally, nursing has extensive skill and experience in coordinating disparate aspects of systems that benefit individuals and society. We now need to have a primary hand in *designing* a coordinated system, rather than trying to make a poorly designed one work.

Politically, nursing leaders need to be involved in taking nursing to the planning tables of legislative initiatives regarding state-level universal access proposals. Washington, New York, Oregon, and Michigan are considering such endeavors. At the national level, nursing leaders need to be actively involved in shaping the initiatives for national *health care*, and not just insurance plans. Clearly, the National League for Nursing, by creating a nursing coalition for a national health initiative, is carrying out important work (Preziosi, 1989). In developing this initiative, it is critical to remember Milio's (1983) exhortation that to "see health as enmeshed in, and sustained by, a socially created web, to view the care of health as a dual strategy — composed in part of primary care with its linked services and also of health promoting public policies — and to accept responsibility for developing and sharing these views is no easier for health professionals than for the public."

A transformed system does not simply add nurses to the list of those receiving fees-for-service, regardless of whether the services are preventive or curative. A transformed system creates a system in which public policy and personal health are fully integrated.

❏   ❏   ❏

Nursing Theories to Guide Differentiated Nursing Practices

Madeleine M. Leininger, Ph.D., L.H.D., R.N., C.T.N., F.A.A.N.

W e are fortunate in the United States to have a number of nurse theorists to stimulate our intellectual and clinical thinking, as well as to give us options in the use of different theories. In the Introduction to this book, Margaret McClure stated that differentiating practice means different things to different people. The members of this conference firmly concur with this statement. The term "differentiated practice," which came into use three decades ago, stood for a way to use associate (technical) and baccalaureate-degree graduates in nursing services. We believe, however, that there is another, far more promising way to interpret differentiated practices and quality nursing services, which is by the deliberate use of nursing theories.

It is the position of the conference participants that nursing theories are a significant and important means to differentiate and improve nursing practice, while at the same time advance the discipline of the nursing profession. This approach is both logical and essential, since any discipline and profession must be primarily grounded in their own knowledge and practices generated from the discipline itself and from conceptual models and theories. It seems rather ironic that this major position has not been fully realized, adopted, and valued by nursing service administrators and clinicians, with the number of theories about diversity developed in the United States during the past three decades. We believe it is time to consider how to help nurses actually use nursing theories, as well as utilize the research generated from the theories to guide nursing practices. With such an approach, we predict many benefits will be forthcoming related to the improved quality of nursing services, decreased costs, and increased work satisfaction for nurses. The purposes of this conference, therefore, are two-fold — namely, to discuss the rationale and importance of using nursing theories to guide differentiated nursing practice, and to present research findings that show how nursing theories can contribute to differentiated, quality-based nursing practices.

In this conference, we take the position that nursing theories and conceptual models are important means for advancing and improving nursing practice. We believe that nursing theories are essential in supporting the discipline and profession of nursing, and in explaining to the public our societal contributions. Some of the major reasons for the use of nursing theories in clinical practices can be highlighted at the outset to help the audience reflect upon them as each theorist and researcher presents her ideas.

First, nursing theories, coupled with research findings, provide a perspective, a common framework, and a sound basis to guide nurse clinicians' thinking, decisions, and actions. Second, nursing theories provide a holistic or comprehensive perspective of human beings under varying life situations or environmental conditions, and prevent nurses from viewing humans simply as organs, body systems, or in other partial, fragmented ways. Third, nursing theories with substantiated and cumulative research findings on nursing phenomena are essential for supporting the judgments and actions of nurses, and for improving nursing care practices. Fourth, nursing theories are a powerful means for stimulating the intellectual, clinical, and humanistic dimensions of nursing practice, so that nursing does not become a boring or highly ritualized technical practice that leads to burnout among nurses. Fifth, with the use of nursing theories, not only will the quality of nursing care improve, but there also will be a decrease in costs and an increase in consumer satisfaction. Sixth, with the use of nursing theories and concomitant research findings generated from the theories, important differences and solutions to current problems in nursing practice will become more readily apparent — alleviating many problems, such as nurse shortages and other concerns. Seventh, the use of nursing theories provides a common referent language which facilitates communication, provides common goals, and plans for nursing care.

Finally, nursing theories can be one of the strongest and most lasting means for identifying and supporting differentiated role practices and role responsibilities in nursing administration. For these reasons, one can predict some highly promising and still largely unknown or unrecognized clinical nursing practices in nursing. Most assuredly, nursing theories can provide a strong position for differentiated or even undifferentiated nursing practice.

It seems ironic that nursing administrators have been so slow, negligent, or disinterested in using nursing theories to guide nursing practice in the United States. It is especially ironic when one considers that in Canada, where only a few nurses are generating nursing theories, nursing leaders have already taken the stand that nursing theories are essential for guiding, justifying, and supporting nursing practice. Why, then, has it been so difficult for nurse administrators in the United States to incorporate theory-directed nursing practices?

The nonuse of such theories in our country is difficult to understand when most of today's nursing programs in the United States — including associate, baccalaureate, master's, and doctoral programs — are using nursing theories or conceptual models. More and more theories are discussed and examined in schools of nursing to help students use them in research and clinical practice. With the development and use of nursing theories in our classrooms for nearly three decades, it would seem that these theories would have pervaded and revolutionized nursing practices. Why, then, has it been so difficult for nursing administrators to use nursing theories to transform clinical practices or as major guides to substantiate nursing practices? I leave you to ponder these provocative questions and challenges during the course of each conference presentation.

❏　　　❏　　　❏

Structure of Knowledge: Paradigm, Model, and Research Specifications for Differentiated Practice

Sister Callista Roy, Ph.D., R.N., F.A.A.N.

What will drive nursing practice in the next century? Nursing practice will be differentiated by the needs of practice and by the knowledge created to meet those needs. And how do we determine the needs of practice and create knowledge? We see the world of nursing practice by way of our paradigms and models. These frameworks give us the language to describe health care practice needs, both for individuals and for society. They also guide our research on the basic phenomena of nursing and the clinical practice related to that phenomena. It would be easy to say that models and theory are unimportant or nonexistent. However, if we examine the last 30 years of progress in this field, we can only conclude that our frameworks for practice will drive the future just as they have structured the current nursing practice.

In the late 1950s, Johnson (1959) noted that to fulfill its commitment as a professional discipline, nursing needed two kinds of information: 1) knowledge of people and how they respond to stress, and 2) theories of nursing intervention which, when implemented in nursing care, would yield predictable and desirable responses in patients.

In the past three decades, various perspectives on the nature of the discipline and the knowledge it contains have been presented, debated, refuted, revised, sometimes partially accepted, and also rejected. One description of the discipline of nursing that received wide recognition was that of Donaldson and Crowley (1978). The authors identified three recurrent themes that scholars use for inquiry, emphasizing the processes and patterns that lead to health. The last 15 years have provided a rich literature on nursing's basic beliefs and focus from which we can explore further areas of common agreement. However, this body of work does not go far enough in providing the energy for the clinical demands of the next century.

One of the highest priorities for creating an appropriate future for nursing is the identification, structuring, and continuous advancement of knowledge that underlies the practices of the professionals (Schlotfeldt, 1988). Schlotfeldt stated that a recurrent concern is the lack of consensus concerning the subject matter that must be mastered by those seeking to practice general and specialized nursing. The position taken here is that the groundwork has been laid for the next crucial step in structuring nursing knowledge. It is based on a common metaparadigm, plurality of models, and intensive research into the basic and clinical science of nursing. From this structure of knowledge, we have the specifications for differentiated practice. The term *specifications* is deliberately chosen, because with a structure of nursing knowledge, we have the detailed description and enumeration of particulars. The evolution of models for differentiated practice is to be based on these specifics, including settings, level of practitioners, quality of care standards, etc.

Paradigms

Currently the commonalities of the discipline can be evaluated according to our view of persons, environmental interactions, and our evolving concepts of health and nursing. By analyzing the scientific processes related to persons in the environment, the following principles are noted in summarizing the thinking of nurse scholars:

- Holism, or integration is assumed.
- Open systems are exchanging energy.
- Patterns emerge from basic life processes.

Some shared concepts concerning health and nursing include:

- Life changes for all people, yet aspects of stability are rooted in human nature.
- Health relates to the expression of a full life potential.
- We have a long tradition of caring that has been called the interpersonal process (Peplau), empathy (Travelbee), and is now defined by such terms as transpersonal (Watson) and transcultural caring (Leininger).

These commonalities have been expanded from our growth in the 1970s and 1980s to an integrated metaparadigm that guides the discipline into the twenty-first century. This metaparadigm focuses on persons within the total ecology — that is, within their human and social environments (Roy, 1988). All persons have internal life processes. At each person's core are human life processes, such as homeostatic regulation, thinking, feeling, and relating. Out of these processes and acting within a given environment, the person develops individual patterns, such as being a sensitive and thoughtful person, or perhaps being an active person with high energy, struggling to master the constant challenges of the environment. The patterns a person develops and their variations are noted by the nurse in human responses. The processes and patterns of groups can likewise be described and studied.

From this metaparadigm two branches of nursing science and a generalized structure of nursing knowledge are derived. These two branches stem from the inner core of the person or group. Basic nursing science deals with understanding these human life processes, which include processes of health promotion; developmental life processes; and life processes related to the stability of patterns, dynamic evolving patterns, and cultural influences as well as group processes. Clinical nursing science enhances, maintains, and promotes the life processes within persons and groups, including clinical nursing judgments about the diagnosis and treatment of the patterning of life processes.

This perspective is the highest level of abstraction where the disciplines share a common focus. Regardless of the population served or the setting in which care takes place, this common focus can provide the perspective for nurse scholars/practitioners to move forward in specifying differentiated practice for the next century.

Complementing this metaparadigmatic unity, we have two strong bases for pluralism in models for differentiated practice. Advanced practitioners contribute to specifications within the common vision by identifying specific phenomena and the contextual setting of their practice. Additionally, they know the research questions to ask in order to develop knowledge for practice. They also possess a unique ability to address these questions. The second basis for pluralism in differentiated practice are the well-established conceptual models for nursing practice.

These conceptual nursing models, developed over the past two decades, have the task of probing the reality of nursing to provide direction, to add to our knowledge of practice through research, and to direct nursing education. Each of the nurse theorists has developed ways of looking at the person as an individual and as a member of society, and at how nursing as a scientific and practice discipline can make a difference in today's society. With such a variety of frameworks, each is a vehicle for developing the basic science of nursing and the practice discipline, thereby adding to the structure of nursing knowledge. They help us define and describe the people we care for in practice and study in nursing research. One such example is that of moving from metaparadigm to model to differentiated practice.

Structure of Knowledge Based on the Roy Adaptation Model

As one of the conceptual models developed over the past 25 years, the Roy Adaptation Model (Roy and Andrews, 1991) is congruent with the common perspective of nursing described herein. Furthermore, it provides guidelines for specific development of the two branches of nursing science — basic and clinical. The model's particular view of the person and environment identifies the basic life processes that enhance health. The concepts of nursing and health related to enhancing these positive life processes then form the substantive knowledge used for nursing judgments and actions that enhance health.

Within the Roy Adaptation Model, the key concept of basic nursing science is the life process of adaptation. Adaptation is both a process and a state (Roy, 1990). It is an active process involving the person-environment interactions (specifically referred to as pooling the focal, contextual, and residual stimuli) that strive for mastery. At any point in time, the adaptive state is the cumulative effect of the ongoing adaptive process. For clinical nursing science, the central theme is enhancing patient adaptation. Some progress has been made on the conceptual level in identifying indicators of effective adaptation (Andrews and Roy, 1986; Roy and Andrews, 1991). The structure of knowledge based on the model, then, presents an outline of the processes and patterns identified.

Within the adaptive processes, basic nursing science considers the cognator (including both cognitive and emotional processes) and regulator (including neural-chemical-endocrine activity) for the individual, and stabilizer and innovator activity for a group; stability of adaptive patterns; and the dynamic of evolving adaptive patterns. These processes promote adaptation within the adaptive modes. In looking at the adaptive modes, one studies development, interrelatedness, cultural, and other influences. The second major category — adaptation related to health — is divided to focus on the person and environment interaction and integration of the adaptive modes.

The clinical nursing science based on the Roy Adaptation Model is divided into changes in cognator-regulator and stabilizer-innovator effectiveness — changes within and among the adaptive modes and nursing care that promote adaptive processes. Clinically, it may be useful to look at the overall effectiveness of adaptive processes. Consider, for example, a cognator process such as problem-solving from which the person has developed an ongoing pattern of being able to meet his own goals. Simultaneously, cognator-regulator effectiveness within each adaptive mode provides a more specific structure of knowledge for clinical investigation and application. The person is seen as a whole, changing with each mode, yet interrelated to the whole picture as in a kaleidoscope.

Further specification of the structure of knowledge is derived from indicators of adaptation within the modes. At the individual level, there are nine components of the physiological mode: oxygenation, nutrition, elimination, activity and rest, protection, senses, fluid and electrolytes, and endocrine and neurologic function. Some examples of the typology of indicators of adaptation within three components of this mode include:

1) Oxygenation
   - stable processes of ventilation
   - stable pattern of gas exchange
   - adequate transport of gases
   - adequate compensatory processes during change

2) Senses
   - effective processes of sensation
   - effective integration of sensory input into information
   - stable patterns of perception (i.e., interpretation and appreciation of input)
   - effective coping strategies for altered sensation

3) Neurological Function
   - effective processes of arousal/attention, sensation/perception; coding, language, memory; planning and motor response
   - integrated patterns of thinking and feeling
   - plasticity and functional effectiveness of developing, aging, and altered nervous system

The model is characterized by three additional modes of adaptation — self concept, role function, and interdependence. The structure of knowledge in these modes includes the following indicators:

1) Personal Self
   - stable pattern of self-consistency
   - effective integration of self ideal
   - effective processes of moral-ethical-spiritual growth
   - functional self-esteem
   - effective coping strategies for threats to self

2) Interdependence Mode
   - stable pattern of giving and receiving
   - nurturing effectiveness
   - affectional adequacy
   - effective pattern of aloneness and relating
   - effective coping strategies for separation and loneliness

Basing a structure of knowledge on patterns and processes allows for the expansion of new knowledge to meet the changing needs of practice in the next century. For example, how will the nurse assist the person with several organ transplants or artificial organs to maintain a stable pattern of self-consistency? On a broader scale, what types of processes will society as a whole focus on to promote health for all socio-economic groups in the coming era of increased AIDS cases, widespread drug abuse, and indiscriminate use of technology? A given focus for the patterns and processes further organizes knowledge for advanced specialty practice and for programs of research targeted within this framework of a basic and clinical science of nursing.

Differentiated Nursing Practice

How does this relate to differentiating practice? The specified structure of knowledge has already provided the basis for distinctions that differentiate practice. For example, in her paper within this book, Frederickson has identified four criteria based on the model that have served as guidelines to differentiate practice. Applying these more specifically to the structure outlined here, we note that the nurse's level of model utilization is based on complexity of cognitive processes used in practice. Basic content of the model has been identified (Andrews and Roy, 1986), yet nurses will vary in the extent and level of content they can apply. The structure also provides for differentiating the complexity of the clinical situation and, thereby, the utilization of nursing resources needed in this area. For example, the extent of process and pattern development and enhancement specifies the numbers and types of nurses to be prepared for that area. The ability to interpret the model to others is another level of differentiation. Such ability qualifies the available nurse for leadership positions as a guide within an already organized practice model. He/she may work on projects implementing the model in a health care setting, as well as teach the model at varying academic levels. Lastly, the model-based structure provides for varying levels of creative knowledge development, for clinical observations to validate the adaptive mode components on a case-by-case basis, and for investigation into the interrelationships of the cognator-regulator and the four adaptive modes.

Another way to view this differentiation for practice is to describe it as a four-tier structure, similar to academic rank. The first level is a general health care aide. Public information, common sense, and basic instruction about persons and their needs related to the adaptive modes can be turned to use in assisting professionals in providing care based on individual pattern maintenance. At another level, the nurse professional may deal more specifically with developing patterns such as growth and development, eating, and sleeping.

At the next level, the professional nurse would be prepared to deal with complex changes in patterns, which are by definition processes — the dying process, for example. This level, which would be equivalent to the associate professor rank, also could specialize in understanding given processes for particular populations — for example, understanding cognitive information processing and how it changes with various neurologic conditions such as head injury and stroke.

Finally, equivalent to professor rank, would be the professional nurse who conducts research related to the structure of knowledge and examines new patterns and processes that emerge in the evolving person-environment interactions. In particular, some nurses at this level would have responsibility for learning about the processes related to changes in society that affect the health of entire populations. Differentiation is not defined by educational level or by institutional definitions. Each practice level described is differentiated according to the structure of knowledge of the model. These descriptions, together with the criteria outlined, are used to derive additional details of differentiated practice based on the Roy Adaptation Model.

Summary

Using this perspective to help guide them as health care professionals, nurses possess the instrument to carry out the task that is theirs — that is, to contribute to the health of each person and to take social responsibility as a profession. As our world goes through incredible changes in eastern Europe and the Middle East, is it not possible that we can initiate changes that promote social order? Nurses can learn from our common beliefs about persons in society and our specialized practice for the common good. Nursing can provide a center point for dealing with the complex issues of our postmodern world. Clinical knowledge structured on our paradigms, models, and research is the particular kind of knowledge most relevant in dealing with the global social and health care concerns of the twenty-first century. Structuring that knowledge provides the opportunity to use our theories and research to create the changes in clinical practice that respond to the social accountability imperative for twenty-first century nursing.

As genetic scientists embark on mapping the entire human genome (every amino acid and nucleic sequence that resides in each human gene), we nurse scientists already inhabit the future with our expectation that we can accomplish the equally significant task of understanding the full measure of the life processes that promote human health.

❏   ❏   ❏

Nursing Theories—A Basis for Differentiated Practice: Application of the Roy Adaptation Model in Nursing Practice

Keville Frederickson, Ph.D., R.N.

A few years ago, as a faculty member, I donned a white uniform and returned to the bedside to provide direct patient care after an absence of 20 years. The purpose for this somewhat radical departure was to regain credibility as a teacher and as a nurse. Having taught a graduate-level theories and models course at Lehman College (in the city of New York) for four years, I found that there were no settings where students could observe the translation of nursing theory into practice.

Returning to practice seemed to be the first step in establishing a theory-based practice unit. Following my humbling experience with direct patient care, a professional practice unit has been established on a neurosurgical unit at Montefiore Medical Center. The unit has adopted the Roy Adaptation Model (RAM) as the basis for practice and other nursing activities. The unit also serves as a laboratory for implementing nursing science as well as a model for retention and recruitment.

My role as clinical nurse scientist for the project was established through a joint appointment with Lehman College and Montefiore Medical Center. Since then, I have become steeped in RAM, using it for research and teaching as well as for clinical practice. Throughout the project, it was important for us to keep in mind that the nursing model's ultimate purpose is to provide the nurse with a structure of knowledge for practice.

In developing the model unit, the project was based on two assumptions about professional nursing practice: 1) that professional nursing practice is autonomous, and 2) that autonomous professional nursing practice cannot exist unless it is based on a nursing conceptual system. From my perspective, for there to be professional practice in nursing, it has to be based on distinct nursing science, just as medicine and psychology are based on their own respective, unique sciences.

After selecting RAM as the framework for practice, the process of change was implemented using RAM for administration. During the conversion to conceptually-based practice, we enhanced the coping skills of the nurses so that they could incorporate the change (or the stimulus) of introducing the nursing model. We also adapted the environment in such ways that conceptually-based practice became part of the environment. At the end of two years, we had some hard data to indicate what occurred on the unit.

For the two years prior to initiating the model, the nursing unit had been losing approximately 10 out of 38 nurses per year. It is estimated that to replace one nurse in this clinical area, it costs approximately $30,000. During the year following the implementation of RAM, no nurses resigned, representing a savings of approximately $300,000 (Frederickson, 1990).

What has been observed about differentiating practice and the use of a nursing model? To date, it has been noted that when using RAM as conceptual basis for nursing practice, a consistency evolves in the approach to all nursing activities; a common language also evolves in the discussion of nursing and patient care. Lastly, knowledge and skills develop that separate the various levels of nursing practice personnel. This last development indicates that RAM offers an opportunity for differences in practice to emerge. More specifically, observations of nursing practice indicate that the use of a nursing conceptual model provides a setting in which differences in nursing practice can develop. These differences can be identified according to the role the nurse assumes — a role enhanced by educational preparation.

Based on observations, conceptually-based practice produces nursing behaviors that can be categorized into four groups. These groups can, in turn, serve as guidelines to differentiate practice based on a nursing conceptual system. The groups are not meant to be exhaustive, but descriptive. For the purposes of this paper, differentiated practice means differences between all levels of nursing personnel producing direct care — from the nursing assistant to the doctoral-prepared nurse, or as Roy has recommended, the "attending."

The first category is the nurse's level of model utilization. This means the extent to which the components of the model are used, as well as the complexity of the cognitive processes required. For example, nursing assistants have used RAM under the clinical nurse scientist's direction as a way to organize information collected during the report. They constructed a report sheet that focuses on the modes and their substructures, with an emphasis on the physiological mode. As the staff development specialist, the master's-prepared nurse uses the model to organize content for teaching and integration of clinical practice with teaching. For example, neuroscience nursing courses are organized and taught using RAM to view the person as an adaptive system. The doctoral-prepared nurse uses the model to integrate practice and/or education with theory development. For example, the model is used as the basis for examining patterns of ineffective adaptation and designing theory-based research to address adaptation (Jackson et al., in press; Strauman, Frederickson, and Jackson, 1987).

The second category is the use of a nursing model to determine the complexity of the clinical situation. This is a frequently mentioned criterion for differentiating practice. The nursing model can be used to consistently identify complex situations and then direct a particular level of nurse to provide care for and/or interact with the patient. For example, using RAM, the number and nature of the stimuli, as well as the number of modes with ineffective coping, serve as guidelines for deciding who should provide which aspects of nursing care to which patients.

The interpretation of the nursing model to others provides another category for differentiating practice. For instance, the doctoral-prepared nurse reaches out to executive-level personnel in other disciplines, such as the chief executive officer of the medical center or the director of the Social Work Association, to explain and interpret nursing. At this level, there must be a full synthesis of the nursing model and its unique value to nursing.

Lastly, practice is differentiated by the level of knowledge development for nursing. For example, using RAM, the associate-degree nurse provides observations within the modes. The baccalaureate nurse observes and questions patterns of behavior and outcomes, relating these outcomes to stimuli and adaptation. The master's-level nurse develops and tests interventions related to patterns of behavior translated into concepts. The doctoral-prepared nurse uses the model to view complex nursing situations and problems, beginning to categorize them and design test studies. One such study probes the role of cognator-regulator and perception, examining significantly different mortality rates among oncology patients receiving toxic chemotherapy (Frederickson, 1991). The model directed the clinical nurse scientist to view patients as biopsychosocial wholes, while developing the theory that guided the research.

In summary, the use of a nursing model such as RAM is extremely valuable in differentiating practice. It provides a common framework so that differences in practice can evolve. The model allows consistency of purpose and execution in all nursing activities. Many of the innovations that we envision for the future will be predicated on such a professional practice model based on nursing science.

❑   ❑   ❑

Insights From Orem's Nursing Theory on Differentiating Nursing Practice

Marjorie A. Isenberg, D.N.Sc., R.N., F.A.A.N

Organizing nursing services to meet the needs of patient and client populations is the prime responsibility of nurse administrators. Essential elements of this structuring process are theories that are content-specific to nursing. By identifying the focus, scope, and boundaries of nursing as fields of knowledge and practice, nursing theories provide the foundation and framework upon which to construct and organize nursing activities.

Theories offer a perspective, a point of view, a way of thinking about and understanding nursing. They provide the substantive nursing knowledge that is vital to structuring nursing practice. In essence, nursing theories identify and describe the nature of nursing as a helping service with a distinct contribution to the health of society.

The specific topic of this paper is a discussion of the ways in which Orem's nursing theory differentiates nursing practice. Before discussing differentiated nursing practice, let's begin with the more general question of how Orem describes nursing. Recall that it was a search for understanding of the domain and boundaries of nursing as a field of knowledge and a field of practice that motivated Dorothea Orem to pursue her theoretical endeavors. She began her work by seeking an answer to the question of what conditions exist in persons when judgments are made about their nursing care. She concluded that the human condition associated with the need for nursing is the existence of a health-related limitation in the ability of a person to provide for his or her own self the amount and quality of care required (Orem, 1985). This insight provided Orem with an answer to the question, "What is nursing's phenomenon of concern?" She identified nursing's special concern as individuals' needs for self-care and their capabilities for meeting those needs. It is this special focus on human beings that distinguishes or differentiates nursing from other human services (Orem, 1985). From this point of view, the role of nursing in society is to enable individuals to develop and exercise their self-care abilities to the extent that they can provide for themselves the amount and quality of care required.

Orem has identified four concepts that best express the properties and actions of persons in need of nursing:

- self-care
- therapeutic self-care demand
- self-care agency
- self-care deficit

Additionally, she has defined the nursing agency and nursing system as concepts that express the properties and actions of nurses.

Self-care refers to the activities that individuals initiate and perform on their own behalf to sustain life, health, and well-being. Self-care is viewed as a form of deliberate action that is learned within a sociocultural context.

Therapeutic self-care demand is defined as the measure of care required at certain moments to meet existent requisites. Orem identified three categories of self-care requisites: universal, developmental, and health-deviation. These three categories of requisites represent the types of purposeful self-care that persons may require at various phases of the life cycle and in various states of health.

The human capabilities for self-care are conceptualized as *self-care agency*. "Agency" is used here in the sense of power or capacity. Thus, self-care agency refers to the complex set of acquired abilities that are specific to the performance of the actions of self-care (Orem, 1985).

The fourth concept in this category is *self-care deficit*, which refers to a specific relationship between the concepts of self-care agency and therapeutic self-care demand in which self-care agency is not adequate to meet the therapeutic self-care demand (Orem, 1985). According to the theory, it is the presence of an existing or potential self-care deficit that identifies those persons in need of nursing. Thus, Orem's self-care deficit theory explains when and why nursing is required and provides criterion measures for identifying those who need nursing. The theory of self-care explains why these forms of care are necessary for life, development, health, and well-being. Finally, Orem's theory of nursing systems explains how persons can be helped through nursing. Clearly, the work of this theorist differentiates nursing from other forms of human service and provides a basis for structuring nursing knowledge and nursing practice.

Let us now turn to the question of whether the theory addresses the issue of differentiating levels of nursing practice. Orem's concept of nursing agency is relevant to the discussion of differentiating roles and role responsibilities in nursing. Nursing agency refers to those specialized acquired abilities that enable nurses to provide care that compensates for or empowers persons in overcoming health-related self-care deficits (Orem, 1985). It is this property that qualifies people to become nurses. It is this "capability" that is activated by nurses as they determine needs for, design of, and production of nursing for persons with various types of self-care deficits. These specialized abilities are acquired through formal educational programs, mentoring by expert clinicians, and experience in nursing situations.

With respect to McClure's question (posed in the Introduction to this book) about what variables should be used to differentiate nursing practice, it would seem that Orem's concept of nursing agency provides an answer by identifying variables for differentiating nursing roles. A nurse's educational preparation, her nursing knowledge and skills, and her orientation toward practice would determine the general roles and role responsibilities for practitioners.

In fact, Orem has divided the roles and responsibilities of nurses according to their nursing abilities into two categories: the professional level of practice and the technological level. The role responsibilities identified for the professional level of practice are to provide nursing diagnoses, clinical judgments, creative design of nursing systems, and design of techniques for attaining nursing results in the absence of validated techniques; to implement and manage nursing operations in complex nursing situations; and to provide nursing consultation. On the technical level, the single role responsibility is to use validated and reliable techniques in implementing and regulating specific aspects of nursing systems (Orem, 1990).

In other words, the technologist performs as an associate of a professional nursing practitioner and contributes specified components to overall systems of care. Furthermore, the technologist works within established protocols in providing nursing care. Orem clearly identifies the professional nurse as possessing the abilities required in creating and projecting designs for nursing systems of care. Designs of nursing systems stipulate:

- The scope of nursing responsibility.
- The general and specific roles of nurses and patients.
- Reasons for nurses' relationships with patients.
- Actions to be performed.

Within this perspective, nurse technologists are expected to possess the abilities required to make adjustments in nursing designs and to implement the design.

The professional practitioner, therefore, is expected to:

- Synthesize and extrapolate knowledge from the theoretical and scientific domain of nursing to the practice domain, and vice versa.
- Diagnose and design nursing systems for covert and complex self-care deficits.
- Develop and validate new or improved nursing technologies when validated technologies are absent or unworkable.
- Supervise the overall implementation of nursing systems of care.
- Contribute to nursing scholarship.

In contrast, the nurse technologist is expected to:

- Contribute to the implementation of nursing systems.
- Identify and endeavor to resolve specific nursing diagnoses of a common, overt nature.
- Use known, validated technologies and work within established practice protocols.
- Work to achieve specified results.

Within Orem's perspective, each level of nursing has a definitive and necessary contribution to make to the whole of nursing practice. However, it is the professional nursing practitioner who is responsible for defining the purpose of the practice, creating the design of the nursing system, determining what level of nursing expertise is needed to implement the care, and delegating responsibilities to members of the nursing team.

Several nurse administrators have documented the usefulness of Orem's theory in nursing service administration (Orem, 1985). Sarah E. Allison, nurse administrator at the Mississippi Methodist Hospital and Rehabilitation Center in Jackson, Mississippi, used Orem's theory as a basis for structuring and organizing nursing practice. The theory, which had been used at the Rehabilitation Center since 1976, was described by Allison as being incorporated within the department's philosophy and objectives and implemented through the organizational structure (Allison, 1985). The theory has proved instrumental in the development of nursing diagnostic and documentation tools. Furthermore, Allison found the theory useful in differentiating the roles and responsibilities of the professional and technical levels of nursing practice. In a case study of a patient with spinal cord injury, Allison illustrated the ability of Orem's theory to provide a basis for differentiating the role focus and the role expectations and responsibilities for the professional and technological levels of nursing practice (Allison, 1985).

In summary, the position that nursing theories play an essential role in structuring nursing practice has been presented herein, through discussion of Orem's nursing theory and its ability to provide a basis for:

- differentiating nursing from other human services,
- structuring and organizing nursing practice, and
- differentiating levels of nursing practice.

❑   ❑   ❑

Parse's Theory of
Human Becoming

Rosemarie Rizzo Parse, Ph.D., R.N., F.A.A.N.

P arse's theory of human becoming posits that humans are
open, unitary beings in mutual process with the world,
cocreating patterns of becoming. The human-world-health
process is the phenomenon of concern to nursing. Parse's theory
focuses on the meaning of lived experiences.

Three major principles identify *human becoming:*

1) Structuring meaning multidimensionally through
imaging, valuing, and language.
2) Cocreating rhythmical patterns of relating through
revealing/concealing, enabling/limiting, and
connecting/separating.
3) Cotranscending possibilities through empowerment
that originates in transformation (Parse, 1981).

These principles guide research and practice. It is my belief
that each nursing theory or framework should have its own unique
research and practice methodology that evolves directly from the
ontology of the theory. Each theory then will have a different practice methodology. Thus, the goals of practice, the outcomes, and the
nurse-person relationship are different. Two different modes of
practice, based on the works of Orem and Roy, have been described

Parse's "Theory of Human Becoming" was originally titled and referred to as "Man-Living-Health: A
Simultaneity Paradigm Theory."

in this book. The theory of human becoming, a simultaneity theory, is very different from these two in ontology and methodology.

For the human becoming theory, the goal of nursing is the *quality of life* as perceived by the person (Parse, 1981). There is no specific, *expected* outcome, since human-to-human interrelationships are not predictable and each person must be guided by his/her values in finding ways of living health. The success of the practice is reflected in the comments on enhanced quality of life from those utilizing the practice:

> Nursing practice from the human becoming view is guided by the theoretical foundation that espouses the human as free agent and meaning giver, choosing rhythmical patterns of relating while reaching for personal hopes and dreams. These beliefs about the human and health lead the nurse to approach the person and family as a nurturing gardener rather than a "fix it" mechanic. To approach a person as gardener, not mechanic, believing that each person lives value priorities, is to be *truly present* to the person as the person changes patterns of health (Parse, 1990).

From this point of view, nursing practice is not a matter of "offering professional advice and opinions stemming from the nurse's own lived value system. It is not a canned approach to care. It is a subject-to-subject interrelationship, a loving, true presence with the other to enhance the quality of life" (Parse, 1987).

The true presence of the nurse is a nonroutinized, nonmechanical way of "being with," in which the nurse is authentic and attentive to moment-to-moment changes in meaning for the person or group. *True presence* surfaces as an intentional reflective love which the nurse shares with the other as the other blossoms according to personal desires and dreams. Intentional reflective love is an interpersonal art grounded in a strong knowledge base reflecting the belief that each person knows "the way" somewhere within self. Each human lives a way — his or her *own* way — which is both alike and different from the "ways" of others. It is like that of others in that it is a personal way of being; each individual has a personal way of being. It is different from others in that it is one's own. It is like a fingerprint in that it belongs to only one human being. While others coexist on the journey of life, each lives his or her own way on the journey. One's own explicit and tacit knowing is the wellspring of moving along the way.

True presence is in the sphere of the inter-human, and this is where the nurse enters the other person's world with an openness, a self-giving, and a strong knowledge base reflecting the human becoming theory (Parse, 1990).

The dimensions of Parse's theory in practice focus on illuminating meaning, synchronizing rhythms, and mobilizing transcendence with the person (Parse, 1987). It is in the true presence of the nurse that the person may realize the meaning of a situation and dwell within the rhythmical patterns of relating that mobilize movement beyond the moment. "Living a true presence with a person is placing the emphasis on the human to-human interrelationship, with the nurse valuing the person as coauthor freely choosing health" (Parse, 1990). The nurse in the nurse-person relationship is a traveler *with* the person, as the person chooses among multidimensional options to change patterns of health.

From the perspective of Parse's theory of human becoming, the traditional nursing process — assessing, planning, diagnosing, implementing, and evaluating — no longer fits. Labeling and objectifying the person through assessment and diagnosing are inconsistent with the assumptions of the theory. The person shares with the Parse nurse a personal description of health and specifies paradoxical patterns of health and desires and hopes in the situation. Persons with whom the theory has been lived have said they experience feelings of dignity and that their own values are honored.

"Nursing practice based on the beliefs of Parse's human becoming theory frees people from enslavement by others' values and enhances quality of life" (Parse, 1990).

❑   ❑   ⊔

Distinguishing Practice with Parse's Theory

Gail J. Mitchell, M.S.N.

P arse's theory offers nurses an opportunity to practice in a way that is very different from the traditional problem-based model (Parse, 1981; Parse, 1987). This approach is structured by unique assumptions and beliefs about human beings and health which distinguish the way in which nurses relate to individuals in practice. My experience with Parse's theory started four years ago in my practice as a clinical nurse specialist in acute care and community settings. I recently completed an evaluation study of this theory-based approach.

Prior to practicing Parse's theory, I had accumulated 12 years of experience in critical care nursing and was considered an expert by most standards. I was technically and clinically skilled in managing and identifying health-related problems. I collaborated and participated in multidisciplinary approaches aimed at managing health according to biopsychosocial norms. Being an expert nurse within the traditional problem-based model was like being one of many — working on the same problems in exactly the same way. I, like other health experts, routinely performed cognitive, functional, and social assessments of older persons so that the team could plan interventions according to what was believed best for the individual. Each of the experts speculated and theorized according to their academic backgrounds and personal experiences, but we all had the same problem-focused approach, with the same expectation that patients should listen to the experts to better understand how to manage health and ways of living.

Several years ago I realized I was not satisfied with the traditional way of practicing. I did not want to continue focusing on human beings and their life experiences as problems, which when identified seemed to serve my needs more than the person in my care. I did not really believe nursing's phenomenon of concern was problem management, and I did not want to practice in a way which ignored, or at best devalued, the individual's perceptions, meanings, desires, and plans.

Parse's theory changed my approach in practice by first changing my values and beliefs about human beings and health. This process of change took time and commitment as I transformed the familiar ways and views of the biomedical model to new ways of viewing and being with people.

For example, a young woman spoke to me recently about the unexpected death of her father. The woman said, "You know, I play games with myself by pretending my dad is still alive. That way I do not have to deal with it." I asked this person to tell me more about the games. She said, "By playing games, I do not have to be with the pain all the time. It gives me a chance to get above the suffering. I don't know if I'll ever be ready to deal with it." In the traditional model, I would have compared this woman's experience of grief to some standard of normalcy. I would have interpreted what the games meant to me as the expert and then taken action according to my goals to move her along in the grieving process. I would have assessed her denial and I may have feared her games reflected ineffective grieving.

Guided by Parse's theory, I considered the woman's games a creative way to be both "with and away from" the pain of her loss. Instead of thinking about a psychiatric consult, I asked her to tell me more about the games and how they helped her to get above the suffering. I asked her to tell me about what it was like "to be above the suffering." Rather than giving advice, I offered true presence to this woman. I went with her, bearing witness to her experience rather than trying to get her to where I thought she should be. I also respected this woman's right to be with her grief as she chose to be without the analysis and interpretation of an outsider. I believed she knew what was best for herself and that she would find that way, for Parse suggests each person knows his own way. My being with her as she moved through her grief was an intentional way of being

— guided by a theory which specifies that, as human beings speak about the meaning of their personal situations, the meanings change and the person moves on in the unfolding process of life.

From Parse's perspective, the patient is not viewed as a problem but as a unitary human being. Having this perspective was the most frequently recurring theme in the evaluation study of Parse's theory at St. Michael's Hospital in Toronto, Canada. This study revealed important changes in nurses' beliefs and actions and patient health experiences when Parse's theory guided practice. A descriptive, qualitative design guided the eight-month evaluation on a 28-bed, acute care medical unit. Data were collected from 23 nurses and the unit manager pre- and post-project through questionnaires, chart reviews and interviews to determine changes in nurses' ways of thinking about and being with patients and of believing about nursing. Data were also collected pre- and post-project from patients and family members regarding perceptions of their health experiences.

Nurses described changes that occurred in their ways of thinking about and being with human beings. The most dramatic differences related to nurses' ways of talking and listening to individuals, because of the different way they thought about them as human beings. Once nurses saw patients not as problems, but as individuals who were the experts in their own lives and who participated in creating their health, and once nurses learned to live these new beliefs, their relationships with patients changed. Nurses stopped labeling and judging patients according to predetermined expectations of biopsychosocial norms. The time spent with individuals was focused on listening to the person's perspective and enhancing quality of life as the person defined it. Adapting to Parse's theory, care plans and charts contained the individual's personal health descriptions and plans for change, rather than traditional nursing goals.

Nurses reported being able to talk to patients about difficult issues for the first time in their careers. This comfort in bearing witness to another's experience echoed Parse's theory that the nurse's responsibility is *to be there* in true presence with the person, rather than trying to fix and control how the individual thinks and feels. Nurses said that in the traditional model they were fearful of talking to patients about difficult things like death or despair because they believed they had to do something with those problems. It was described as opening up a can of worms that they could not handle, so it was easier to ignore the people and their pain.

The traditional problem-based model presents a tremendous burden for nurses because they are taught to believe they can fix and control human beings by manipulating or managing the environment or the person.

In addition to the new way of relating to individuals, nurses in the evaluation study described a difference in the way they related to members of other disciplines. Nurses guided by Parse's theory said they knew the uniqueness of their contribution to the individual's health because no other health care provider presented the person's perspective, meanings, plans, hopes, or dreams. The other members of the health care team presented their own expert interpretations of patient and family situations.

Other common themes that resulted from Parse's theory revolved around enhanced morale in nurses and enhanced quality of the nurse-person relationship as perceived by individuals and their family members.

Nurses on the unit that evaluated Parse's theory have adopted it as their permanent theoretical guide. Ten other units at St. Michael's have expressed a desire to evaluate this unique approach, and the family practice and labor and delivery units are presently investigating how Parse's theory distinguishes nursing practice in those areas. Parse's theory also has been evaluated on long-term psychiatric, pediatric, and surgical units at other hospitals in Canada. Preliminary findings from these other centers are consistent with findings from the research on the medical unit.

Parse's theory in practice makes a difference to quality of life for persons and clarifies practice for nurses. The traditional problem-based model does not clearly differentiate nursing practice from other disciplines and actually confuses nurses about the focus and direction of their actions. Nursing frameworks are the proper guide for nursing practice. Differentiation among practice methodologies is expected within the discipline as nurses continue to define and distinguish nursing science and its unique theoretical applications.

❏   ❏   ❏

PART II

Models of Differentiated Nursing Practice in Hospital Settings

Building on Shared Values: The Dartmouth-Hitchcock Medical Center Approach

Linda Cronenwett, Ph.D., R.N., F.A.A.N.
Kay Clark, M.A., R.N.
Susan Reeves, M.S., R.N.
Laura Easton, M.S.N., R.N.

Mary Hitchcock Memorial Hospital (MHMH) is one component of the Dartmouth-Hitchcock Medical Center, located in Hanover, New Hampshire. The hospital has 411 licensed beds, 416 full-time equivalent (FTE) registered nurse (RN) direct-care providers, 91 nonprofessional nursing staff members, a ratio of 1.65 RN FTEs per occupied bed, and nursing services that are organized into 22 nursing units.

Our experience with different roles for RNs began in 1987, when Laura Easton worked with the staff of our 26-bed orthopedic/urology unit to develop a new nursing care delivery model. That unit, prior to the initiation of the pilot project, had used a total patient care delivery system. Licensed practical nurses (LPNs) had received *patient* care assignments instead of assignments to work with an RN. The staff nurse vacancy rate was 25%, morale was low, and clinical nurse specialists (CNSs) and others expressed concerns about the quality of nursing care.

Over the next two years, the nursing staff designed and implemented a case management nursing care delivery model called the Patient Care Management Model. Four patient care managers, who were salaried and worked varying hours depending on patients' needs, held 24-hour and length-of-stay accountability for the nursing care of the patients in their caseload. The caseloads of the patient care managers matched the caseloads of one or more attending physicians, so that collaboration between nurses and physicians was facilitated. Patient care managers were responsible for initial assessment and care planning, teaching, evaluation and revision of care plans, preparation of the patient and family for discharge, timely coordination of all services the patient needed while hospitalized, and the documentation of these activities.

Although direct hands-on care activities were frequently performed by patient care managers, the responsibility for ensuring that all required direct care activities on a shift were accomplished belonged to RNs in the role of patient care coordinators. Patient care coordinators had a geographically-based caseload and worked with other RNs, LPNs, and nursing assistants in the provision of direct care.

Past attempts at providing RN length-of-stay accountability through primary nursing on this unit had failed for many reasons:

- lack of a sufficient number of RNs who worked enough days of the week to provide continuity in patient care;
- lack of ability and/or willingness among a number of RNs to be accountable for the assessment, planning, and evaluation components of nursing care; and
- inefficient or inappropriate use of assistive personnel when RNs provided patient care to primary patients while trying to provide professional components of care to another set of patients.

With the change to patient care management and differentiated RN roles, LPNs could be used effectively because every patient had an RN who was accountable for the management of nursing care. In the length-of-stay accountable role, RNs worked full-time, five days a week. One patient care manager worked each weekend. The nurses also covered each others' patients during vacations and other absences.

The success of the transition to this new model was due, we believe, to the strength and vision of the nursing managers and their commitment to involving the staff in all decisions. They organized multiple retreats for the staff as a whole and separate retreats for persons in the three different roles. During the retreats, managers led the staff in values clarification and helped to develop communication and conflict resolution skills. The transition was not easy, either on this unit or on the neuroscience unit that implemented a similar model a year later. Major issues were:

- Fears about the relative value placed on each role.
  Was there a dichotomy between "thinkers" and "doers"? Would patient care managers be valued if they were doing work that had received the lowest priority from nurses for decades (documentation, education, discharge planning) — the work that some stayed to do after the shift was over? Were managers going to value the assessment of RN coordinators and providers? Were persons in one role going to have to work harder than persons in another role?
- Fears about how nurses would be chosen for patient care manager positions.
  Were nurses without BSNs going to be excluded from consideration? (Nurses with BSNs seem to be advantaged in the competition for positions — all staff participates in the hiring decisions — but we used an assessment-based, not education-based, approach to hiring for different roles. Most of the nurses who have been successful in the patient care manager role either have their BSNs or are in school finishing their degrees.)
- Resentment over the splitting of responsibilities for patient care.
  Although nurses on this unit recognized that patients had not been assured a standard of care that included RN assessment, planning, and evaluation, some RNs still wanted to try and do it all for just their patients. They did not want to be forced to work with someone who could delegate a plan to them or to whom they would need to delegate care responsibilities.

As the first year came to an end, attitudes of the staff on the unit changed. RNs with shift accountability were able to finish their day's work on time. Per diem and float nurses expressed greater satisfaction in caring for patients because they could work with the patient care manager and be assured that the plan of care for the day matched the patients' needs. For the first time in the unit's current history, BSN-prepared nurses were seeking to work on this unit. Staff perceived that the overall quality of nursing care had improved, and these perceptions were supported by first-year evaluations from CNSs, social workers, discharge planners, and quality assurance data. Patients wrote appreciative letters, and the length of stay from the more complex surgical groups decreased.

Attending physicians embraced the concept once they saw the impact on patient care. Adjustment problems were related to the fact that they were used to doing all their planning with a head nurse. Now the head nurse no longer performed that role, which was sometimes inconvenient. Some MDs were threatened by a stronger nurse role in terms of clinical decision making. By the end of one year, however, these physicians were participating in the hiring process, and some refused to consider moving their patients to a new unit unless they could be assured of the same nursing care delivery model there.

Problems with the house staff persisted, however. The new alliance between attending physician and patient care manager caused resentment among the house staff. Because of deficits in the medical teaching model, attending physicians did not always go on rounds with the house staff; therefore, situations arose where patient care managers knew more about the attending physician's plan of medical care than the house staff did.

Generally, the reaction of nurses throughout the rest of the hospital was not positive. Other RNs heard about the difficulty of role transition. It was feared that the feature that fit the ortho/uro unit — planned use of LPNs in the new model — would spread to other units. Part-time nurses resented that full-time people were in manager roles. The usual threat of professional/technical distinctions were discussed with little knowledge of the values that had guided the development of the model or the outcomes.

In the meantime, MHMH applied for and received a planning year grant from the Robert Wood Johnson/Pew initiative, "Strengthening Hospital Nursing: A Program to Improve Patient Care." A major objective of that proposal had been to restructure nursing roles, both in terms of creating different roles for direct care providers and creating a career advancement program that would be compatible with differentiated roles.

The American Nurses Association had just undergone a consensus-building process to determine the form of its new organizational structure. We decided to use the same type of process for consensus building to determine the basic values that would be the framework for nursing care delivery models in our hospital.

A group called the Nursing Professional Practice Council (NPPC) accepted responsibility for guiding our work on the Pew grant objective to restructure nursing roles. This council was (and continues to be) composed of one staff nurse representative from each nursing unit and representatives from each group of managers and support personnel. It is the body with formal authority and accountability for standards of nursing practice. The NPPC appointed a Role Development Task Force to begin the brainstorming processes and procure the first draft of ideas about potential values and standards that might guide the development of nursing roles. This task force, and the NPPC as a whole, read article after article about current concepts related to differentiated practice, nursing care delivery models, peer review, and career ladders.

Two consultants, Dr. Linda Aiken and Margaret Murphy, spoke to MHMH nurses, administrators, and physicians about their views of the changes required to meet current and future needs for nurses. At a critical juncture in the process, JoEllen Koerner told Sioux Valley's story as part of her keynote address at the 1989 New Hampshire Nurses Association convention. Outside authorities, all pointing out the need for change, were extremely helpful.

At the same time, the hospital's senior management team was struggling with problems that resulted from a lack of continuity of caregivers. They were attempting to influence both physicians and nurses to adopt the standard that every patient admitted to MHMH would have an identifiable nurse and physician who remained accountable for the nursing and medical plans of care throughout that patient's stay.

Many forces came together to influence the way the values and standards were first defined by the Role Development Task Force. The group was strongly influenced by the fact that we had one successful pilot unit where the purpose of RN role differentiation was to provide the same standard for accountability and continuity that senior management desired.

Other potential goals for role differentiation were considered during readings and consultations. The task force found that some hospitals provided a case manager or primary nurse for only a certain subset of patients and that some hospitals planned care delivery models with all-BSN primary nurse concepts in mind. They also found that some hospitals' goals for differentiation were to provide a role for every nurse commensurate with that nurse's education, experience, and competence, regardless of the time of day or number of days per week she worked. The task force rejected these options in favor of value statements reflecting the overall goal desired by senior management and demonstrated in our pilot project. No one knew if nurses in our department would agree, but these statements were discussed during retreats.

We used about $30,000 of our Pew planning year grant to pay RN salaries for retreats. All RNs were invited to attend, at minimum, a three-hour retreat. Some units held eight-hour retreats. The retreats were attended by 89% of the RN staff.

Each retreat opened with a presentation about the health care environment and the issues related to nursing supply and demand. Presenters described the methods used to develop 31 value statements on role development and a list of 57 possible characteristics for reward in a career ladder. The remainder of each retreat was used to discuss the implications of each value statement and career ladder reward system. Each attending nurse indicated the extent to which he or she agreed with each value statement on nursing roles, choosing the 10 most valued characteristics in a career advancement system.

The processes I have just described were not as linear, rational, or precise as they might sound. Never before had all our nurses been exposed to concepts so potentially divisive and controversial. Never before had nursing administration gone to the staff as a whole for direct guidance on a project that had so much potential impact on nurses' lives. Testing continued as nurses decided whether their collective opinions would, indeed, make a difference.

As a member of the NPPC, the senior vice president for nursing assured staff on many occasions that their decisions would be implemented. Complete survey data, including negative comments, were circulated to NPPC members and directors, and then to staff. Our consensus — the opinion held by 80% or more of the staff — had to remain consistent throughout all processes. Ideas, values, or standards that were not endorsed by 80% of the staff were dropped.

From the beginning of the planning process, anger and value conflicts that would normally be elicited only after a completed proposal was on the table were out in the open. It was an uncomfortable time for everyone, particularly the retreat leaders, front line managers, and NPPC members. Some staff suspected that a fully developed plan had been predetermined by the authority figures ("them"). NPPC members, who were reading literature and discussing ideas at length, had an advantage over their peers in terms of dealing with the emotions related to differentiated practice and career advancement programs. Nonetheless, they began to feel inadequate because some of their colleagues were upset or indifferent.

The people leading these discussions had to continually remind themselves and each other that this was a new process for our department. In the past, staff had always been presented with a finished product; therefore, it was logical that some staff would be suspicious of a new approach. Likewise, nurses who had developed proposals in the past were used to thinking through most details, implications, and structures of an innovation. They could describe exactly how a new plan would work. In our process, retreat leaders had no such ready answers because the vision of the ideal world had yet to be created by the staff as a whole. Leaders, as well as staff, sometimes lost perspective in the middle of heated discussions. It was emotionally difficult to be attacked, to not have the answers, and to be unable to promise what the outcomes of new programs might be.

At the same time, a growing number of staff members were excited about the planning process and the issues being raised. Their enthusiasm and participation kept the process moving. NPPC members began to find colleagues who wanted to try to improve the delivery of nursing care on their units. Staff who had been resistant to the process or critical of retreats began to hear things differently when the issues were discussed a second or third time.

Over the course of the year, trust began to evolve. Nurses who had not yet attended retreats asked retreat leaders to meet with groups of staff from their units for preretreat discussions of the issues and process. Nursing units that had held retreats early in the year asked for continued discussions with retreat leaders in unit-level committees. The senior vice president for nursing and the Pew grant project directors were invited to speak to groups of nurses at meetings inside and outside the institution. Every request for interaction was granted. Differences of opinion were recognized as valid, and all persons were free to influence others.

The goal, nevertheless, was to reach consensus on as many values and standards as possible. Conflict was acceptable, but it could not stop the planning process and the movement toward consensus. The reasons why we could not go on with business as usual were continually reinforced. Eventually, nurses began to believe their views would make a difference — not all nurses, of course, because not all views prevailed — but enough to make the discussions productive.

Six months after the first retreat was held, the data from 89% of the RN staff were analyzed (see Table 1). Seventeen value statements received a response of "strongly agree" or "agree" from more than 80% of the staff.

At this point, a validation survey was mailed to all RNs. The 17 value statements were printed and nurses were asked to indicate whether or not they agreed with the role development issue, and whether or not they could live with it. In keeping with the consensus-building approach, the object was to know how many nurses were comfortable with the outcomes.

NPPC staff nurse members distributed and collected the surveys. They were disappointed to learn that only 60% of their colleagues returned the questionnaires (although that was the best response rate we had ever achieved to a mailed questionnaire). Many NPPC members encouraged their colleagues to participate. Others left it up to the staff entirely. The percentage of respondents who indicated that they could live with the 17 values surveyed ranged from 92-100%.

In the validation survey, we asked when nurses would be willing and ready to go about the process of patient care delivery system assessment and redesign to incorporate departmentally-shared values. Although critical care nurses were not as ready as other groups, the number who were ready within the next year was phenomenal (76%), given this group's initial resistance to the concept of a length-of-stay accountable nurse, either within or outside of their units.

Staff struggled long and hard over the issue of titles for nurses in different roles. The terminology we will probably use is *clinical nurse* for nurses with shift accountability, and *attending nurse* for nurses with length-of-stay accountability.

Many options were considered about how role differentiation would affect the design of a career ladder. One of our assumptions for the career ladder component of the salary structure model is that experts in either role will be able to earn similar incomes. That means that the hourly salary level of the attending nurse would be higher due to the salaried status, but the total income of an expert clinical nurse who worked rotating shifts and/or weekends would approximate the salary of the attending nurse. In our experience, it took only a few months for clinical nurses to agree that attending nurses should be earning higher hourly wages for the amount of responsibility they were willing to assume.

The reason for supporting relatively equal potential incomes for nurses in each role is that we may achieve our departmental values without differentiated roles on all nursing units. The intensivist nurses in the emergency department, the post-anesthesia care unit, and perhaps even some of the ICUs are not likely to differentiate roles due to the short-term nature of the patient stay. Instead, these nurses will work with other units' attending nurses who are responsible for coordinating nursing care throughout the length of stay. The level of professional responsibility and decision making on the part of expert intensivist nurses is high, though taking on different dimensions than those of the attending nurse. Reaching the expert level of the clinical nurse track, then, may represent the only career option for nurses on units where patients stay a short but critical time during their hospitalization.

Where are we now? Our current efforts are focused on management development, nursing care delivery model redesign, building nurse-to-nurse collaboration skills, developing competencies for each level of the differentiated career ladder structure, and experimenting with systems of peer review. A third patient care unit, the surgical subspecialties unit, developed their new nursing care delivery model this fall. A number of additional proposals are in the planning stage. Given the necessity of developing nursing care delivery models that are budget neutral, considerable planning and effort are involved at each stage.

The development of nursing managers is crucial to progress. At the same time that the staff retreats were going on, we held a discussion that lasted more than 10 hours for all nursing leaders in the department. In retrospect, the retreats should have been held before the first two units implemented differentiated roles. They might have lessened resistance to the models on the part of other directors and supervisors and more support might have been available to the pilot units.

Further management development is needed. Although we have staff nurses with the vision and motivation for change, the process slows considerably when the managers are not able to follow through. Managers need to be able to develop concrete budget proposals for the desired models, deal with the stresses of role transition on the part of nursing and medical staffs, and make the transition to letting go of whatever clinical care management might have been part of their role. Fortunately, the more units that have a differentiated practice model in place, the greater the variety of models for others to emulate. Clearly, education for nursing managers needs to include content on interactive planning processes, how to manage role change transitions, and basic content on the goals and potential models of differentiated practice.

Although education would certainly help, it may not be the total answer. This particular magnitude of change requires the commitment and vision of leaders, be they staff, managers, or nurse executives. Someone has to be available to cheerlead, to keep the group focused on goals, to reiterate rationale for changes 1,000 times a month, to be flexible and yet steady in dealing with each individual staff member's personal reaction to change, and to constantly evaluate the unit outcomes and share them with internal and external groups.

On that note, what did we learn about evaluation of outcomes? That it is very difficult. On the first pilot unit, we monitored the traditional outcomes — length of stay, patient satisfaction, nurse/MD/other professionals' judgment of the outcomes, quality assurance outcomes, and cost. We documented the maintenance or improvement of these outcomes, as nurses have done in many other institutions.

Other outcomes are convincing our nurses that differentiated practice models are good for patients; however, these outcomes have not been studied. We would like to know if the patient care management models resulted in less skin breakdown; fewer wound or respiratory infections; fewer readmissions; faster identification and attention to acutely confused states; less depression; better pain management; better coordination of care between clinic, hospital, and home; etc. In relatively small hospitals like ours, with only one of each type of unit, the threats to the validity of our study designs are overwhelming. We support the need for multisite studies of patient outcomes to better help us answer questions concerning the effectiveness of differentiated practice.

What do attending nurses — whether primary nurses or case managers — need in the way of education? We are currently duplicating the process we used to identify what characteristics staff thought were most important for a career ladder. However, this time the target nurse is the attending rather than the clinical nurse. To date, our observations are that these nurses need educational content in physical assessment, diagnostic reasoning, methods of research use, the concepts behind nursing standards and evaluation of outcomes, and nursing and health care economics. They need clear, efficient, professional documentation skills; conflict resolution skills; and knowledge about principles of delegation, supervision, collaboration, and accountability. Finally, they need experiences with peer review, ethical decision making, and patient advocacy. When knowledge and skills are the focus of the BSN nurse's preparation, there will be no obstacle to moving into an education-based role differentiation.

What information would have been helpful when we began this process of change? We should have been prepared to put this change in perspective. In order to be involved in the decisions about practice, staff and managers need education and time to discuss feelings before any true problem solving can occur. There is little to be gained by a sense of impatience and much to be gained by letting everyone involved have their say.

As with any change, we also had to learn again that you can never please all the people involved. The 20% who oppose the change will be the loudest voices; therefore, the use of surveys for all staff members is crucial in determining staff opinion. We will continue to use this process as the career ladder evolves.

Finally, we would do it again. An intimacy has evolved among departmental nurses during this last year that is rarely experienced. That intimacy involved conflict as well as closeness, but it was professionally stimulating and exciting for many people. Both the process and the outcomes have been worth the investment.

❑   ❑   ❑

Table 1
Values Statements in RN Validation Survey

Mary Hitchcock Memorial Hospital Department of Nursing
April 1990

1. Nursing care delivery models should be chosen based on what will provide the best outcomes for patient and families.

2. Patients and families would have better outcomes if one RN was accountable for planning, coordinating, and evaluating the nursing care of each patient and family during their length of stay (LOS).

3. Patients and families would have better outcomes if one MD was accountable for planning, coordinating and evaluating the medical care of each patient and family during their length of stay (LOS).

4. All patients deserve/require assignments to RNs who are LOS-accountable for nursing care during the patients' hospitalizations, regardless of whether this accountability is maintained by one nurse or passed to another when a patient is transferred.

5. Patients and families would have better outcomes if the LOS-accountable RN and MD worked together on the same caseload of patients.

6. There should be built-in mechanisms for regular face-to-face communication between the patient's LOS-accountable RN and MD team members.

7. Goals for medical plans of care and nursing plans of care should exist and be known by all members of the health care team as well as patients/families.

8. Under some conditions, accountability for medical and nursing care planning and evaluation should be transferred to another RN/MD team.

9. When accountability is transferred during one hospitalization period, the original accountable RN/MD team retain a consultative role to the new attending RN/MD team.

10. Assistive to professional nursing roles should be defined to use the skills and talents, within legal boundaries, of LPNs, CNAs, monitor technicians, and mental health workers where appropriate to nursing care.

11. Nursing care delivery models may differ from unit to unit, but they should be structured to accomplish the same goals and values.

12. For any nursing care delivery model, the selection of persons to fill different roles should be based on self, peer, and supervisor assessment of competence and on self-assessment of current goals.

13. For any nursing care delivery model, there should be mutual valuing of the skills and expertise required to perform each RN role.

14. Discharge planning should begin on or prior to admission and should be completed by the RN who has primary accountability for the patient throughout hospitalization.

15. Learning needs of all patients should be assessed by an RN in a deliberative, noncoincidental manner, and should be reflected in the plan of care from admission to discharge.

16. All patients should be able to identify the RN who is accountable for the planning and coordination of their nursing care and should know how to contact that RN or an identified substitute, if necessary.

17. Nurses who accept roles that involve accountability over a patient's length of stay should work shifts that facilitate collaboration with families, physicians, off-shift nurses, CNSs, and other members of the health care team.

Building on Shared Governance: The Sioux Valley Hospital Experience

JoEllen Koerner, M.B.A., R.N., C.N.A.

Webster defines a healer as "one who makes whole, one who restores integrity" (Webster's, 1991). We are all healers within the nursing profession — individuals who are brave in encouraging a wholesome existence for ourselves and others. Our focus historically and appropriately has been on the clients we serve. The healing I am referring to today is of equal importance within the nursing profession — the healing of ourselves. For too long we have been a profession overcome with class and gender issues, resulting in segregation of colleagues through multiple educational pathways, isolation of education from service, and a host of other issues which create fragmentation and discontent. We can only provide clients with that which we inherently possess. Thus, if wholeness is our goal, we must first be whole in order to manifest that quality to the public we serve.

During the past three years, Sioux Valley Hospital (SVH), Sioux Falls, South Dakota, has implemented an extensive project involving their design of professional nursing practice. Our primary goal was to expand the role of nursing to that of professional business partner (Koerner, 1990). Balancing clinical and business competencies would help integrate nursing into the decision-making arena of the health care industry. Achieving that goal required the implementation of differentiated practice and case management, along with the creation of a shared governance environment built on individual autonomy and accountability. This activity was a very challenging process for our nursing practice. During the change effort, several themes kept reappearing; eventually, they became the guiding principles for our process. I would like to share these principles in an effort to communicate the essence of what differentiated practice may offer any nursing practice in the country.

The Context Surrounding Change is Everything

In her compelling novel, *The Handmaid's Tale*, Margaret Atwood (1985) depicts the universe after a nuclear holocaust. Certain women are kept for breeding purposes while the men plan ways to recreate the universe. In one scene, a woman is taken to a man's room where she is invited to play chess. The man asks her, "Why can't you laugh?" Later, after their sexual encounter, he says, "Why can't you be more responsive?" To each query she replies with the haunting theme of the book, "The context is everything."

Today nursing has been offered a context for change that is unparalleled in our professional history. The health care industry is in such a state of turmoil that individuals and groups with the most innovative ideas have the greatest chance of implementing the changes needed to maintain viability. Why should we consider differentiated practice during times of shortage and role confusion? Because it is the only answer to an increasingly fragmented health care environment, to changing career expectations of college graduates seeking progression and advancement based on educational levels and experience, and to changing methods of reimbursement which demand coordination of care to maximize productivity while maintaining quality.

The American Nurses Association began setting the national stage for differentiation with their 1965 *Position Statement on Entry into Practice* (American Nurses Association, 1965). It called for two distinct levels of registered nursing based on educational preparation and the resulting competency acquired. Several years ago, the National Commission on Nursing Implementation Project (NCNIP) thoughtfully examined the issue of differentiated practice and created a time frame in which to reach this goal (National Commission on Nursing Implementation Project, 1986). This conference offers a collage of the wonderful work being done nationwide on an idea whose time has come. Nursing is creating a solution to the health care delivery crisis by redesigning the roles and responsibilities of care providers through the differentiation of practice. Again, "the context is everything."

At the state level, collective activities are also underway. In South Dakota, a nursing shortage prompted the legislature to propose the reopening of six LPN schools in response to the lack of qualified personnel. The nursing community organized the State-wide Project for Nursing and Nursing Education. Armed with only a commitment to offer an alternative solution to the issue, a demonstration project to test two levels of registered nurse practice was established in four regional centers. These were comprised of large and small hospitals, long-term care, and home health agencies. The outcome of that work generated $800,000 from the legislature to open one LPN school and heavily fund ADN and BSN education (Statewide Project Steering Committee, 1988). A significant victory for organized nursing had been achieved.

Within Sioux Valley Hospital, a project was designed to construct a professional practice model for nursing. The goal was to create a "magnet hospital," such as those evaluated in a comprehensive study completed by the American Academy of Nursing (1983). In reviewing that work, the practice at SVH identified four components as essential to professional practice: a participative management structure, a comprehensive care delivery system, collaborative professional relationships, and opportunities and rewards for professional growth. Redesigning nursing roles and responsibilities was the primary goal. At the same time, the Statewide Project emerged and Sioux Valley was positioned to successfully pilot the concept of differentiated practice (Koerner et al., 1988).

As the Essence of a Concept is Grasped, the Form May Change

Our initial exposure to differentiated practice came through Dr. Peggy Primm, who assisted with the Statewide Project. From her work, we viewed the role of the nurse in three domains: provision of care, communication, and management of care (Primm, 1987). Differentiated practice was presented as a care delivery system which provided two distinct roles for nurses — case manager and case associate. It formalized nursing diagnosis and nursing process as the communication mechanisms which unified the activities of these various care givers.

Dr. Margaret McClure introduced us to the work of Lawrence and Lorsch, two members of the faculty at the Harvard University School of Business. Lawrence and Lorsch (1967) studied the notion of differentiation and integration in various corporate, educational, and health care settings throughout the United States. From their work, we came to view differentiation more broadly as a basic philosophical viewpoint regarding one's work. The differences vary around the time frame, structure of boundaries, scope of interpersonal relationships, and orientation to lifelong learning. At this point we began to enlarge the definition of expanded practice beyond the role of case manager to include other more complex roles, such as charge nurses who manage systems issues, or the home health nurse who works in a nonstructured setting. Staff changed the titles to *registered nurse* (reflecting the current RN role) and *primary nurse* (reflecting the enlarged scope of responsibility) to maintain the identity of "nurse." One-third of the practice moved into the expanded roles which formalized and rewarded individuals demonstrating broader initiative and leadership (Figure 1).

The Harvard study also stated that differentiation alone can increase fragmentation within any setting. People have a tendency to see only their world as the total entity. The success factor in complex, differentiated settings was a strong integrative force which unified the various components around a common vision and goal. Thus, the nursing practice named their revised care delivery system "Integrated Care," positioning primary nurses as the integrative force within the institution.

Integrative pathways were designed as a working tool to facilitate client movement throughout their acute episode of illness by coordinating the activities of various health care providers with the needs of the client. Primary nurses were the critical force in providing managed care within the hospital setting.

As nurses became more skilled in longitudinal thinking and discharge planning, it became apparent that care needs extended well beyond the hospital walls. Case management was perceived as advanced nursing practice. The CNSs would design a unique pathway for each client needing specialized services to support their modified existence in the presence of life-altering disease (Figure 2).

Clients needing case management included those with chronic illness, financial or knowledge deficits, or lack of support in the home setting. Care needs were matched with available resources through integrative functions which assisted client movement through the health care delivery system. Quality outcomes and significant cost savings were being realized through the implementation of this integrative care delivery mode (Figure 3).

Change is Messy, Noisy, Energizing, and Liberating

Erik Erikson observed that timing is critical to change. He proposed that there have been many leaders as great as Lincoln, Gandhi, and Napoleon. What made these particular men exceptional, however, was the fact that each man, his ideals, and the needs of his country came into perfect alignment at the same time in history. Erickson believed that the changes occurred almost in spite of the leaders because the time for change had come. Conversely, when there was no alignment of these factors, no change could occur.

Planning a change project of significance is much like remodeling a house. In estimating the time and cost involved, the old rule of doubling one's figures is appropriate. Nurses within the organization are ready for change in varying forms, at varying rates. Forcing a change will not achieve the same results as creating readiness for change and facilitating its movement.

During the change process, focus is usually placed on movement of the innovation. "How to" activities are developed along with timeliness and strategies for change. The initial point of importance, however, is the area of nonmovement, as the focus at this point is on "the why" of change. A recent workshop on transitions asked participants to list their ages by each year since birth, noting the years of significant transition in their lives. The group was then challenged to focus on the "white space" — the time between the transitions when inner work was being done. A great deal of support and information regarding change and the consequences of various choices should be given to individuals making a shift in their personal and professional career definitions, which may have spanned many decades. Voluntary movement denotes completion of some internal processing, which is essential if one is to move into a new way of "being."

Support to facilitate the change process on nursing units must be provided through clear communication and feedback as staff struggles with internalizing the major concepts. A helpful strategy to facilitate the internal struggle is the notion of "revisiting." We discovered that one in-service on differentiated practice is not enough to teach staff the concept. After repeated in-servicing every few months, staff had the opportunity to review the concept, experience it in their work, return to the concept with a deeper understanding based on their lived experience, and modify their behavior and definition of the concept.

Support also comes from connection among the various units as they experience the impact of major change. A rule for the South Dakota Statewide Project was that each institution had to have a minimum of two units participating in the demonstration project. We found that change is not neat and linear, but rather a matter of taking two steps forward and one step back. During transition, parallel systems are running — the old way and the new. In times of crisis or stress, it is very tempting to revert to old, well-known behaviors. This can cause, great dissonance within the unit. When one unit "hits the wall," the other may be on course, and vice versa. Thus, partnership among units is critical as nurses experience the joy and frustration of innovation and change.

The rate of change varied among nursing units at SVH. Those that moved more quickly had a history of innovation — a tenured unit manager who had strong credibility and trust in her staff, and a staff composed of nurses who were involved in committee work, continuing education, and professional organizations.

The rate of change also varied among the clinical divisions of practice. When a practice can see the value and relevance of the proposed change in their work, change comes quickly. If the concept is seen as superfluous, the change effort will quickly dissipate. The maternal-child health area at SVH, known for a strong preference for meaningful interpersonal relationships, quickly recognized the value in primary nursing and was the first department to adopt differentiation. The medical-surgical area discovered its value for discharge planning and client teaching, and adapted quickly as well.

The area that saw little relevance to its work was critical care. The nurses here, more focused on technical skills, saw their work as comprehensive, in need of no reform. Through the development of integrative pathways with receiving units, as well as dialogues in committee work, they gained a new awareness. Acuity, as they had experienced it, was associated with critical multisystem failure.

Complexity, as experienced in the world of chronic illness, presented another type of nursing challenge. An 82-year-old diabetic with cataracts, needing education on insulin self-administration and dietary modification within a three-day length of stay, was as challenging to the professional nurse as the trauma client admitted to critical care from the emergency room. The maternity unit, with a 24-hour length of stay, was faced with the difficulty of educating a first-time mother in breast feeding and parenting techniques while she was recovering from delivery. A new understanding of the challenges facing all professional nurses emerged, and a sense of collegiality was enhanced.

As their world view expanded, critical care nurses began to identify a need for broader relationships with other units, physician specialty groups, and client families in the waiting room. Thus, better communication with these groups was woven into the expanded primary nurse role in critical care, extending differentiated practice throughout the practice.

Management had to stay one step ahead of the staff in order to lead and support the change process. A series of four management development classes was designed, with two completed before implementation of differentiated practice began. These classes focused on creativity and communication, management and leadership skills, as well as personal and professional issues surrounding change. The management team established new criteria for situational leadership, negotiation and conflict resolution, and partnerships among themselves. Consultation between front line managers of the nursing units was a major force in successful housewide implementation of the project.

As understanding increases, so does the energy and commitment to the task at hand. Proper support and guidance are essential to directing this energy into productive channels which support the goals of the change project. However, it also is important to note that as the units internalize the concept, it can take varying forms. A key component for management is the need to "maintain the vision, but embrace the hybrid." This concept will work best for the group that knows their specialty and the clients they serve.

Finally, change is noisy. A model based on competency and choice was designed by the staff to assist nurses with placement into the nursing roles. If nurses demonstrated the requisite competency, they could choose to move into the primary role. Some nurses quickly chose to either move into the expanded role or remain in the current RN role which gave them great professional satisfaction. The group that experienced the greatest difficulty was comprised of those who had trouble selecting a career option.

It became very clear in evaluating the dissension within the system that those with the greatest difficulty with the new model often demonstrated low self-esteem and had a history of negative behavior. I believe that the movement toward differentiation of nursing practice stimulates the self-esteem issues of all practitioners within the field. Organizations must address personal and professional development issues through their continued education offerings as nurses are called upon to increase their autonomy and accountability.

Changes in Application of Role Competencies Mandate Changes in the Socialization and Education of Nurses

The paradigm for nursing practice is changing. Differentiated practice does not build on increased technical skills, but rather on communication and the critical thinking competencies of the nurse. In her innovative theory, "Health as Expanding Consciousness," Dr. Margaret Newman proposed that professional nursing is primarily relational (Newman, 1986). She envisions emerging professional roles and responsibilities which call for innovation and creativity, empathy and caring, and powerful interpersonal skills to influence and negotiate on behalf of the client as well as the professional.

Initially, the practice at SVH identified skills necessary for effectiveness in the primary nurse role. These skills included: clinical competence, business competence, surveillance skills, diagnostic reasoning, human interaction, and communication skills. However, as we moved further into the project, it became clear that prescriptive thinking was very hampering to the nurse. A current pilot project being tested by an innovative BSN program which values differentiated practice is addressing this problem.

RNs moving up through their program receive clinical training on their unit of employment during working hours, rather than migrating to a unit of specialty study in the student role. This school operates on the assumption that all client populations offer real or potential nursing diagnoses. Therefore, when a functional health problem is being studied, such as impaired skin integrity due to penetration of skin barrier, it is to be assessed and addressed while the nurse is on duty in his or her place of employment. The focused learning occurs during faculty-led grand rounds. Each nurse gives evidence of assessment of the client and this is mapped on the board. The ER nurse might assess a laceration, the OB nurse an episiotomy, the OR nurse a surgical incision, the pediatric nurse a tracheotomy, and the long-term care nurse a decubitus. Thus, multiple examples based on age, disease process, and geographic location expand the nurse's awareness to be able to diagnose the conditions in places other than the surgical floor. Further, the process establishes an expectation that one is always learning on the job, and not only in a circumscribed "student-faculty" experience on a "student rotation." We have found that the interspecialty networking has had a profound impact on collegial relationships. Class projects have strengthened the practice of nursing on the student's unit of employment.

In a short length-of-stay, high acuity environment, rapid and accurate assessment and intervention are crucial. Nurses are called upon to make effective decisions regarding patient care and allocation of resources in a timely fashion. Where we once had weeks to care for a client, we now have days. Getting to the root of problems quickly in order to assure a rapid turnaround is essential. A second, related challenge is the need to expedite the learning process. While students in an academic setting are given material over a period of time, continuing education of adult staff is meted out in shortened time frames because of the organization's demands and fiscal constraints. The need to grasp new concepts or reframe old ones quickly and comprehensively is imperative to continued competence and job satisfaction.

A local college offering a BSN degree assisted with the design and delivery of a three-credit course on change. Based on the adult learning principles, we created classes for staff, emphasizing experiential learning. Each concept was introduced through an experience which captured its essence, followed by dialogue and application on a work-related project.

The issue of grief and loss accompanying change began with a burial at a local funeral home. On decision points surrounding change, our class traveled to the state penitentiary where we experienced solitary confinement — reviewing self-imprisoning behavior and attitudes. A class on values, judgement, and self-esteem began in a jury box at the county courthouse. Team-building was studied at a wellness center, with a coach as our instructor. The impact on staff was transformational — demonstrating that relevant learning can be dynamic, even when compressed in time.

We are now designing a learning experience for nursing students in a differentiated environment that will facilitate collegial and collaborative relationships. Clinical experience for ADN and BSN students from programs committed to the philosophy of differentiated practice will be held simultaneously on one unit. The ADN students will perform in the traditional registered nurse role. BSN students will work as primary nurses, collaborating on the care plan with ADN students. These BSN students also receive home health experience by following their clients into the home, thereby strengthening their longitudinal awareness. A physician from the medical school has asked if he could teach an interdisciplinary class where nursing and medical students attend grand rounds together. He and the primary nurse providing care will focus on pathophysiology, medical and nursing interventions, as well as ethical and philosophical issues surrounding the care of the client. Thus, collaboration begun in the student socialization process, may become a reality in future practice.

Legal Implications of Advancing Practice Opportunities Must Be Addressed by Experts Who Understand the Work

Nursing has always governed its own, as have all the other true professions. This has been our fortunate history, and must be maintained into the future. State boards of nursing are given the dual charge of protecting public safety through monitoring entry-level activities and maintaining legal/ethical practice. As the definition of competence continues to expand, so too must understanding and evaluation.

In a provocative editorial, Barbara Barnum relayed an observation made by medical sociologist Hans Mauksch (Barnum, 1989). He stated that nursing and medicine hand out knowledge with a different focus. According to Mauksch, medicine says, "Here is knowledge, and it is power. The more you know, the more powerful you are." Nursing, on the other hand, says, "Here is knowledge, and it is dangerous. If you don't use it right someone will be hurt." Thus, medicine views knowledge as an asset, while nursing experiences it as a burden.

My own lived experience as executive secretary of the South Dakota Board of Nursing affirmed that observation. I constantly saw the medical board review practice privilege requests with an inclusionary interpretation: if it is not addressed in the law, it is perfectly legal to perform. Nursing, on the other hand, views the law with a more exclusionary interpretation: if it is not addressed in the law, it can only be done with elaborate demonstrations of how competency will be obtained and maintained. This can be a particularly limiting approach during a time when nursing and medical roles are being redefined, with multiple boundary issues emerging.

While nursing practice and nursing education are experiencing the challenges and opportunities inherent in redesign, it is imperative that our legal arena do the same. Many state boards are composed of political appointees rather than experts in the field who can best interpret what is appropriate nursing practice. I have seen outstanding nursing leaders and creative nursing projects designed to meet the changing health care needs of clients penalized by a board that does not fully understand the innovation. If nursing boards are to be effective and supportive of advancing nursing practice, one of two options should be considered. Ideally, all boards would be composed of experts in the field of nursing education and nursing service so that public safety and nursing innovation to meet their changing needs would be given mutual consideration.

If the first strategy is impossible, a second strategy is essential. In emerging practice issues, a panel of experts could be convened to study the proposed innovation and make recommendations to the board as in expert witness testimony. In either scenario, the balance between protection of the public and advancement of nursing could thus be maintained.

This is Nursing's Moment ... And It Must Be Acted On Now

We live in a privileged time and place. The civil rights movement, the feminist movement, and the overall advancement of humankind has given a profession consisting predominantly of women the momentum for healing and growth. Economic and demographic changes have given nurses a public mandate that fits their agenda. The shortage of qualified personnel has added economic power and influence to the health care arena. Thus, the factors necessary to support our evolution are present.

The essential ingredient needed for nursing to capitalize on this opportunity is the courage to move forward in unison and harmony. The power of our collective efforts was demonstrated in the recent defeat of the registered care technician (RCT) proposal. We must maintain that momentum as we redesign our reality to fit today's needs. This requires each of us to reevaluate emerging career opportunities and the manner in which we carry out the work being done in the education, service, and legal arenas.

The opportunities offered through differentiated practice; case management; changes in education, administration, and politics; and employment advancements are a double-edged sword. These opportunities force people to be accountable for their own destiny. With that discomforting reality comes a certain amount of "noise." I have seen many wonderful nursing leaders and organizations react to that dissonance, fearing that the idea is not good or that they will create chaos within the organization if they pursue innovation. They pull back and modify a wonderful design, hoping to quiet the dissension. The tragedy is that the hybrid is not as effective as the original, and the noise will continue due to the inherent discomfort brought on by any change. Further, the momentum for change will have been lost and is difficult to recover.

A group of supervisors at SVH were meeting to redesign their career goals as their roles were eliminated from the organization. Though some were eager to participate in redesign, many were angry and resistant. Then one of the supervisors told a story which had significance; it became the metaphor for the entire group:

> When lions go out to feed, they place the oldest lion with the fewest teeth at the entrance to a cave. He roars fiercely and loudly in the direction of the forest. All the little creatures hear him and scatter in the opposite direction, only to run into the clutches of the young, strong lions positioned behind them, waiting for their arrival. The moral of the story is "run to the roar." Your safety and your strength lie in facing the noise or threat and conquering it.

This group of supervisors became very creative and innovative as they reviewed the multiple needs of clients and the organization. Many have moved into rich and meaningful new roles, while several left the profession to pursue careers more consistent with their talents and abilities. I believe that not all nurses are prospering in their current professional career. Some feel "stuck," while others are disillusioned. These people need to be assisted with career counseling as changing career options emerge. Some will find answers within the profession, while others will leave it for other opportunities.

Changing the old myth that "a nurse is a nurse is a nurse" is what differentiated practice is all about. It is an idea whose time has come. We have wonderfully capable leadership in nursing education and service and the legal arena to help us evolve into our full potential. To do that we must support and celebrate each other at all levels of practice as we evolve toward wholeness.

❑   ❑   ❑

Figure 1
Framework for Differentiating Practice Roles of Nursing

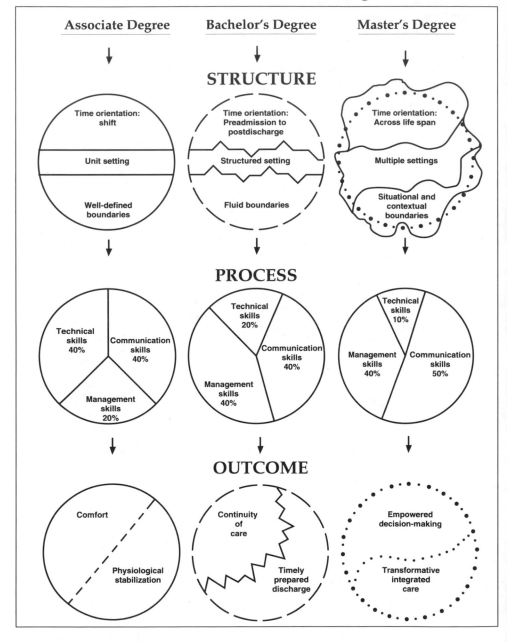

Figure 2
Continuum of Health Care Services
and Integrating Factors

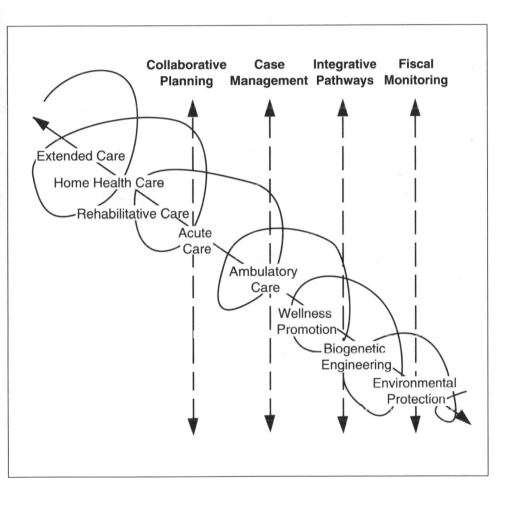

Figure 3
Hospice Program Funding

Total Payment/Client	$8,500.00
Average Cost/Client	3,720.00

Hospice Utilization Review

	1988–1989	1989–1990
Medical Supplies	$1.01/day/pt	$ .58/day/pt
Lab	2.46/day/pt	.08/day/pt
DME	.53/day/pt	.07/day/pt
Pharmacy	2.95/day/pt	4.31/day/pt
Radiology	.87/day/pt	.40/day/pt
Other Total		50.59–ER
		106.20 Enteral

The Nursing Initiative Program: Practice-Based Models for Care in Hospitals

Jean Marie Ake, M.A., R.N.
Susan Bowar-Ferres, Ph.D., R.N.
Toni Cesta, Ph.D., R.N.
David Gould, Ph.D.
Jeannine Greenfield, Sc.D., R.N.
Pamela Hayes, Ed.D, R.N.
Greg Maislin, M.S., M.A.
Mathy Mezey, Ed.D., R.N., F.A.A.N.

Overview

Documentation of a shortage of professional nurses receives constant mention in both the professional and lay press. Despite the fact that more nurses are now employed than ever before, the nursing shortage remains acute. And, while adequate salary compensation is clearly a factor in the recruitment and retention of RNs, several studies have documented work conditions, burnout, and inadequate advancement opportunities as substantially influencing job retention (Aiken and Mullinex, 1987; Aiken and Hadley, 1988; American Hospital Association, 1988; Nursing Restructuring, 1990; The Commonwealth Fund, 1990).

In 1987, the nursing shortage in New York, New York hovered around 16%. Seeking to demonstrate its commitment to resolving

This work was partially supported by grants from the United Hospital Fund, New York, and the Aaron Diamond Foundation.

the severe shortage, the United Hospital Fund invited hospitals in the New York metropolitan area to submit proposals for two-year trials to test new approaches to the organization and support of nursing services. In mid-1988, the fund awarded grants to five hospitals. Three of these (Brooklyn Hospital, New York Hospital, and Columbia-Presbyterian Medical Center) also received a partnership grant from the Aaron Diamond Foundation. The foundation was interested in these projects' potential for creating significant opportunities for career advancement among minority health care workers.

The basic premise underlying all five projects was that the hospital environment can be restructured in such a way as to increase RN productivity and satisfaction without jeopardizing patient care. The overall objectives of this two-year project were to improve working conditions for registered nurses, and to more clearly define professional and nonprofessional nursing roles (see Table 1).

The five participating hospitals, representing major medical centers and large teaching hospitals in the New York metropolitan area, were: Brooklyn Hospital, Long Island Jewish Medical Center in Queens (LIJ), and three hospitals in Manhattan — New York Hospital (NYH), New York University Medical Center (NYU), and Columbia-Presbyterian Medical Center/Neurological Institute (PH/Neuro) [see Table 2]. These five hospitals represented diverse institutions. Yet, prior to beginning the project, LIJ, NYH and NYU were remarkably similar as to the percentage of staff that were RNs, the size of nursing staff, and number of RNs per hospital bed. At Brooklyn Hospital, a smaller percentage of staff were RNs, and PH/Neuro had a smaller ratio of RNs per hospital bed than any of the other four (see Table 3).

The program in four of the hospitals involved a total of 294 beds on nine units: eight medical-surgical and one neonatal ICU. This represented a range of from 8% of the total beds at Brooklyn Hospital to 20% of the beds at PH/Neuro. There were a total of 330.5 FTE nursing staff on these units — 72% were RNs, 4% LPNs, and 24% nursing assistants. The project at NYU involved all units and approximately 200 RNs. At the time of the program's inception, the participating hospitals' RN vacancy rate was between 7 and 43% (see Table 4).

With the exception of the NICU at LIJ, the percentage of nursing staff that were RNs was lower on the participating units than in the hospitals as a whole. This is consistent with national data which

90

indicates that 40% of hospital R.N.'s work in specialized units (United Hospital Fund, n.d.) [see Table 5].

Project Evaluation

The sites funded under this initiative constituted five "case studies," in that they were not chosen to conform to a preconceived model. The plan for evaluation attempted to respect the differences among participants while drawing on the commonalities across programs to capture a sense of the project's overall success.

The evaluation was quasi-experimental, multidimensional, and prospective. Each site submitted data at three time points: baseline data were collected within one month of each site's start-up, called their "birthday" (Time 0); mid-point data were obtained within one month of their first birthday (Time 1); and end-point data were collected approximately 18 to 22 months into the project (Time 2). Data were standardized as to time frame, definition of terms, and use of standardized instruments, when feasible.

The evaluation instruments are summarized in Table 6. Descriptive hospital and unit data, including bed capacity, occupancy, and nurse staffing were collected using hospital and unit description forms. Data collection included budgeted and actual positions, and turnover and vacancy rates for RNs, LPNs, and nurses aides.

The Nursing Job Satisfaction Scale, a valid and reliable instrument originally developed by Brayfield and Rothe and modified by Atwood and Hinshaw (Atwood and Hinshaw, 1981; Atwood and Hinshaw, 1984) was administered to all RNs on all shifts at all three time points. Quality of care was assessed through site-specific data on four quality of care indicators: infection rates, falls, decubiti, and medication errors. Finally, the Hinshaw and Atwood Patient Satisfaction Scale (Hinshaw, 1982) was administered to all patients within 36 hours of discharge at each data collection point at each site, with the exception of NYU.

Data analysis consisted of computing descriptive statistics for each site over time, making comparisons between Time 0 and Time 2 using paired t-tests and chi square statistics, where appropriate. The RN satisfaction global and component scores were summarized by unit within each hospital by computing means and standard deviations at each time point. For LIJ, two groups (patient care managers, yes and no) were compared at each time point using pooled t-tests, unless the variances differed significantly. In those cases, Welch's t-tests were used. For NYU and NYH, because data were collected at three time points (before, during, and after intervention), we were able to compare mean changes over time using a repeated measure of analysis of variance (ANOVA) to assess the statistical significance of differences.

For each participating unit, global and component patient satisfaction scores were summarized for each data collection point. Since the samples constituted independent random samples, we were able to use a one-way ANOVA to assess the significance of changes in means over time.

Description and Project Outcomes from the Four Sites Implementing a Differentiated Practice Model

While each site took a somewhat different approach to enhancing professional nurse practice, four of the projects focused on a "differentiated practice model," which redefined nursing roles and work environments (see Table 7). First, nursing tasks were stratified into those requiring direct RN involvement and those which could be safely delegated to nonprofessionals or technical staff under RN supervision. Next, necessary administrative changes were identified and implemented. Educational modules prepared nonprofessional providers to perform new tasks, and RNs to delegate and supervise nonprofessional and/or technical staff. Lastly, project participants established mechanisms for ongoing communication.

Introducing an Augmented Role for Expert Nurses: Long Island Jewish Medical Center

The goals of LIJ were primarily to improve the match between professional nurse capability and patient needs, and to enhance the skills of nurse attendants as a means of freeing the RN to concentrate on professional tasks. Three nursing units from LIJ participated in the project: a 39-bed medical neurology unit with 24.8 FTE RNs and 16 nursing attendants; a 32-bed surgical/orthopedic unit with 15 RNs and 11 nursing attendants; and one 40-bed neonatal ICU from Schneider Childrens Hospital with 80 FTE RNs.

Based on clinical expertise and willingness to participate, experienced nursing staff on each unit were chosen to assume new positions of patient care managers (PCMs) [see Table 8]. By the project's completion, 20 PCMs were in place on the participating units, representing 20% of the units' RN staff. In addition to regular staff functions, the workload of the PCMs was adjusted to allow them to care for one to three patients identified through a patient acuity system as requiring comprehensive coordination of services, teaching, and discharge planning. In order to underscore the role of PCMs as being the focal point of care for patients, families, physicians, and other hospital staff, PCMs distributed business cards to patients. Simultaneously, an educational curriculum was implemented to upgrade the skills of nurse attendants on the pilot units. In addition to their regular job responsibilities, nurse attendants were trained in taking blood pressure and changing dressings, and were included in walking rounds with the RNs.

The average nursing hours per patient at LIJ and all other projects was similar at the beginning and end of the project. The reorganization of nursing personnel, however, was associated with increased professional nurse productivity, as evidenced by declines in the number of RN hours per patient, and fewer RNs on the units (119.8 FTEs at start-up, as compared to 113.7 FTEs at 18 months). Yet, despite fewer RNs, there was substantial evidence of improved RN satisfaction (see Table 9). The RN vacancy rate decreased from 8% to 0% on medicine, and from 23% to 0% on surgery. The NICU had no RN vacancies throughout the project.

RNs also indicated increased job satisfaction on all three units (see Table 10). Response rate to the RN Satisfaction Scale ranged from 89-90%. Because of changes in RN staffing, statistical analysis comparing groups over time was not appropriate, but the trend for improved RN satisfaction at 18 months in comparison to start-up is readily discernible. Of particular note were the significant ($P = .0008$) improvements in job satisfaction from the beginning to the end of the project between nurses selected as patient care managers in contrast to other RNs (see Table 11).

These changes in professional nurse responsibility and improved satisfaction were associated with moderate improvements in quality of care. While patient falls increased on the medical unit, infections and medication errors declined both at the midpoint and the end of the project.

Overall scores on the Patient Satisfaction Scale remained relatively unchanged. However, the scores of patients cared for by PCMs at 18 months showed significantly smaller variance ($P<0.05$)

than those cared for by other RNs, suggesting a consistency of satisfaction among patients (see Table 12).

Based on feedback from patient care managers that patients on the medical unit were too complex to manage in addition to other direct patient care responsibilities, the medical unit introduced a full-time PCM to manage the care of 15 patients with no additional bed-side responsibilities. Length of stay on this unit decreased .5 days from start-up to completion, in contrast to increases of from .2 to 2.1 days on comparable units.

Changing the Role for Nursing Assistants: the Brooklyn Hospital Medical Center and the New York Hospital Projects

While augmenting the role of nursing assistants was a secondary objective in the LIJ project, it was the central focus of the Brooklyn Hospital and the New York Hospital projects.

The major impetus for the Brooklyn Hospital Medical Center project was to upgrade the role of nursing assistants and to modify the professional to nonprofessional staffing mix to reduce the number of RNs, thus addressing an RN vacancy rate of 21%. A 39-bed medical unit was restructured to introduce a model of team nursing. A seven-session management curriculum prepared the RNs on the unit to augment their administrative skills to include assessment and planning of care, delegation of tasks, and supervision and evaluation of delivery of patient care (see Table 13).

A new, eight-week, 240-hour, performance-based curriculum prepared nursing assistants in skills such as blood pressure monitoring, tube feedings, suctioning, and simple dressings changes. Through publicity within the hospital and surrounding community, Brooklyn Hospital received over 75 applications for each of three nursing assistant training sessions. Of the 41 persons who enrolled, 36 completed the program. Upon finishing, assistants were given a certificate and recruited for new nursing assistant positions within the hospital. Interviews and career counseling encouraged nursing assistants to enter RN programs.

As predicted, over the course of the project the total number of RNs on the unit declined and the number of nursing assistants increased (see Table 14). RN FTEs decreased from 15.2 at start-up to 11.5 at 22 months, while the number of nursing assistants increased from 9.7 to 13. These changes in the mix of professionals to non-professionals were not reflected in major changes in patient satisfaction or clinical care indicators.

Rather than adding to the responsibilities of nurse assistants, New York Hospital sought to restructure the work environment so that RNs and nurses aides on three hospital units worked in concert instead of independently (see Table 15). The project involved three experimental and three control units. It specifically addressed age, ethnicity, education, and longevity of employment differences between the RNs (most of whom were young, white, baccalaureate-prepared, and employed at NYH for less than five years) and the nurses aides (who were primarily middle-aged, African-American, high school educated, long-term employees).

Before the project began, RNs worked 12-hour shifts and practiced modified primary nursing. Nurses aides, on the other hand, worked 7.5-hour shifts, five days a week, and covered the whole unit, often in pairs and with no consistency of assignment. The project divided each unit into two geographical districts, created permanent team assignments for RNs and nurses aides, and created clear expectations that RNs and nurses aides were to work together (see Table 17). Nurses were to give nurses aides specific instructions, both groups were to communicate frequently during the day and at change of shift, and both were to acknowledge each others' contribution to patient care. Based on responses to an RN satisfaction questionnaire, head nurses attended an educational program on management, task delegation, and conflict resolution. Staff nurses and nurses aides on all shifts participated in team building sessions.

At the completion of the project, each of the three units had been restructured into two RN/nurses aide teams, and primary care assignment for personnel in these teams increased from rarely to 90%. From the beginning to the end of the project, RNs on the experimental units significantly increased their management of nurses aides, in comparison to the control units (see Table 16).

Moreover, as expected, the findings confirmed that RNs on the experimental units had less need to structure the work activities of the nurses aides, primarily because the two groups worked out more trusting team relationships (see Table 17).

While having a moderately positive effect on the nurses aide vacancy rate, changes in the mix and relationship of professional and nonprofessional providers at Brooklyn Hospital and New York Hospital were not associated with improvements in RN satisfaction. RN satisfaction in the two sites either remained the same or declined, although the erratic RN response rates at both hospitals makes interpretation of these findings difficult (see Table 18). The

RN vacancy rate at Brooklyn Hospital was unchanged, while at New York Hospital the vacancy rate increased.

Creating New Roles for LPNs on Acute Units: The Presbyterian Hospital Partnership in Transitional Nursing Practice Program

In contrast to the Brooklyn Hospital and New York Hospital projects, Presbyterian Hospital focused on creating a new role for licensed practical nurses. Looking creatively at nurse staffing was imperative, as eight beds on a 36-bed unit had been closed for 16 months due to a 43% RN vacancy.

New positions were created for LPNs enrolled in RN programs (see Table 19). Nursing practice was differentiated, and partnerships created between professional and technical nurses. Consistent dyads of professional and practical nurses cared for groups of 12 patients. Managerial changes included dividing the unit into three districts, establishing performance standards for RNs and LPNs, and revising the procedures for monitoring patient outcomes. Classes, workshops, and ongoing "coaching" helped augment RNs' managerial and communication skills.

Creating new positions for LPNs on the unit substantially increased flexibility of nurse staffing. The project created nursing positions which can "swing" between LPN and RN positions, thus accommodating the needs of LPNs in transition to becoming RNs, LPNs who become RNs and wish to remain on the unit, or LPNs who complete an associate or baccalaureate nursing program but fail RN boards (see Table 20). During the course of the project, four from the original LPN group did, in fact, become RNs and remained on the unit. The project was associated with the re-opening of the previously closed eight beds, and a decrease in patient length of stay from 21 to 19 days.

At the project's completion, and for the first time since 1984, all RN leadership positions were filled, and the RN vacancy rate had declined from 43% to 26%. Moreover, 25% of the RNs on the unit were enrolled in either undergraduate or graduate programs. The relationship of these changes to RN satisfaction is unclear (see Table 20). Despite a notable improvement from a low of 69 at the project's inception, RN satisfaction scores remained low at the completion of the project (the RN satisfaction questionnaire response rate was 95% at all three data collection points).

Patient satisfaction appeared to fluctuate in accordance with changes in RN staffing, with high satisfaction occurring at the time of high RN staffing, and low satisfaction evident at time of low RN staffing. The changes in patient satisfaction between the project's beginning and completion may, however, have been influenced by other factors, such as a change in administrative leadership and the unit's move to a new facility. As in the other projects, quality indicators showed modest improvement. Falls and medication errors declined, while infection rates and the number of decubitus ulcers remained unchanged.

Reducing Stress in the Workplace: New York University Medical Center's Professional Self-Development Program

In contrast to the other projects, the New York University Medical Center and NYU Division of Nursing developed and tested a program, "Professional Self-Development Program for Nurses," which was implemented as an in-service education program to help decrease the high level of work-related affective stress, thus encouraging nurses to remain in hospital-based practice.

A voluntary sample of 175 full-time RNs in staff positions or in management positions directly concerned with patient care were randomly assigned to one of three intervention groups — the program, comparable time off the unit, or no intervention. Participating RNs represented 58% of the 336 who met the study criteria. RNs were primarily Caucasian, female, single, Christian, and baccalaureate-prepared. Their ages ranged from 21 to 61 ($x = 31$), and they had an average of 7.5 years of experience (range = 1-40 years). There were no significant differences between groups on any demographic characteristics.

Program content consisted of information and experiential exercises delivered over a 16-week period in 12 classes, each 1.5 hours long (see Table 21). The project produced a manual which provides information about the program in sufficient detail that it may be replicated by any department of nursing.

The major program outcomes were measured using five self-administered questionnaires: the Maslach Burnout Inventory, the Nursing Distress Scale, the Personal Views Survey, the LaMonica Empathy Profile, and the Personal Orientation Inventory. In addition, the program tracked RN absenteeism and turnover. Data were collected at three data points: prior to assignment to an intervention group, at the completion of the intervention 16 weeks later, and six months after the intervention began.

Nurses who completed the stress reduction program showed significant decreases in perceived job stress, and significant increase in personality hardiness and self-actualization when compared with the two control groups. Repeated measures of ANOVA indicated that the job stress levels of RNs who participated in the stress reduction program decreased significantly compared with RNs who did not participate in the program (see Table 22). There were no significant differences between the time-off and nonintervention groups.

Similarly, an ANOVA indicted differences among groups in sick time, with the program group having significant decrease in sick time as compared to the time-off and nonintervention groups (see Table 23). There was no significant difference between the time-off and nonintervention groups. Retention rates for RNs in the program were 97%, in comparison to 90% for the time-off and nonintervention groups.

Summary

The major conclusions to be drawn from this project are shown in Table 24. The project provides convincing evidence that differentiated practice can be an effective means of improving RN job satisfaction, increasing retention and recruitment, and improving RN productivity. Findings also support that when carefully supervised and incorporated, the role of nursing assistants and LPNs can be successfully expanded without jeopardizing patient care.

Lastly, all sites found that they needed to respond to deficiencies in the management and supervisory skills of the RNs, a message which should be explored further with schools of nursing. The project has created models for training of nonprofessional providers which could be widely disseminated and replicated.

❏   ❏   ❏

Table 1
Project Goals

- Improve working conditions for professional nurses.
- Improve professional nurse productivity.
- Create new roles for nonprofessional providers.
- Maintain or improve quality of care.

Table 2
Participating Sites

- Brooklyn Hospital (Bklyn)
  A 682-bed teaching hospital

- Long Island Jewish Medical (LIJ)
  A 825-bed regional teaching hospital

- New York Hospital (NYH)
  A 1,092-bed teaching hospital

- New York University Medical Center (NYU)
  A 870-bed teaching hospital

- The Neurological Institute (PH/Neuro)
  A 183-bed institute in the Presbyterian Hospital/
  Columbia-Presbyterian Medical Center

Table 3
Staffing at the Participating Hospitals

Site	Number of Nursing Staff per Hospital Bed	Number of RNs per Hospital Bed	% of Nursing Staff that are RNs
Bklyn	1.50	.80	63%
LIJ	1.70	1.20	73%
NYH	1.75	1.35	77%
NYU	1.55	1.17	75%
PH/Neuro	1.29	.93	73%

Table 4
Description of the Participating Units (Start-up)

- Total Units 9
    - Types:
        - Med-Surg 8
        - Neonatal ICU 1
- Total Beds 294
- Beds in Demonstration Units as %
  of Total Hospital Beds (Range) . . . . .8 to 20%
- Total FTE Nursing Personnel 330.5
    - % RNs 72%
    - % LPNs 4%
    - % Nursing Assistants (NAs) 24%
- Unit RN Vacancy Rate (Range) . . . . .9 to 43%
- Hospital RN Vacancy Rate (Range) . . . . .7 to 33%

Table 5
Percent of Nursing Staff that are RNs

Site	Total Hospital	Participating Units
Bklyn	66%	56%
LIJ	73%	81%
NYH	77%	70%
PH/Neuro	73%	61%

Table 6
Evaluation Instruments

- Descriptive data . . . . • Hospital and unit description forms
- RN productivity
  and work conditions . . . . • RN/patient ratio
    - • RN turnover and vacancy
    - • Hinshaw and Atwood Nursing Job
      Satisfaction Scale
    - • Number of open beds
- Non-RN provider role . . . . • Non-RN/RN ratio
    - • New nursing positions
- Quality of care . . . . • Clinical indicators
    - • Hinshaw and Atwood Patient
      Satisfaction Scale

Table 7
The Differentiated Practice Model

- Differentiation between professional and nonprofessional tasks
- Administrative changes
- Educational modules
- Mechanisms for ongoing communication

Table 8
LIJ Activities

- Select expert RNs as "patient care managers" (PCMs)
- Assign PCM to coordinate care of 1-3 complex patients
- Decentralize unit decision making for RNs and MDs
- Introduce new tasks, certification, and assignment of NAs
- Establish walking rounds

Table 9
LIJ Vacancy Rates

	Vacancy Rates (%)		
	Start-up	12 months	18 months
Medicine	8	13	0
Surgery	23	8	0
NICU	0	0	0

Table 10
LIJ Nursing Satisfaction

	Start-up		12 months		18 months	
	n	*mean score*	*n*	*mean score*	*n*	*mean score*
Medicine	20	87.3	26	90.2	19	93.7
Surgery	13	90.0	16	97.9	15	96.9
NICU	79	103.1	69	104.8	59	105.3

Table 11
Global RN Satisfaction Score*

	Start-up		12 months		18 months	
	n	*mean score*	*n*	*mean score*	*n*	*mean score*
PCMs	26	98.9	17	104.1	20	108.1*
Other RNs	86	99.3	94	99.7	78	100.3

*p = .0008

Table 12
Comparison of Patient Satisfaction Scores Between Patients With and Without PCMs at 18 Months

	PCM		Other RNs		DF for Welch's Test for differences in means**
	mean	*s.d.*	*mean*	*s.d.*	
Professionalism	29.0	1.7	29.8	3.8	41.1*
Education	30.1	1.9	31.2	4.2	39.2*
Trust	33.6	2.2	34.0	4.2	33.1*
Global	92.7	4.0	95.1	10.7	49.4*

*F-test for differences in variance p<.05
**No difference in means was statistically significant

Table 13
Activities

- Implement a new 8-week, 240-hour, performance-based curriculum to teach nurse assistants new skills
- Recruit nurse assistants from the community
- Create a model 39-bed medical-surgical teaching unit
- Implement a management curriculum (7 sessions) for RNs
- Develop protocols for RN/NA teams
- Create a career path for NAs and RNs

Table 14
Registered Nurse and Nursing Assistant FTEs

	Start-up	12 months	22 months
• RNs (actual FTEs)	15.2	13.0	11.5
• Nursing assistants (actual FTEs)	9.7	15.1	13.0

Table 15
Activities

- Team assignment of RNs and NAs
- Permanent geographic districts
- New patterns of authority between RNs and NAs
- Curriculum on communication skills for unit staff
- Management workshops for head RNs
- Team building for RNs and NAs
- Decentralization of decision making
- New role for head nurse

Table 16
Comparison of RN Management of Nurses Aides on Experimental and Control Units

Group	n	1988 RN mean score	s.d.	1990 RN mean score	s.d.	sig.
Experimental	24	13.4	4.8	16.0	3.2	.02
Control	15	16.9	3.3	15.8	3.9	n.s.

Table 17
Comparison of Need for RNs to Structure Nurses Aides' Work Environment on Experimental and Control Units

Group	n	1988 RN mean score	s.d.	1990 RN mean score	s.d.	sig.
Experimental	24	24.0	7.4	36.0	7.9	.004
Control	15	42.7	6.1	41.6	10.4	n.s.

Table 18
RN Global Satisfaction Scores

	Bklyn n	mean score	NYH 1 n	mean score	NYH 2 n	mean score	NYH 3 n	mean score
Start-up	11	75.6	13	76.2	14	78.3	20	87.8
12 Months	6	73.2	12	79.7	11	72.1	16	89.1
18 Months	8	70.1	14	74.9	12	76.9	10	79.9

Table 19
Activities

- Introduce LPNs enrolled in AD/BSN programs onto the unit
- Create 6 pairs of principal (RN) and associate (LPN) partners who work flex-time.
- Establish performance standards for RNs and LPNs
- Refine procedure for monitoring patient outcomes
- Establish educational programs to improve RN management skills

Table 20
PH/Neurological Institute Outcomes

	Start-up	12 months	18 months
• Average nursing hours per patient	4.9	4.9	4.8
• RNs (actual FTEs)	15.5	12.1	18.0
• LPNs (actual FTEs)	4.0	9.6	5.6
• RN vacancy rate (%)	43%	37%	26%
• Mean global patient satisfaction score	99.7	89.2	122.8
• Mean global RN satisfaction score	69.0	90.7	76.6

Table 21
Program Components

- The nature of nursing
- The meaning of nursing in society
- Reduction of affective stress
- Promotion of self-awareness:
  — meditation
  — relaxation
  — guided imagery
- Development of personality hardiness
- Cognitive restructuring

Table 22
Composite Nursing Stress Scores Over Time
and by Group

Group	Pre-Intervention		Post-Intervention		6 Months Post-Intervention	
	m	*s.d.*	*m*	*s.d.*	*m*	*s.d.*
Program	45.2	14.3	41.3	13.9	39.1	14.8*
Time-Off	49.5	13.4	50.5	17.3	52.1	16.0
Non-Intervention	44.9	12.6	45.3	14.3	57.0	12.2

*Wilks $(4,342)$ = .149, $p,.001$

Table 23
Sick Time Hours Over Time and by Group

Group	Pre-Intervention		6 Months Post-Intervention		Adjusted
	m	*s.d.*	*m*	*s.d.*	*m*
Program	10.4	20.6	3.1	5.9	1.9*
Time-Off	9.3	15.3	8.8	12.8	8.2
Non-Intervention	5.2	10.5	8.3	19.4	9.8

*$F (2,171)$ = 8.27, $p,.001$

Table 24
Implications for Deployment of
Nursing Resources and Patient Care

- Differentiated practice:
  — improves RN productivity
  — enhances RN retention/recruitment
  — maintains RN satisfaction
  — provides model for changing roles for LPNs and NAs
  — does not appreciably affect patient care
- A stress reduction program decreases stress and improves nurse satisfaction and observations
- RNs found to be deficient in managerial/supervisory skills
- Patient satisfaction appears sensitive to changes in nurse staffing
- LPNs and NAs respond enthusiastically to new opportunities

Hartford Hospital's Patient Care Delivery Program

Joy Ruth Cohen, M.S.N., R.N., C.N.A.,A., editor
Doris M. Armstrong, M.Ed., R.N., F.A.A.N.
Beverly Koerner, Ph.D., R.N., F.A.A.N.
Maurita Soukup, R.S.M., C.C., D.N.Sc., R.N.

Introduction

Hartford Hospital (Hartford, Connecticut) has been selected as one of 20 recipients of a five-year implementation grant by The Pew Charitable Trusts to develop within this institution a state-of-the-art, futuristic vision of what health care delivery should be. The end-point vision is an innovative, hospital-wide patient care delivery program that is patient/family centered and will maximize quality of care while utilizing system resources cost-effectively.

The purpose of this paper is to describe the interactive and multidisciplinary planning process from 1988 to 1990 that resulted in a blueprint for action and total restructuring of hospital-wide systems. Three principal innovations will be addressed, including the redesign of collaborative practice, the organization, and information systems.

Making It Happen

In the fall of 1989, Hartford Hospital's Interactive Project Planning Group (IPPG) made a decision to learn, model, and use interactive planning. The interactive process served as a dynamic catalyst and continues to be a major impetus during project implementation. Patients/families made a significant contribution to the planning process by offering a dimension of reality. Through interactive planning, the board of trustees, chief executive officer, physicians, management, and multiple and/or paraprofessionals made a commitment to effect a hospital-wide organizational change.

The innovations to be implemented are defined in the following discussion.

Collaborative Practice Redesigned

This will result in the integration of functions of nurses, physicians, and other professionals. The design is to include concurrent and retrospective multiprofessional patient record reviews, implement patient care team coordinator roles, and utilize advances in automated information systems. We will initiate interactive collaborative practice and management to include teams and triads, the newly developed differentiated practice model, and a clinical ladders program.

Differentiated practice will be derived from an assessment-based model using outcomes of formal nursing education, professional competencies, and a work experience profile. Delineation of responsibilities is being formulated through a range of programmable to complex interventions. Staff nurses, clinical nurse specialists, and nursing leadership have been interactive in creating the initiative. It is hypothesized that differentiated practice will provide a better way to assure quality and cost-effective patient outcomes, offer nurses roles that match their competence and attributes, and improve nurse utilization and retention.

Career ladders are being refined to accommodate differentiation of practice and program redesign. Combining and cross-training of selected personnel are planned within the project's educational endeavors. In addition, we will explore other ways to provide coordinated care at a higher level by extending opportunities for patient care involvement, cross-training, and job enrichment for a wider variety of technical personnel. Predictable patient patterns will be described in standardized protocols to make care more efficient and effective. All caregivers will be accountable for achieving quality patient care outcomes based on the predictable nature of illness, course of treatment, and anticipated length of recovery.

Organizational Redesign

The proposed design will focus on three organizational levels:

1) Tactical (at the nursing unit level).
2) Operational (involving multiple units/support services).
3) Strategic (at the hospital-wide level).

This hospital-wide restructuring will be directed toward our end-point vision. It will be ever-evolving and redefined, using our evaluative data and a decision-tree model for contingency planning.

At the unit level, there will be an interactive multidisciplinary team composed of nurses, physicians, and other professionals and support personnel in new roles. These team members, with strong allegiance to the unit program and line responsibility to their department directors, will be authorized to coordinate resources in a manner that is in the best interest of the patient/family. Team members will be consistently assigned to the same units; large units may have more than one team. Team membership may fluctuate and some professionals (such as pharmacists and social service personnel) will be part of several teams or units to assure economy of scale and avoid over-specialization. At the highest level of clinical competency, professional nurses will participate in increased clinical decision making regarding the patient's admission process, hospitalization, and discharge. They will be designated as patient care team coordinators. The head nurse will have increased management accountability as opposed to direct care involvement.

Integral to this initiative is the interactive collaborative management component. This is a modified vertical/horizontal matrix which integrates multidisciplinary teams and a clinical patient care coordinator role at the unit level, triads at an administrative level (e.g., clinical nursing director, MD chief of service, and the administrator of that service), and a multidisciplinary interactive project group (MIPG).

Organizational restructuring will address all of Hartford Hospital's services and programs within three years.

Information Systems Redesign

This system will affirm advances in technology, monitor productivity, and provide necessary information relating to patient assessments, outcomes, and decision making. Decisions pertinent to priorities of programs to be implemented will be guided by the executive information committee. Information derived from our implementation investigation will be used in the design of an information system geared specifically to facilitate patient care.

The active patient record will change to an automated, integrated document with patient-centered quality improvement indicators. Personal computer work stations in patient care units are proposed as the vehicles for integration. By adding disease-specific protocols to the personal computer, which would be algorithmically invoked, all health care providers will use the same protocols/templates for patient care and outcomes.

Multivariate Systems Matrix

The essence of our project is patient-centered, surrounded by an interactive network of people, processes, and systems. In our model, we envision three interactive resources within a matrix of clinical decision making (see Figure 1).

These key resources include multiprofessionals, the patient/ family/community, and interactive systems. Examples of interactive components which influence outcomes for clinical decision making are identified within each of the three dimensions of the matrix. Conceptually, these examples are offered from the perspective of integration and synthesis to increase understanding that is consistent with interactive planning.

For example, continuity is a component of the matrix that is interactive among all key resources. The hospital's patient care delivery program focuses on the patient/family in the pre-admission (input) phase, the admission and hospitalization (throughput) phase, and the discharge (output) phase. Clinical decision making involves the expertise of various multiprofessionals using a scope of patient practice, based on outcomes and multiprofessional patient-focused standards. Continuity, pre-, intra-, and post-hospitalization will be coordinated to optimize patient outcomes using advances in computer technology (e.g., electronic medical records, common and shared databases, estimated advanced billings, and coordination of community services).

Education

Within the project, on-site educational programs on organizational redesign and financial and management skills will be offered.

Additionally, the hospital will continue to provide educational opportunities (i.e., work-release time for selected professionals, scholarships, and tuition reimbursement) so that employees will be able to assume positions for which they were not qualified previously. Thus, the hospital seeks to use the project as a means to overcome some of the internal and external barriers originally identified in the planning grant proposal. The outcomes will allow for appreciation of breadth and depth of accountability, enhanced continuity of patient/family care, improved quality of care, increased job satisfaction for all team members, commensurate improvements in recruitment and retention, and improvements in cost effectiveness.

An outside project consultant will provide hospital-wide assistance to senior management in continuing to assess the dynamics of the relationship between project implementation and the hospital's strategic plan. Through this ongoing educational thrust, the project consultant will guide major changes in the organizational structure and decision making in all systems. Concomitantly, he will educate team members regarding concepts and skill development in organizational structure, culture, development and change; coordination mechanisms and processes; conflict management; negotiation; function of the middle manager; obtaining and using power; management and communication styles, group structure and process; and creative problem solving.

The education and discussion processes will be enhanced by retreats, team building, creative problem-solving techniques, and other organizational development methodologies. Senior management and others from within the hospital infrastructure will be included in ongoing education for systems changes. To strengthen collaborative practice and collaborative management and to support change within the organizational redesign, all supervisors and managers from a given clinical program will participate in multidisciplinary educational programs. Opportunities for health care curriculum review and revisions within the multiple academic programs that provide classroom and clinical educational opportunities to practitioners will be identified and maximized.

Significant management components essential to the efficient, effective practice of professional nursing need to be deliberately integrated into the curriculum of multiprofessional health care professionals. Multiskilled nonprofessional workers will be identified and prepared for the broadened scope of work responsibilities and assignments. Selected personnel will be educated and qualified to perform specific direct patient care tasks through cross-training methods. Assessment and evaluation of the work they currently perform will provide the baseline data essential for the determination of retraining outcomes, with the expectation of greater productivity.

It is hypothesized that the improved utilization of these multiple skill level personnel, as well as the delegation of lower level tasks to less skilled personnel, will result in measurable changes in at least two dimensions. The first dimension will be evidenced by nurses' increased and appropriate intervention in direct patient care with concomitant opportunity for increased clinical decision making. The second dimension will reveal evidences of more efficient use of nurses' time, reducing the overall number of nurses required per patient day. To support these new dimensions of employee development, the nurse manager must become skilled in leading, directing, negotiating, supervising, and assessing professional performance.

At the unit level, an educational problem-solving program will be implemented. Education will be integrated across all programs, units, and services to accomplish the objectives of the project.

A special task force of the Connecticut Department of Higher Education (which includes the vice president for nursing, as well as other state-wide administrators and educators) will articulate opportunities for academic and clinical advancement from the LPN to the RN level of professional practice.

Inherent in the developmental education dimension is the realization that any differentiation of roles on behalf of patient care, as well as worker satisfaction, will be addressed and accomplished through interactive processes and at multidisciplinary levels of integration. Thus, differentiation of practice will be evidenced at all levels and across all disciplines.

Evaluation

During the planning year, the evaluator and project staff met with key individuals in quality assurance and with hospital personnel to determine the crucial elements for evaluation. The evaluation consultant was the dean of the University of Connecticut School of Nursing. He had acted as Hartford Hospital's evaluator for the previous collaborative practice project in 1982.

Elements critical to the evaluation of this project were determined to be:

- care
- continuity
- cost
- quality
- communication

Formative evaluation will be presented to the MIPG on a quarterly basis using a decision-tree model with contingency planning format. This methodology displays the appropriate logical and temporal sequence for decision making related to problems in systems change. The likelihood of chance events is represented by explicit probability values, while the desirability of outcomes is expressed by utility values. Using this structure, the component parts of the problem are analyzed and recombined in a systematic way, and the expected outcomes of potential strategies can be analyzed and compared. The formative evaluative data can be used by the MIPG and chief executive officer to implement alternative strategies to support a project environment which is responsive to both internal and external changes and dynamics within the hospital.

In order to assess summary outcomes, evaluation themes have been defined for each of the five years of the project. These focus on the major elements of the reorganization. During the first year, reorganization of the patient care delivery program will be a major theme for summary evaluation. Additionally, the first two years of evaluation will focus on the educational component. The theme of the second year will be evaluation of management/governance, decision making, and corporate policies. During the third year, the focus will be communication flow throughout the enterprise. Interactive boundaries of relations and systems will be the theme of the fourth year. The overall project evaluation and recommendations will occur in the fifth year. These themes identified for summary evaluation are derived from the conceptual model of the project (e.g., input, throughput, and output) and are consistent with the project's overall objectives. Lastly, the evaluation methodology will track achievement of projected objectives, and any changes made in planned innovations and strategies.

To begin the evaluation, a patient career profile format will track a random sampling of OB-GYN patients from the clinic or private MD office, through the admissions process, and into the OB-GYN units. The patient/family also will be followed through the discharge process and reintegration into the community. Management engineering personnel will coordinate data collection. This methodology will provide a profile of patient experiences prior to the implementation of new systems. As the hospital is restructured, data will be collected from patients to determine differences in quality, communication, efficiency, coordination, and continuity of care.

Quality of care will be measured by analyzing variables such as clinical expertise, accountability, risk taking, professional attitudes, and interdependence. Group decision making, communication, negotiation, and conflict resolution will be key elements in evaluating horizontal management and governance issues. Whenever possible, the project effectiveness will be linked to the hospital's ongoing quality improvement programs and JCAHO standards of quality of care.

A variety of other strategies to determine cost data will include time estimates of direct and indirect work and productivity. For example, the cost of adding multidisciplinary services in relation to the benefits derived by the patient from the established template/ protocols of patient care can be obtained from the medical records. Costs associated with deviations from the established templates also can be analyzed using analysis of variance. The ultimate challenge is to orchestrate the entire patient care delivery program so as to minimize the use of resources within the context of cost constraints, while at the same time optimizing patient outcomes.

Research also is a crucial element in the overall success of the project. The project director will receive proposals from a variety of disciplines that may evolve from the redesign of the patient care delivery program. Faculty members, clinicians, graduate students and post-doctoral fellows will be encouraged to participate in a variety of research and evaluative projects that will be disseminated through publication.

Summary

This project will result in an institution-wide change, empowering caregivers closest to the patients. It has potential for replication in other health care institutions. It is anticipated that changes will make a major difference to the future of the health care industry in:

- quality, continuity, and cost of patient care;
- management and retention of scarce human resources;
- hospital-wide communication, problem-solving, and decision-making activities that will enhance responses to a rapidly changing environment, and
- dissemination of project data to insurers, regulators, providers, and academicians.

❑   ❑   ❑

Figure 1
Matrix of Clinical Decision Making

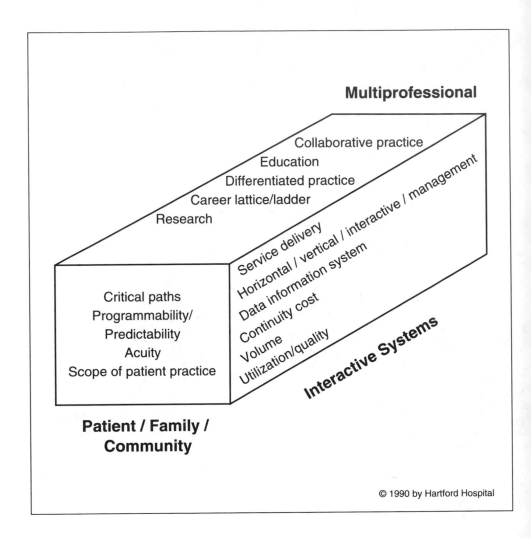

© 1990 by Hartford Hospital

A Community Hospital Experience: The Maryvale Samaritan Medical Center Approach

Kathleen Malloch, M.B.A., R.N., C.N.A.

Maryvale Samaritan Medical Center is a 256-bed community hospital in Phoenix, Arizona. Two-and-a-half years ago registered nurse role differentiation was implemented on two inpatient units. A transitional model of differentiated practice was chosen to utilize the current knowledge and skill base of each nurse. In this model, experienced registered nurses selected roles based on an assessment of their knowledge level and skill base. New graduates were assigned the role for which they were educationally prepared.

After the decision was made to use the transitional model, evaluative criteria were selected. We selected criteria related to patients, nurses, and finances. Baseline, interval, and tracking data were collected and continue to be monitored. Patient indicators included nosocomial infections, medication errors, patient falls, and length of stay. Indicators that measured quality or positive outcomes, such as patient and family management of illness and level of health knowledge, were more desirable, but not easily measured.

In view of nursing concerns related to autonomy, working relationships, and pay, we selected job and work satisfaction instruments with these subscales. We also tracked retention rates,

turnover, position vacancies, nursing documentation, and participant profiles. Financial indicators included hours per patient day,
overtime, and supplemental agency and salary costs per patient
day. Salary costs per patient day represented the most comprehensive indicator, while the others were only partial indicators of financial impact. Evaluative results from the first 18 months of our project,
reflecting positive outcomes, were published in the February 1990
issue of the *Journal of Nursing Administration* (Malloch, 1990).

Planning Philosophy

Once the indicators were selected, a planning philosophy was
developed that had three critical elements: collaboration, change
theory, and commitment.

Collaboration

Role differentiation has far-reaching implications for baccalaureate and associate degree educators, nurse managers, nurse
researchers, staff development coordinators, human resource directors, and administrators. To facilitate these groups working together
to create change in education and practice settings, a task force was
formed with representatives from each area. Active participation by
key members in decision-making positions was essential in guiding
this project and achieving the desired long-lasting changes. Therefore, task force meetings have been held at least monthly for the last
three years. Attendance varied, but membership was stable and
interest remained high.

Knowledge of Change Theory

Awareness of change theory phenomena has been most helpful
in maintaining our focus. Throughout the project, we were enter-
tained, and at times frustrated, as our colleagues became caught up
in various stages of the change process.

The "status quo champions" have pleaded with us to leave
things the way they are, and the "organizational powerbrokers"
have been angry and frustrated at the thought of losing authority.
The most challenging have been the "expert bargainers," who work
diligently to compromise the change out of existence. Finally, there
are those who "remember the good old days" and cannot understand why we need to change. We have also learned that not every-

one automatically resists change. Nurses who require additional information or clarification of misinformation should not be considered resistant.

Personal Commitment to the Change

There is a need for all involved not only to understand the definition and theory of role differentiation, but also to articulate what they need to support it. As all task force members began to clearly understand the nature of their participation, a vague commitment to a professional ideal became a strong personal commitment to implementing differentiated practice.

This "Three Cs" philosophy — collaboration, change, and commitment — provided a solid foundation for implementation planning. For presentation purposes, I have organized our planning by days of the week. While the steps are presented as distinct, in reality they are overlapping and interrelated.

Implementation

On the first day, Monday, we began with manager and unit selection. Two unit directors, representing two distinct patient populations, were asked to participate in the project. Both directors were cautiously interested, but for very different reasons. The medical unit director was experiencing high turnover and declining staff morale, and was willing to try anything to improve the situation. In contrast, the surgical unit director had a stable staff, high morale, and low turnover. She was interested in being a part of designing the future of nursing, but not at the cost of upsetting anyone on the unit.

On Tuesday, day two, we focused on staff preparation. A total of 36 registered nurses on both units completed baseline job and work satisfaction questionnaires. The concept of role differentiation was then introduced. We held formal and informal sessions on all shifts. Each session focused on the rationale for the project and incorporated specific examples of the differentiated roles using patient scenarios from each unit. These patient and family situations were most helpful in demonstrating the reality of the concept of differentiation. At the completion of these sessions, nurses were asked whether or not they wished to proceed with this project. Once again, responses were mixed. The decision of the nurses on both units was to pilot this project for a three-month period. Over the course of time, three distinct groups of nurses emerged: those who were active supporters, those who tolerated the project until something better came along, and those who were not sure if anything was happening.

On Wednesday, day three, job descriptions and position titles were selected. Job descriptions from the ICON (Rotkovich, 1986), WICHE (Western Interstate Commission for Higher Education, 1985), and MAIN (Primm, 1986) models were examined in depth. The MAIN job descriptions were selected because of the ease with which they guided the delineation of roles on the two units. Title selection for the two roles became a very emotional issue. Nurses struggled with position titles because titles needed to reflect both actual role expectations and their mutual values. Eventually, the titles of *case manager* and *case associate* were selected.

On Thursday, the fourth day, every nurse became actively involved. This was the day for nurses to select their roles. The role selection process was the first tangible step for many nurses in the implementation of differentiated practice. The purpose of role selection was to delineate for each nurse the scope of practice and performance expectations based on an assessment of knowledge and skill base, regardless of formal education or years of nursing experience. This selection process also was used to identify both areas of strength and areas needing improvement as a basis for developmental goal setting.

Nurses selected the role of their choice, collected documentation to support that choice, and reviewed this information with a nurse trained in role differentiation. Our experience indicated that this review process can take from 30 minutes to 1½ hours, and is probably the most productive of all time spent in professional development activities. Nurses continue to submit materials on a regular basis for evaluation of how well they meet the performance expectations for their selected scope of practice. The opportunity to change roles is limited to once a month and, in 24 months, only three nurses have changed roles.

On Friday, day five, we addressed student nurse experiences. Rather than continuing to randomly assign students to the RNs, we had an opportunity to provide experiences that related more directly to educational program objectives. With the assistance of nursing faculty, students from baccalaureate programs were precepted by a nurse functioning in the role of a case manager. Students from associate degree programs were precepted by a nurse functioning in the role of a case associate. Students now had learning experiences with nurses functioning in the roles they would be expected to assume after graduation.

On Saturday, day six, we selected Monday, February 15, 1988, as the day that differentiated practice would begin on both units. One week before implementation, task force members encouraged us to consider postponement. Not all the policies were written, nor had all the nurses completed the role selection process. Lastly, the project was not widely understood by other hospital departments. After much discussion and hesitation, task force members realized that we would never be fully prepared. If just one nurse began to function in the case manager role for one patient, the change process would have begun. We proceeded with the February 15th implementation date.

After six days of extensive collaborative planning, we were hoping to rest on Sunday, the seventh day — at least in the spiritual sense. Not only were we denied rest, but the issues and challenges that arose will probably keep us busy well into the future.

We found that we needed to reconsider whether or not this was a "project" in the traditional sense, with a pilot phase and a terminal point. We now realize that role differentiation is more than a change project. It is the first step in an evolutionary process to form a professional practice model.

We also realized that we need assistance and support from professional peers in two major areas: role clarification and recognition.

Role Clarification

With role clarification — as it relates to service, education, research, and productivity systems — there needs to be an intensified focus on deciding what nursing is and what it is not. To support the transfer of non-nursing responsibilities and eliminate the substitution of registered nurses for other health care workers, we must accelerate the development of assistive roles and the two roles of the registered nurse. To facilitate and support nursing and non-nursing roles, nurses need expertise in delegation, a skill not frequently used in total patient care or primary nursing models. This is necessary to avoid slipping back into the composite registered nurse role.

We also need research assistance in the form of more sensitive tools and instruments to measure the quality of our changes, not just the decrease in negative outcomes. Researchers also could assist us in the development of a second generation patient classification system reflecting both registered nurse roles. An effective system would validate the demand for more baccalaureate-prepared nurses, as well as provide tools to effectively assign patients. The definition of the role of the registered nurse, the role of assistive personnel, enhancement of delegation skills, and patient classification systems require changes in practice and education. We need to begin now.

Recognition

If we are to continue to progress with role differentiation, we need recognition for our efforts, which are not always perfect. We need recognition not only at the verbal level, but also at the financial and programmatic levels. All nursing organizations and practice settings should mobilize their resources and breathe life into role differentiation. We need to provide resources for staff development time, seminar attendance, audio-visual aids, and computer support for data management. Most significantly, redesigning the clinical ladder to recognize both roles and resources for restructuring the salary program, and to appropriately compensate the two roles is of utmost importance.

We have been fortunate for the consistent and enthusiastic administrative support our organization offers verbally, programmatically, and financially. The commitment of resources to and ongoing recognition of our efforts have been an essential part of our project.

One exciting event at Maryvale is the annual differentiated practice celebration we sponsor to review our progress and recognize nurses. Most notably, we recall Dr. Martha Rogers (1989), the keynote speaker at our first anniversary celebration, when she said, "I have waited all my life to praise nurses for actually practicing nursing based on educational preparation."

Summary

We believe that we have improved the practice of nursing. We also believe that the anticipated change in nursing requires performance and response resembling that of the phoenix. This fabled bird, known to sacrifice itself to the fire and then rise from the ashes, can be an inspiring symbol of the change we believe is necessary for nursing. We have a strong sense of the direction we need to take to continue the evolution and rebirth of nursing.

Yes, it may be Sunday, but there is no end in sight and hopefully there never will be. We are rising from the ashes of the phoenix. The process of role differentiation is dynamic. It is evolving to meet the twenty-first century with open arms.

❑   ❑   ❑

Development of a Differentiated Practice Model

M.A. DiMola, M.A., R.N.
Stephen Burns, M.B.A., R.N.

The Planning Phase

The process of designing the future at St. Vincent's Medical Center in Jacksonville, Florida, began in December 1988, when a group of nurses met to generate ideas to improve patient care. These ideas took shape and eventually became a grant proposal.

St. Vincent's Medical Center (SVMC) then received a one-year planning grant of $50,000 — jointly funded by the Robert Wood Johnson Foundation and The Pew Charitable Trusts. It was part of a $26.8 million project called "Strengthening Hospital Nursing: A Program to Improve Patient Care." Securing the funding served as a catalyst for beginning the process of change at SVMC.

The Strengthening Hospital Nursing program was born out of a need to deal with the severe national nursing shortage. The appeal of a project such as this was evidenced by the fact that a total of 1,120 hospitals responded to the call for proposals. Although only 80 hospitals received planning grants, and 20 of those were implementation grants, the project caused hospitals throughout the country to begin generating ideas about the future of health care and redesigning the hospital workplace to meet the challenges of the '90s.

One assumption of the planning process was that the hospital of the future will be very different from the current acute care environment. Of course, the trend to more outpatient services will continue to decrease the number of inpatient beds. Inpatients, for the most part, will be older and progressively sicker. Jeff Goldsmith, a well-known health care economist, predicts that in the next 10 to 20 years hospitals will admit only acutely ill elderly and trauma patients (Goldsmith, 1989).

We have witnessed the beginnings of this trend in our own institution, where Medicare patients now comprise 53% of our patient days, a percentage that has steadily climbed over the last five years.

The cost of caring for patients also has grown exponentially, yet federal reimbursements do not begin to cover expenses. Administrators are dealing with issues which face many hospitals and that will have a global effect on patient care. There was a general lack of knowledge about diagnosis-related groups (DRGs) among the patient care staff, due partially to the fact that a majority of DRGs were not assigned to the patient until discharge. Of concern was the fact that length of stay in top DRGs exceeded the national mean. There was no consistency in how nursing care was delivered to patients from unit to unit.

It was believed that nonprofessional staff could be utilized differently, and could have a positive impact on the professional staff shortage that we were experiencing in the lack of nurses and respiratory and physical therapists.

Many innovative ways to use paraprofessionals continue to evolve, and their effect on the nursing profession must be evaluated (RCTs, for example). In a recent survey, however, 70-80% of chief executive officers from all types of institutions predicted that paraprofessionals will continue to be used extensively to replace professionals (Hudson, 1990).

It soon became obvious to us that not only were we dealing with a professional staff shortage, but also with a true health care crisis. In order to make progress in resolving these issues, we needed to redesign our patient care delivery system with quality, efficiency, and cost containment as priorities.

This effort needed to be institutionwide. We wanted to have a model designed to include optimum delivery of care and organizational change, since one without the other would mean reverting back to old practices and habits.

The practices and methods in our health system today are in need of reorganization. Often, it is not until one steps back and carefully evaluates the situation and its alternatives that one sees the inefficiencies and realizes the need for changes.

An idealized model was used as a planning framework, so that we planned for what we wanted, and not for what we did not want. This framework was popularized by Russell Ackoff, professor of systems science at The Wharton School at the University of Pennsylvania, and a health care and business consultant (Ackoff, 1974). We also experimented with scenarios of "if we could . . . then we would. . .", rather than merely "fixing up" our current system.

We made the following recommendations regarding reorganization:

- Eliminate some of the traditional boundaries between specialized departments, with a goal of satisfying patient care needs versus departmental needs.
- Make managers responsible for cost and quality.
- Redesign work so that new patterns of staffing and task assignments would emerge.

Our planning was extremely interactive and occurred at all levels within the institution. Staff representing all disciplines and all levels in the organizational hierarchy became involved. This part of the process cannot be underestimated because, aside from creating a plan for innovation, the collaboration, *esprit de corps*, and enthusiasm generated were significant byproducts of the process. All participants had a stake in the outcome, engendering some degrees of ownership and acceptance of change. An advisory board was created as a consulting group which included top hospital executives, physicians, and community leaders such as the dean of the University of North Florida, and a Daughter of Charity representative who also happened to be the president of the National Health System. The core team was composed of the top hospital staff — the CEO, COO, vice-president for nursing, chief of medical staff, and project director. It was the approving body and ultimate decision-making group. There were additional focus groups made up of physicians, staff, and patients.

The steering committee included representatives from all patient care departments and other key service areas such as finance, medical records, and education. Since this group was fairly large, some splinter work groups were developed. These often split further into extended work groups that added personnel in the process, so that the ideas for differentiated practice evolved from a grass-roots approach.

The steering committee examined many issues and collected baseline data. In a study conducted on six of our medical-surgical units to evaluate how nursing staff (specifically, RNs, LPNs, NAs and UCs) spent their time, we found that only a small percentage (13.8%) of RN time was spent in the actual nursing process. We found we were using our valuable nursing resources to accomplish a host of other activities.

These statistics were very consistent with findings in the literature. Not surprisingly, we wanted to increase the percentage of actual nursing process time so that it represented the majority of the nurses' time. Additionally, we needed to make distinctions between the kind of nursing care required and the appropriate resources to deliver it.

We began to develop ways to do this. The results of this work remain in progress which, ideally, will never be truly completed. We wanted a model that was flexible enough to respond to unforeseen events and changes the future would bring; therefore, we will frequently redesign and enhance it. Our model was called "patient-oriented delivery."

Traditionally, many physicians practice on a given unit. Although patients often share a common pathology, such as neurology or pulmonary, they are very diverse human beings. A typical patient is usually assigned a DRG on the third day of hospitalization or at discharge. He or she is transferred up to five times during hospitalization (resulting in an average of 2,100 transfers a month at SVMC). There is a narrow range of patient acuity. As the patient becomes sicker he/she is transferred to another unit, and then back again as he/she improves. The support services are departmentalized, and the unit is generally 30-40 beds.

We proposed a modular unit, or pod, of 16 beds for ease of staffing and clustering of patients who are homogeneous (admitted by limited, specific physicians). The DRG was assigned on admission and the patient remained on the unit unless critical care was required. Telemetry capability was available in all rooms to limit transfers and enhance continuity of care. The range of acuity, therefore, was much broader. The support departments were integrated with the functions.

The traditional "team" seldom goes on group rounds. It is composed of numerous caregivers so that the patient may interact with gibility for Medicaid there while eliminating coverage of some treatments.

But President Clinton and Health and Human Services Secretary Donna Shalala will impose stringent conditions on Oregon to try to limit federal costs and at the same time prevent sharp reductions in services for poor people and those with disabilities, the officials said.

Under the plan, which needs federal approval because it would be financed partly with federal Medicaid money, the number of Medicaid recipients in Oregon would rise to 360,000. There are 240,000 now.

The plan, which was revised after the Bush administration rejected a similar proposal last year,

OREGON: *Page A17 Col. 4*

coercion by public offic.
complained privately that i

Clinton May
For Computer

By T.
Associ

Washington

President Clinton, whose computer screen name is "Clinton Pz," may sit down soon at a White House terminal for a live "on-line town hall meeting" with home computer users.

The hint from White House officials comes as Clinton's team of young, high-tech specialists ponders new ways of communicating directly with Americans.

☑ **'CREATIVE PROSECUTIONS'**

Second-Degree Murder

By Harriet Chiang
Chronicle Legal Affairs Writer

Irving Mouton is serving 15 years to life in prison for murder even though prosecutors admit he did not fire the fatal shot.

In July 1990, 19-year-old Mouton accompanied a friend to an East Palo Alto apartment. A fight erupted, guns were drawn, and a bystander was killed.

In finding Mouton guilty of second-degree murder, a San Mateo jury decided that he helped create the violent atmosphere that led to the death of Beatrice Jackson.

Several defense lawyers and legal scholars regard the Mouton case as one of the most flagrant examples of a growing tendency of prosecutors and judges to stretch the definition of murder. The Mouton conviction "flies in the face of the bedrock principles that guilt is personal," six law professors wrote recently in a legal brief with the state Court

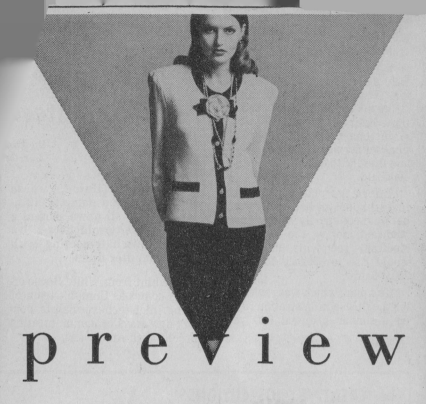

preview

THE ST. JOHN SPRING 1993 COLLECTION
WILL BE PRESENTED THURSDAY THROUGH SATURDAY,
MARCH 18TH THROUGH 20TH FROM 11 TO 4
WITH INFORMAL MODELING.
ST. JOHN'S FASHION DIRECTOR, HELEN DZO DZO
WILL BE ON HAND TO ASSIST WITH
YOUR SELECTIONS.
ST. JOHN BOUTIQUE, THIRD FLOOR.

Post & Powell Streets, San Francisco. 986-4300.

SAKS FIFTH AVENUE
SPRING

up to 30 individuals a day. Nurses are very task-oriented and give their technical assistants minimal direction. The courier/transport process is fragmented, and often nurses or other professionals provide this function.

We proposed nursing partnerships where a nurse and a new level of technician, an ACP (*ancillary care provider*, which includes the LPN), agree to work as a team on a fairly permanent basis. The nurse hires, fires, and supervises the ACP. Team rounds are made daily at a specified time, caregivers are limited, couriers are centralized, and the nurse becomes accountable for patient outcomes. Documentation is integrated, meaning that all disciplines chart on the same form, and it is moved to the bedside. The family is strongly encouraged to actively participate in care rather than being passive observers.

The "team," as we use the word here, includes the patient, the RN (BSN, ADN, and diploma), the physician, the family, allied health professionals, the ACP (including LPNs), a hostess who provides guest services, and a registrar who admits the patient and provides financial consultation to the family.

The model is patient-focused rather than department-focused. It uses a case management approach, which emphasizes discharge planning and patient teaching and incorporates the family as much as possible. There is a case manager who tracks patient progress, a hostess and a registrar for every 16 beds, and a pharmacist and a unit manager for every four 16-bed pods. The allied health professionals are assigned to specific pods and their assignments are consistent. The ratio of these professionals to units or pods depends on patient type. For example, a respiratory therapist may be assigned to only one pod depending on the need, or cover several if the need is not as great. The FTEs from various hospital departments — such as lab, EKG, admitting, and ECS — will be assigned to the appropriate pods to compensate for those functions that will not be performed by the team members. For example, the ACPs will carry out phlebotomies and EKGs, and the hostess will clean the patients' rooms.

Our model provides certain contrasts to our current organization — i.e., there is no head nurse, assistant head nurse, or charge nurse, as we currently define these roles. There is no unit clerk; nurses carry vibrating beepers to enhance communication, save steps, and reduce overhead pages. Telemetry capability in each room limits transfers and improves continuity of care.

In December 1990, we implemented the patient-oriented delivery model on a former general medical unit. After evaluating our top medicare DRGs, we realized that our impact would be greater if we began our mode with cardiovascular patients — specifically internal medicine, since heart failure patients comprised our top DRG, with a length of stay that exceeded the national mean. Any impact made in reducing length of stay while maintaining or improving quality would have major financial benefits.

We collected baseline data over a six-month period on one cardiovascular unit where there were an average of 31.6 Medicare cardiovascular DRGs for an average of 153 total Medicare days allotted per month. On an average, in only 2.3 cases per month did the days allotted actually equal the length of stay, which left an average of 75 days per month in excess of allotments. We believed our model could significantly improve these statistics.

Development of the team for our demonstration model included the recruitment of two physicians, case managers, and a multidisciplinary staff. Obviously, the relationships that were formed and the collaborative groundwork were essential to the success of this model.

It was also particularly important for the RNs to differentiate technical and professional categories of practice in the new model, as they have traditionally functioned under one nurse practice act and job description.

The cost benefits were based on five-year projections done by the finance department and resulted in a savings of $1.2 million per year, with a payback to the institution in three years. This was reflective of costs associated with renovation and equipment, and savings from the change of staff mix — i.e., the ratio of professional to nonprofessional staff. Our model decreased the needs for RN staff by 7-10% of the current demand. Cost benefits were also realized by the decreased length of stay, which we projected would lower our current means by 10-15% during the first year. Improved documentation should occur since the charts were moved to the patient room, allowing immediate access to care providers, and furthering an integrated approach to documentation.

Putting Innovation Into Action

Phase 1 of project implementation involved physician renovation and construction of the demonstration unit; training of staff;

and development of job descriptions, policies, procedures, and critical paths.

Although the project management plan progressed as scheduled, there were expected and unexpected pitfalls, such as communication issues based on semantics. For example, the use of the term "case manager" alarmed physicians so much that the local medical association newsletter published an editorial on the subject. It stated that "physicians should not relinquish their control over directing all aspects of their patients' care under any circumstance" (Gilbert, 1989). Other terms which caused confusion with the medical staff were "quality," "collaborative practice," and "patient outcomes." Even the term "discharge planning" meant one thing to nurses and another to social workers.

Another pitfall encountered was the RNs' perception of their role. With the traditional RN role changing in the demonstration model, they were fearful and anxious about role transitions, delegation to technical staff, and the different expectations others would have of them. This made recruiting RNs to the model unit difficult and created challenges in implementing the differentiated roles. The nursing staff had no role models or experience with differentiated practice, making exhibition of the desired behaviors impossible. This was an anticipated obstacle and a process was systematically implemented which included education, observation, and group sessions to define the concepts and associated behaviors of each role.

Physical barriers within the institution posed a host of unforeseen problems due to the layout of the unit and its difficulty in meeting codes and other state requirements. With a little ingenuity, budget exceptions, and a lot of hard work, these barriers were eventually overcome.

Phase 2 of implementation began in December 1990, when the first patients were admitted to the model unit. Although only a short time has passed since the 12 beds opened, preliminary data are very encouraging. Revision and refinement of the conceptual model has been the mode of operation. The evaluative phase will be comprehensive and thoroughly explored prior to expansion of the patient-oriented delivery concept.

Planning and implementing a differentiated practice model is a significant undertaking. This project has raised the consciousness of not only administrators and nurses, but of all employees regarding important aspects and outcomes of the care we deliver. Differentiated practice has enabled us to provide our staff with opportunities to develop new skills, refine old ones, and stretch talents to achieve new practice patterns. Although this growth has been difficult, it is rewarding to both the individual and the health care environment. It has been like waking a sleeping giant and watching him come to life.

❏　　　❏　　　❏

Part III

Differentiated Nursing Practice in Community-Based Care

Three Differentiated Practice Models for Ambulatory Care

Fay W. Whitney, Ph.D., F.A.A.N., editor
Maureen Hazen, M.H.A., R.N.
Kate Fleming, M.S., R.N.,C., C.R.N.P.
Beth Ann Swan, M.S.N., R.N.,C., C.R.N.P.

Abstract

The tremendous fiscal and demographic pressures in health care have changed the face of hospital ambulatory care practice. In response, nurses at the Hospital of the University of Pennsylvania have developed three dynamic differentiated models of nurse-managed practice that have revolutionized the delivery of health care in the emergency department. The three models currently in place are:

- an emergency room walk-in clinic,
- a managed care clinic for Medicaid patients, and
- an occupational health service.

The three practices employ various levels of nursing personnel. Nurse practitioners, registered nurses, and nursing assistants are the primary providers of health care in these settings. Physicians and other health providers are used in consultative roles. The expansion of nursing roles and the increased demand for nursing services requires a broad, flexible nursing base; an increased responsibility for care of patients and their families; and an accountability for continued care throughout the visit, planning for discharge and needed home services. Most importantly, it requires careful delineation of roles among nurses and optimal use of skills and educational preparation.

Differentiated practice, with clear role definition, has made a significant contribution to patient satisfaction, cost containment, efficient care and increased access at the Hospital of the University of Pennsylvania. The models described herein can be useful in designing similar ambulatory services elsewhere.

Introduction

Emergency department use, especially for nonurgent care, has steadily increased during the past 25 years (Coates et al., 1988; Epting, Haddy, and Schaler, 1987). While the rising trend has occurred in all settings, it has been more prominent in inner-city hospitals with large indigent and minority populations. Patterns of utilization of services by the poor indicate their reliance on episodic and sporadic care, obtaining access to the health system through emergency rooms and public health centers (Hurley, Freund, and Taylor, 1989).

In 1988, it was estimated that 85% of emergency room visits were for non-life-threatening conditions, with poor individuals disproportionately represented as consumers of primary care in this setting (Coates et al., 1988; Hurley, Freund, and Taylor, 1989).

Appropriate access to primary health care has long been a concern of federal and state governments and third-party payers (Freeman et al., 1987). But reform has been slow and uneven. Politically, denying services at any point of access is unpopular, thus, elected officials have been slow to change points of entry. Even the prepayment reforms in inpatient care have not yet been applied to ambulatory care entry and treatment. Economically, allowing universal, uncontrolled access to costly services (such as hospital emergency rooms) has further exacerbated the problem of ever-escalating health care costs, resulting in increased unpaid debt pools for hospitals. Therefore, the poor and indigent, or those who simply lack primary care services, arrive in emergency rooms for care and encounter a system not designed to deliver first contact, comprehensive, continuous, or family-centered care.

In many hospitals, employee health is handled by using emergency room access for treatment of acute problems. For continuing chronic problems, referral is made within the hospital or to community-based practices. The system does not necessarily serve the needs of the employees with regard to comprehensive work-related health and safety programs, but it does fulfill the need for access to care for work-related sickness and injury. It also provides liability coverage to the hospital as employer.

Nurses at the Hospital of the University of Pennsylvania (HUP) have solved the problem of the poor and indigent who use their hospital, and the resulting need for expanded occupational health services, with a new design of three interconnected services. These dynamic, differentiated models of nurse-managed practice have revolutionized the delivery of health care in the emergency department. They are currently in place in the emergency room walk-in clinic (WIC), the managed care clinic for Medicaid patients (PCG), and the occupational health service (OHS).

This paper is a combination of three original conference papers presented by the nurses who were instrumental in the development of the practices at HUP. Each section contains background about the populations served, description of the physical set-up and services offered, and the model of differentiated nursing practice used. These practices have made a significant contribution to patient satisfaction, cost containment, efficient care, and increased access at the Hospital of the University of Pennsylvania. It is hoped that the models described here can be useful in designing similar ambulatory services elsewhere.

The Emergency Room Walk-In Clinic (WIC): The Multidimensional Nursing Role Within an Ambulatory Care Setting

Maureen Hazen, M.H.A., R.N.

As the use of emergency departments has steadily increased in the last 25 years, the incidence of true emergencies has not (Coates et al., 1988). More patients are using hospital emergency facilities for nonemergency care, but this episodic form of health care provides neither continuity nor comprehensive care. Ultimately, it is more costly to both the patient and society as a whole.

There are many reasons for the increased use of emergency rooms for primary health care. Among them are:

- provider-related issues of specialization, decreased availability during "off hours," and geographic mobility;

- reimbursement policies that limit poor and indigent patients entering private practice;
- insurance reimbursement that covers primary care treatment in hospitals, but not physician's offices; and
- public expectation that health services should be responsive on a 24-hours-a-day basis (Epting, Haddy, and Schaler, 1987; Habenstreit, 1986).

Reducing reliance on the emergency department (ED) as a major source of primary health care would be beneficial. Hospitals could more efficiently allocate their human and capital resources to respond to true emergency needs. Emergency personnel could then concentrate professional skills on those patients in the greatest need. Purchasers of care would avoid costs that are excessive in relation to the level of care required (Freund, Hurley, and Taylor, 1989). Experiments in providing special services for nonurgent patients through EDs have been successful in showing that waiting time is decreased, patient satisfaction increased, and alternate services can exist within busy teaching hospital EDs (Clark, 1988; Jalowiec, Powers, and Reichelt, 1984).

The Clinic Operation

The Hospital of the University of Pennsylvania is a 700-bed urban teaching institution and tertiary medical center. The walk-in clinic was opened in 1974, a fast track for nonemergency ED patients and episodic care patients.

The purpose of the WIC was to act as the portal of entry into the health care system for the surrounding community of southwest Philadelphia. Services were meant to provide high-quality episodic care within a primary care framework, while assuring appropriate education, follow-up, and referral services. Sources of referral were to be from self-referral, the acute section of the ED, occupational health services for nonoccupational related problems, specialty clinics within the hospital for urgent episodic care, or from private physicians. The majority of patients were expected to be relatively healthy individuals with episodic, self-limiting conditions.

Four examination rooms and a physician's office comprised the total complex. The WIC was originally staffed by a physician, an LPN, and a secretary. It was open from 8:00 a.m. to 4:30 p.m., Monday through Friday. Patients were registered by the secretary as they arrived. She then performed some primitive triage based on the entering complaint and the apparent degree of distress. She alerted the LPN and MD about patients who might need early intervention. Later, a registered nurse was added to the staff based on a need for more formal triage procedures and increasing patient demand for services. The nurse essentially acted as gatekeeper and identified patients who would be evaluated more appropriately in the acute emergency room section.

Four years later, as patient volume increased, both the ED and the WIC were relocated to a new facility. Since then, the WIC has grown considerably. Today, it is conveniently located adjacent to the ED. Patients can physically access the clinic from the main lobby of the hospital, from the ED, and from occupational health services. The waiting area can accommodate approximately 25 patients. While patients await evaluation, they have access to educational literature, bulletin boards, and videos. There are five examination rooms, a provider's office for note writing and consultations, a triage room, and a patient consultation/teaching room.

The present staffing is interdisciplinary, with three levels of nursing personnel. There are two full-time RNs, three nurse practitioners, one full-time and one part-time nursing assistant, one attending physician, one to two interns who rotate on a daily basis, three full-time receptionists, and a nurse practitioner and medical students who rotate weekly. All RNs, nursing assistants, and receptionists are cross-trained to work in the ED and WIC. The RNs assigned to the WIC are required to have previous ED experience and to be excellent triage nurses.

The WIC offers patients several advantages:

- convenient hours (8:30 a.m. – 9:00 p.m.);
- a central location near public transportation;
- a liberal billing policy allowing indigent people to receive care; and
- location within a tertiary center with access to specialists, radiology, social service, and high technology.

Conditions that may result in triage in the WIC include upper respiratory infections, urinary tract infection symptoms, soft tissue injuries of the extremities without neurovascular compromise, suture removal and wound checks, sexually transmitted diseases, rashes, psychiatric problems without suicidal/homicidal ideation, social problems, dental complaints, headaches, pain syndromes, crisis situations, or incision and drainage procedures. The needs are varied and the patients have multiple problems, but the WIC acts as a point of entry where nursing personnel can administer total patient care.

The emergency department averages 50,000 patient visits a year, with the WIC accounting for approximately 13,000 of those visits. Because of its central location within the emergency department complex, the WIC acts as a hub for nonemergent services and provides access to special services for patients who require them.

Differentiated Practice in the WIC

The division of nursing at HUP implemented a system for levels of practice in 1982. The goals of the program included:

- promotion of job satisfaction and career mobility,
- increased nursing professionalism through recognition of increased responsibility and accountability,
- personal compensation for expertise in practice at different levels,
- improved clinical assessment through matching staff nurse expertise with patient need, and
- financial compensation for actual clinical behaviors (Hospital of the University of Pennsylvania, 1985).

Differentiated practice has grown out of the levels of practice.

There are four nursing level positions at HUP — staff nurse positions are classified as Level I, II, or III; Level IV is a clinical nurse specialist/nurse practitioner role. The registered nurses, nurse practitioners, and nurse assistants presently working in the WIC bring strong, varied backgrounds to their positions. Both RNs are Level III nurses, one with 16 years of experience and one with 12. One is working toward a BSN and the other holds a master's degree in health administration.

The nurse practitioners are master's-prepared, with a range of one to nine years clinical experience as NPs. A doctorally-prepared nurse practitioner acts as a consultant/provider on a part-time basis. The nursing assistants have an average of 17 years clinical experience, the majority of which is in the WIC/ER.

The registered nurses are responsible for the intake and outflow of patients, the coordination of staff, and for the triage that moves patients between the levels of service. They are the operations managers. As such, they are vital to the way in which the WIC fulfills its mission. In the present clinic, the RNs maintain a follow-up clinic for episodic patients who may need a single return visit to the clinic for a recheck of their condition (i.e., wounds, stitches, blood pressure). The RN also supervises the nursing assistants' practice.

The RN maintains a multidimensional role while interfacing with various departments and personnel through the triage process and everyday occurrences. The combination of strong clinical expertise, appropriate educational background, and good relations within the hospital community make this multidimensional role functional and rewarding.

The nurse practitioners are direct primary care providers, working between the WIC and the HealthPASS Clinic (described later in this paper) on a rotating basis. In the WIC, the nurse practitioners developed practice parameters to facilitate the movement of patients through the system. Working with the physicians and RNs, they developed a triage category of "nurse practitioner-appropriate patients." This included most minor complaints or those related to chronic, stable illnesses. Generally, these patients would not require physician intervention except for brief consultation, and could be moved more quickly through the system. The attending physician then worked with medical students, house staff, and more difficult patients. Examples of problems that are not considered NP-appropriate are new chest pain, acute abdominal pain or abdominal pain in older adults, joint taps, head trauma, or onset of new neurological symptoms.

The RN is responsible for triaging the patient to the appropriate provider, using clinical judgement during the triage process to do so. The interaction between the nurse practitioner and RN is collegial and interactive. Each seeks advice and help from the other as they go about their different but related tasks.

The nursing assistants have fairly traditional roles in ambulatory care. They stock rooms, escort patients to examining rooms, take vital signs, prepare patients for medical examinations, and supervise pelvic exams. They also teach these patients to use crutches and canes (they are excellent patient advocates), and help the other nursing staff communicate more effectively within the cultural parameters of the population. The RNs and NPs maintain ongoing interactions with the nursing assistants about patient conditions and patient flow.

In this model, the differentiated levels of nursing practice are compatible and reinforce one another. Individual strengths are also accommodated so that each nurse feels expert in an area of clinical competence. In the WIC, the RN is the major organizer of services, and the nurse practitioner is the major provider. The nursing assistant is the adjunctive provider who blends all the services together. The physicians work with the nurses to provide care, but are not involved directly in the management of the unit and patient flow.

Summary

The walk-in clinic is part of the emergency services department at HUP, and works in conjunction with all other services. It is the hub of ambulatory services and receives and refers patients within the many services of the hospital.

Nurses in the WIC provide stability and continuity to a group of inner-city patients who have limited access to ambulatory care services. Where the physician providers can only offer discontinuous coverage, nursing personnel are always available within the area.

Throughout all levels of nursing, each professional brings a different approach and expertise to the WIC. They blend together to implement a nurse-managed clinic that optimizes available care and makes efficient use of resources and personnel. This model is stable, and is being increasingly used at the Hospital of the University of Pennsylvania. It is a model that can be used in other busy emergency rooms for nonurgent care.

HealthPASS Preventive Care Group (PCG):
A Nurse-Managed Primary Clinic for
Medicaid Recipients

Kate Fleming, M.S., R.N.,C., C.R.N.P.

The HealthPASS Preventive Care Group (PCG) was opened in 1986. It is a nurse-managed clinic for Medicaid recipients at HUP. Located in emergency services, its purpose was to provide services that would improve the delivery of care to Medicaid recipients who live in a designated area of Philadelphia.

It developed in response to a state-mandated insurance experiment to bring case-managed, prepaid health care to a population that historically has experienced difficulty gaining access within the traditional Medicaid system. Its focus is on the provision of comprehensive care at a facility that otherwise provides acute, episodic, emergency care.

The health care needs of the poor are well recognized (Mundinger, 1985). Among poverty-level populations, there are increased barriers to care and increased needs (Hohlen et al., 1990; Freeman et al., 1987). Specific health problems include malnutrition, increased contact with sexually transmitted diseases, lack of prenatal care with resulting low birth weight babies, nonresponsive prevention strategies, inadequate immunizations, and high levels of chronic diseases such as hypertension and diabetes. Efforts to control health care costs may further jeopardize this population by decreasing access to high quality, affordable, comprehensive health care resources (Inglehart, 1982; Inglehart, 1985). As the number of uninsured individuals approaches 30 million in the United States (Inglehart, 1985), access to quality health care becomes a serious national health problem.

Reimbursement mechanisms for Medicaid recipients have discouraged open access to private care and have compounded urban hospitals' problems in providing indigent care with dwindling resources. The Omnibus Reconciliation Act of 1981 introduced "programmatic waivers" to permit states to experiment with program designs to reduce costs which did not fit normal Medicaid guidelines (Freund, Hurley, and Taylor, 1989). Section 1915 of the act provides flexibility for state Medicaid programs to contract with prepaid health plans for total health care management of enrollees.

In the last 10 years, many states have experimented with alternatives to Medicaid, among them "managed care" demonstration projects. In general, primary care providers act as managers of care and gatekeepers for referral to other health care services. As of October 1985, 59 managed care programs existed in 28 states (Freund and Hurley, 1987).

Although these experiments have yielded mixed results, some positive results are available. Case-managed care has been shown to improve access (Temkin-Greener, 1986), and significantly reduce the number of Medicaid recipients seeking primary care from emergency rooms (Hurley, Freund, and Taylor, 1989). The major concern is that state agencies have had difficulty in implementing and managing these programs effectively (Freund, Hurley, and Taylor, 1989).

In Pennsylvania, a fixed monthly fee is paid to a private insurance firm, which then subcontracts with physicians, hospitals, and other providers to deliver ambulatory services, monitor the referral of patients to subspecialties, and provide inpatient services from a hospital-pooled fund. The Hospital of the University of Pennsylvania is the largest provider of adult primary care services in west and southwest Philadelphia. It is one of the primary HealthPASS sites in the state. Approximately 6,000 of 95,000 possible adult recipients are registered with HUP as the source of their primary provider.

When the program was first implemented at HUP, two departments were designated as care sites: the medical clinic, the main training site for medical residents, would see the chronically ill, unstable patients; and the preventive care group (PCG), a nurse practitioner group in the emergency room area, would see the younger, largely female population who would generally be well, but in need of episodic care. Approximately 2,000 of the 6,000 adult recipients were assigned to the preventive care group.

The PCG location, next to the walk-in clinic (WIC) and adjacent to the emergency room, has been beneficial in channeling patients into the managed care clinic. The WIC and PCG share a waiting area and the same receptionists. Since the nurse practitioners are providers in both clinics, there is a greater chance that patients in the managed care system will be streamlined into the PCG for a walk-in appointment, rather than into the more expensive, noncompensated care of the WIC.

The nurse-managed PCG clinic now includes many patients with chronic health problems, some men, and some older women. Contrary to projections, this population of inner-city women is not as healthy as predicted, and the nurse providers find themselves faced with many complex health problems. In addition, the patients have been reluctant to transfer care to the medical clinic after a relationship has been established with PCG, where they feel they receive less fragmented, more personal, and more consistent care from providers who are more readily available.

The PCG practice accommodates 200 to 250 patients per month (for fiscal year 1989, total patients equaled 2,460). The average age of the population is 30 (range, teen to 60 years). 86.5% of the patients are female, and over 90% are black. Many patients are young, unmarried women raising children alone. These figures are not surprising considering eligibility requirements for Medicaid in Pennsylvania that determine HealthPASS coverage. Although health maintenance activities comprise the largest component of care provided, hypertension ranks fourth as the most frequently seen problem.

Differentiated Nursing Care in the PCG

The clinic is staffed by three master's-prepared nurse practitioners who also provide cross coverage for the walk-in clinic. These
Level IV nurses, hired by the nursing department, report to the
clinical director for medical nursing and the head nurse for emergency services. Administration of the clinic is the primary responsibility of one of the practitioners. The nurse practitioners function as
independent providers. Physician colleagues act in consulting roles,
with one emergency room attending physician available at all times.
They have responsibility for dispensing medical care and observing
protocols mutually agreed upon by the nurse practitioners and collaborative practice arrangements. They see patients only on referral
by the nurse practitioners.

A full-time nursing assistant is an integral member of the PCG
clinic. In addition to the regular duties of most nursing assistants,
she schedules consultation appointments, participates in phone
triage, provides lab retrieval, and, in many cases, begins to collect
the health history. The nursing assistant's skills are maximized.
Patients trust her knowledge and skill in assisting with their care.
She is involved in counseling and patients seek her advice. The
nurse practitioners trust her judgement and share new skills and
education with her as she develops. She reports to the nurse practitioners who are responsible for her evaluation.

A full-time receptionist/secretary is responsible for scheduling
appointments, limited phone triage, chart management, and scheduling referrals. She also assists with patient registration and acts as
a part of the "waiting room team" who sit with and help manage the
patients waiting to be seen in both the WIC and the PCG. Team-
work is essential in this setting. Many of the day-to-day tasks are
shared by the nursing assistant and the secretary.

The interrelationship of the WIC and the PCG nurses is maxi-
mal, enhancing both settings. The WIC nurses help to stem the flow
of patients into the area where PCG patients are waiting, thus teaching this population the value of a consistent care provider who
knows them. The nurse practitioners who work in the WIC help the
PCG nurse practitioner when the HealthPASS walk-in population
becomes overwhelming, reinforcing the same type of care in the
WIC as they receive in PCG, and encouraging patients to keep
appointments and use the managed care system to their advantage.
The WIC now has HealthPASS patients who are able to participate

in their own health care because they have learned to do so under the managed care concept of PCG. There is better follow-up from the WIC for patients needing short-term follow-up. The interaction of the two sets of nurses has strengthened the unique contributions each has to make to this difficult but rewarding population.

Clinic Operation

The PCG clinic is open from 8:30 a.m. – 5:00 p.m, Monday through Friday. Evening and weekend coverage is obtained through the emergency department. There is one primary examination room and access to a secondary one three afternoons per week. Additional rooms can be borrowed from the WIC, but it is difficult to do so. Usually, only one nurse practitioner is seeing patients in the PCG at one time. The other two are doing rotations in the WIC, fulfilling other clinical responsibilities, handling phone follow-up, and consulting on problems relating to case management of a large practice.

The clinic's location in emergency services allows for immediate x-ray and laboratory results when needed. Although the clinic was originally designed to avoid duplication of services offered in other areas of the hospital, the practice provides comprehensive care. Prior to the start of the HealthPASS program, many patients had a long history of going to specialty clinics for problems that could be readily managed within a primary care setting. Now, at considerable cost savings, they are handled in a single visit to the PCG clinic.

As case managers, the nurse practitioners provide primary health care, with an emphasis on self-care, education, continuity of care, and a holistic approach. Preventive care and the management of acute and chronic health conditions require coordination and development of interdependent services. For example, to provide mental health services, pregnancy prevention, and drug and alcohol services for these patients, a series of formal and informal contacts are established for early referral and consistent relationships, regardless of ability to pay.

Managing this type of care is demanding, time-consuming, and intricate. But the PCG clinic has made significant advances in preparing the way for acceptance of patients in other clinics/systems. For example, patients now receive prenatal care that, prior to the preliminary screening and early intervention of the PCG in prenatal care, was often lacking. They also receive subsequent referral to the existing prenatal/obstetrical system. When the complexity of the patient's health status requires frequent physician involvement or

146

hospitalizations, the patient is usually transferred to the medical clinic HealthPASS group.

The clinic is not without problems. At the present time, accurate studies on the cost-effectiveness of PCG are unavailable. Information on patient utilization rates, hospitalization, and other vital statistics have been lacking since the program began in 1986. Similar failures to follow cost and utilization have led to the demise of other experimental Medicaid programs (Aved, 1987). The program has always been under financial threat. The first corporation chosen to manage the program went bankrupt in 1989, due partly to over-expansion in the HMO market outside Pennsylvania. The second managing corporation was under scrutiny for showing favoritism in awarding their contracts, but has subsequently signed a second contract with the government. These fiscal disruptions left participating practices and hospitals with unpaid bills (some to be settled in bankruptcy court), and caused rampant confusion and fear among patients and providers alike.

A paucity of quality assurance programs has been notable within clinics as well as the contracting firms. Without appropriate monitoring of the new managed care concept, it will be impossible to tell whether the Medicaid population can benefit from this type of program in the future. This information is vital for policy makers and program managers alike.

In evaluating this nurse-managed practice, there are many positive aspects. The primary care approach has flourished by decreasing fragmentation of care, improving quality of care, and increasing access. Nurses excel in prevention, education, and health maintenance activities. They also complement the access to tertiary services available in the hospital. A collegial, collaborative relationship has developed among physicians, nurses, nursing assistants, and other personnel working in the area. The clinic has been successful at expediting care, and patients have learned the value of making and keeping appointments.

The clinic provides endless opportunities for teaching and learning for nurse practitioners and medical students. Within a context of managed care, students learn to value collaborative, cooperative care — where patients exert both control and responsibility. A strong link to the school of nursing at the University of Pennsylvania has been fostered, with a faculty member and a nurse practitioner sharing part-time responsibilities in each setting. The nurse practitioners lecture and teach physical assessment at the school. A formal peer review program among all nurse practitioners assigned to the area (a total of nine) is in place. A research proposal to study utilization and outcome variables has been designed and submitted cooperatively by the schools of nursing and medicine — to study whether the clinic actually makes substantial differences in patient care through the nurse practitioner, case management model.

While no single health care system can solve the myriad of problems seen in poverty situations, the PCG has made progress with a group of patients often thought of as difficult and resistant to taking part in their own health care. Because of the success of this nurse-managed clinic and its usefulness to the west Philadelphia population, nursing has incorporated the nurse practitioner role in the acute section of the emergency department. Hopefully, the patients discharged from the ED can be integrated into the PCG when appropriate, continue to receive coordinated care through cooperation with the WIC, and improve long-term health in a coordinated nursing system.

Differentiated nursing practice in the emergency department uses the best of every nurse to care for its community population through the integrated models described herein. As this continues, nursing practice becomes increasingly sophisticated, integrated, and successful. This maximizes our image and promotes good feelings about ourselves as professionals.

Occupational Health Services (OHS): Delivery of Occupational Health Services to Hospital Employees by Nurse Practitioners

Beth Ann Swan, M.S.N., R.N.,C., C.R.N.P.

Occupational health nursing has its roots in the post-Civil War industrial boom. But the profession, as we know it today, is truly "a product of a high-tech world barely a decade old" (Bodner, 1988). For several years prior to 1980, the Hospital of the University of Pennsylvania had an employee health service (EHS) that provided primary care services and managed work-related illnesses and injuries, free of charge, to all HUP employees. Providers were residents in medicine who rotated through the service on a short-term basis. There was little continuity of care, often resulting in inappropriate referrals and follow-ups which were costly to both the employees and the hospital.

In the early 1980s, it was agreed that an expanded program, using a nurse practitioner as a main caregiver, could reduce duplication of services already provided through the health insurance plan and develop a more organized, comprehensive approach to injury prevention and management. The goal of the new occupational health service (OHS) would be to increase cost- effective care for HUP employees and to contract with other employers to provide work-related services, thereby increasing ED revenues. The services to be offered would include health assessments, counseling, health education, health and hazard surveillance, injury prevention, and work-related injury and illness management. Today, the OHS provides care for occupationally-related illnesses and injuries to the employees of HUP, the University of Pennsylvania faculty and staff, and several other industries located in the area of the hospital, resulting in approximately 7,000 visits per year.

The development of the present program began with the education of an emergency room nurse in a year-long nurse practitioner certification program at the University of Maryland. She has been joined by two master's-prepared adult nurse practitioners, one prepared as an occupational health nurse practitioner. An attending ED physician who shares time with the WIC and the acute emergency department section has been added as a part-time provider and consultant to the nurse practitioner staff. A full-time receptionist and secretary also work in the area.

Clinic Operation

The OHS offers 24-hours-a-day coverage for employees in conjunction with the acute ED. Non-work-related injuries or illnesses are referred either to the WIC or to the employee's own primary care provider. In some cases, patients are seen in the PCG. Thus, nursing personnel in these areas administer to the care of employees in collaboration with the OHS nurse practitioners.

The mission of the OHS includes a commitment to:

- clinically excellent care of employees;
- education of staff through inservices;
- academic development of students from the school of nursing in primary care, occupational health, and community health programs; and
- clinically-based research to solve problems related to patient care.

The OHS integrates clinical practice, education, and research to provide cost-effective care. It does not interfere with the relationships employees have with their personal physicians, but supplements and complements those relationships by providing on-site management of work-related health problems and the teaching of injury and illness prevention.

According to an American Association of Occupational Health Nurses (1988) position statement:

> The employment of well-qualified occupational health nurses to develop and implement a comprehensive health program promotes better employee health, decreases costs, improves employee morale, increases productivity, and facilitates continuity of care.

It is the occupational health nurse practitioner who determines real and potential health problems and hazards; develops and implements programs to deal with identified health problems and hazards; verifies that health programs comply with federal, state, and local regulations; evaluates and monitors outcomes; and promotes and facilitates continuity of care. As shown by McGrath elsewhere, this OHS has demonstrated that qualified and competent nurse practitioners can produce cost- effective care (McGrath, 1990).

A major cost-saving initiative has been to reduce hospitalization by transferring care and procedures to the less expensive outpatient setting. Preventive health care programs and early treatment of illness and injury can reduce the number of days lost at work. Follow-up of work-related problems can be handled in this setting without costly referral to specialty care. The nurse practitioner can readily expand the programs of care and embrace cost-containment measures by "doing more with no more" (Sovie, 1985). The nurse practitioner has been a revenue generator in the emergency department at HUP, bringing new business to the ED through its contracts with outside employers. For this hospital, the nurse practitioner practice has been both cost-effective and efficient.

Differentiated Practice in the OHS

Differentiated practice exists among the three nurse practitioners in the OHS with regard to educational background, experience, and individual expertise. The original nurse practitioner, educated in a continuing education program, is a diploma nurse with 35 years of clinical experience, including many years of emergency nursing at HUP. Her experience was invaluable in setting up the original OHS program. She has helped develop the outreach programs to educate employees about hepatitis B vaccine, helped develop standards for protection from bloodborne pathogens, and contributed to the AIDS awareness program offered in the hospital. Her activities are largely patient-centered, and she spends about 95% of her time in direct patient care.

One master's-prepared adult nurse practitioner has seven years of experience as a nurse practitioner. She divides her time between direct patient care, education, administration, and research. The educator role includes developing and teaching employee education programs, and functioning as a clinical preceptor and clinical lecturer for graduate and undergraduate nursing students at the University of Pennsylvania School of Nursing.

As an administrator, she is responsible for staffing the OHS, coordinating the activities of personnel, updating and maintaining policy and procedure manuals, acting as the spokesperson for OHS on committees both outside and within the ED, coordinating various hospital programs (i.e., annual visit programs, medical reentry programs for self-disclosing substance abuse employees, preemployment evaluations), and supervising the development of new programs.

As a participant in research, she defines clinical problems in OHS and pursues their investigation in collaboration with nurse colleagues and other health professionals. Examples of some projects under investigation include:

- a study of needlestick and blood/body fluid exposure,
- a protocol for early intervention in back injury, and
- compliance with return for the hepatitis B vaccination series.

These studies affect current hospital policies and programs. For example, the needlestick study identified a need for increased health care worker education as well as a need for improved engineering controls; the back injury study helped introduce a limited duty policy that sends people back to work earlier while treating the injury.

The nurse practitioner who is master's-prepared as an occupational health nurse practitioner is involved in direct patient care, education, and administration. Her unique contributions utilize her educational preparation and skills in surveillance programs and outreach programs for on-site evaluations of potential employer contracts, and as a consultant on work site and worker-related health issues. She is a member of the hospital's safety committee.

Her administrative role includes development of new services for contracted companies and new program development. She is involved in developing new protocols (i.e., a pesticide protocol for the University of Pennsylvania groundskeepers, and a smoking cessation program to maintain the hospital's "smoke free" status) and educating employees about hazards and methods to avoid illness and injury. She coordinates the care of several special populations, such as the University of Pennsylvania lab animal researchers, Monell Chemical Senses Center animal handlers, and phlebotomists from a local private company.

She also is active in the school of nursing as a clinical preceptor, class lecturer, and a member of the advisory board of the occupational health program. In addition to clinical expertise, her particular background in occupational health makes her a valuable resource in industrial health and safety surveillance.

The practices of the three nurse practitioners are differentiated by educational preparation. Additionally, the division of labor is based on individual interests and special competencies.

Summary

The occupational health service is an excellent example of a nurse-managed ambulatory service where differentiated practice within a single level of practice makes a well coordinated, diversified clinical practice possible. As part of the total ambulatory offerings within the emergency department, it provides a model of autonomous, yet interactive, nursing practice — where nurse practitioners share collaboratively with both intra- and interdisciplinary colleagues. Employees are the chief beneficiaries of this model of care.

Conclusions and Directions

Nursing practice is diverse. To optimize individual strengths, educational backgrounds, clinical experiences, and abilities, nurses practicing together need to develop models that complement and enhance each other's backgrounds. The emergency services department at the University of Pennsylvania is a model based on three separate but interwoven practice areas where nurses have taken the leadership in management and provision of services. It has resulted in increased access for poor and underserved populations (HealthPASS, PCG, and WIC), efficient and cost-effective care for employees (OHS), increased patient satisfaction in the ED, and successful modeling of nursing case management. Physicians in the emergency services department have developed satisfying collaborative practices with the nurses and, as they have become more interactive in the care process, the patients have received better medical and nursing care.

The differentiated nursing model recognizes the need for practice to be fluid. Whether nurses continue to grow and control those areas of patient care where nursing is the predominant need depends on how well they are able to define and delineate individual practices within service settings. Where nurses can develop both inter- and intradisciplinary practice relationships that maximize individual contributions and concentrate on the needs of patient populations, success stories will continue to abound.

At the time of this writing, a differentiated model of practice is developing in the acute emergency department using nurse practitioners, experienced emergency nurses, and nursing assistants. It is modeled on the WIC successes. In the medical clinic, a nurse practitioner has been hired to provide case management and primary care for the chronically ill HealthPASS population, following the design of the PCG group. New referral patterns, developed by nurses in the three clinics, have facilitated better communication among the clinics and increased specialty clinic access for the patients who enter the emergency department. There are some isolated but promising instances of interdisciplinary teaching/learning in the three areas where student nurses and doctors are assigned the same patient to determine needs, and where residents in training engage in mutual practice with the nurse practitioner providers. Cooperative behaviors are learned as care is provided.

The three practices described herein are a beginning. The future holds great possibility for change in health care delivery. Nurses who have defined their roles, have implemented differentiated practice models, and practice the philosophy that patients will best improve under the coordinated care of all nursing providers, not only will survive, but will become the leaders of the future.

❑   ❑   ❑

Integrated Care in the Home Health and Hospice Settings

Sandy Young, M.S., R.N.

Sioux Falls is a city in South Dakota. It has approximately 100,000 people and is surrounded by rural towns. The city borders the states of Minnesota and Iowa, so referrals are also received from these areas. South Dakota has a population of 715,000, one-third of which lives east of the Missouri River, where Sioux Falls is located. Sioux Valley Hospital (SVH) is a 512-bed hospital. The home health and hospice departments are a part of the hospital.

In January 1987, the SVH nursing department selected units to participate in a statewide project for nursing and nursing education. This project differentiated nurses into two categories based on experience and competence. The difficulties and trials of the project have been discussed previously. After we participated in the project, however, we knew we could never go back to the former way of practicing.

With the problems inherent in rising client acuity, the fragmentation of health care, the DRG system, etc., we could see that, as a practice, we needed to change. Our vice president of nursing, JoEllen Koerner, posed a question earlier in this conference which helped to clarify why our nursing practice needed to change. She asked, "How many of you have updated your wardrobe in the last 20 years?" Obviously, 100% of us indicated that we had altered our wardrobe in some way to keep up with fashions and trends.

Just as we update our wardrobe, nursing practice must also be updated to stay current with the trends occurring in the health care system. We expanded differentiated practice into integrated care and built upon the knowledge we gained through participation in the differentiated practice project.

We no longer have to follow the pack. We do not have to deliver nursing care in the same manner as everyone else. We can modify our present system to meet the needs of the health care system. The experience was often very isolating for us, but the thrill and excitement of creating and implementing a new care delivery system was very rewarding.

In February 1988, Sioux Valley Hospital termed *differentiation of practice* as "integrated care," and defined it as:

A system of patient care delivery that integrates the allocation of resources (human and material) over a variety of settings within appropriate time frames and through the differentiation of nursing practice. Differentiation implies expansion of patient care management beyond physiologic stabilization to the entire episode of illness from pre-admission to post-discharge.

The elements of this definition say that integration is a process for which care is delivered to the patient using both available human and material resources in all settings. When a patient is transferred from the oncology unit to hospice, we are able to maintain that continuity of care. For example, the oncology nurse shares with the hospice nurse the care plan developed on her unit, as well as the data base and admission sheets. No longer is that wealth of information lost, requiring the next nurse to start from "ground zero" again. The same sharing of information occurs when a pediatric or intensive care infant is discharged from the unit to home health for private duty nursing. The case manager in the home setting is often one of the ICN nurses who has been working closely with the patient and family. Trust and continuity, therefore, are maintained, even as the care settings change.

The SVH definition of integrated care also says that, as nurses, not only are we concerned with treating and maintaining the patient's physiological status, but we also are moving into encompassing the entire episode of illness. In addressing the causative factors that precipitated the illness, we are concerned with the coping strategies that must be mobilized to enable the individual to remain at home without repeated hospitalizations.

To integrate the client's care, nurses must assume broader responsibility in allocating the human, fiscal, and material resources. To do this, we differentiated the nurse's role into two types or categories: *RN case manager* (at SVH, the term "primary nurse," rather than "case manager," was used, as it was less threatening to physicians), and *case associate nurse* (SVH calls them "RN in the associate role"). We also added the role of the clinical nurse specialist to hospice, which is the master's-prepared nurse.

The nurse was able to choose in which role (either case manager or case associate) he/she preferred to function, based on:

- preference (perhaps the nurse's home life was such that taking on more responsibility was not feasible),
- experience (a strong background in nursing typically indicates a case manager candidate),
- competency (according to Benner's [1984] ranking of nursing levels from novice to expert, the nurse who is the most proficient is the case manager), and
- availability of positions (executive management has allocated funds for 35% of the nurses to be in case manager or primary nurse roles).

We believe that, in the future, education will be a criteria for determining the role, with the BSN being the requirement for the case manager role.

In defining roles and responsibilities of the case manager and case associate nurses, we discovered that the roles differed based upon time frame, structure, and interpersonal relations.

Regarding time frame, the case associate nurse is one who focuses vertically. In other words, this individual works a specific shift. The nurse case manager focuses horizontally to coordinate care for the client throughout the episode of illness. For example, when a client is transferred from hospice to the oncology unit for acute care, the hospice case manager continues to coordinate the care for the client, working closely with the nurses on the oncology unit. The case manager will develop an ongoing nursing care plan using nursing diagnosis that incorporates mutually-established goals identified by both the client and nurse to coordinate the necessary resources to deliver client care. To achieve the identified goals, the case associate nurse will deliver care to the client on the scheduled shifts following the established care plan. The case manager and case associate nurse must work closely together. They need to develop a high level of trust so that all information is shared and quality care is delivered.

In defining structure, the RN in the case associate role works with established policies and has access to the support of a wide range of services. The case manager works in both structured and unstructured settings, and may or may not have a set of well-defined policies. The case manager must be skillful at problem identification and resolution, and must possess clinical competence.

In the area of interpersonal relations, the case associate nurse resolves conflicts and issues concerning client care on the shifts worked. The nurse case manager expands the role to negotiate solutions surrounding the client to achieve a more comprehensive outcome. The RN in the associate role focuses on the client and family, whereas the case manager's focus includes all members of the health care team.

Briefly, the clinical nurse specialist functions in the roles identified in the literature — consultant, researcher, educator, and clinician. The major task for the hospice CNS in implementing integrated care is to educate and mentor the case manager and case associate nurses in their respective roles. The CNS did have a caseload on which she modeled the case manager role.

When examining the two nursing roles further, we tried to determine if each role had different components, and resolved that each role had the same components:

- The *technical skills* area included what we already do — i.e., start IVs, perform assessments, etc.
- The *communication skills* area included the ability to interact with clients, departments, etc.
- The *care management* area included the nurse's ability to think critically and plan the care.

In looking at these three nursing roles, we stressed how much we valued each of the competencies identified in the case manager and case associate roles (see Figure 1).

Planning, communicating, and doing — critical thinking, interpersonal, and technical skills are all equally important for the nurse to have, whether he/she is acting in the case manager or case associate role (see Figure 2). The time allotted to each of these skill areas varies, depending on the role in which the nurse is functioning (see Figure 3).

In other words, the case associate nurse spends much of his/her time communicating and performing technical duties, whereas the case manager spends most of his/her time planning and communicating. However, all three areas of competency are valued equally in each of the roles.

The goals of our integrated care in hospice and home health services were threefold:

- to enhance job satisfaction by empowering the nurses in home health/hospice to practice professionally,
- to enhance quality of care, and
- to do both in a cost-effective manner.

The level of nursing job satisfaction at SVH has improved. There has been less turnover in our department and more expression of satisfaction with the care the nurses are delivering. If they meet the criteria, nurses now have the ability to move between the roles of case manager and case associate. For example, one of our nurses moved into the case manager role. After assuming the position, she found that, due to the responsibilities she had in her personal life, she could not assume the responsibility and accountability for the case manager role. She then transferred back into the case associate role, enabling us to maintain her in the department without losing her to another unit or hospital. This flexibility enhanced her job satisfaction. Nurses now have the opportunity to expand the clinical role at the bedside without transferring into a management position.

The positive responses we are receiving to questionnaires sent to physicians and our clients indicate that we are giving quality care. Our closely monitored quality assurance program offers the same response. Patients and families express satisfaction in knowing there is an accountable person they can go to with questions or concerns.

The last area examined was our cost effectiveness. Hospice is not a moneymaking department, so linking quality care to cost effectiveness was a priority. We conducted a utilization review comparing the years 1988 and 1989 (see Figure 4).

As integrated care matured in the hospice department, we could see a direct correlation to an increase in cost effectiveness. Pharmacy costs did increase, but they were directly related to a substantial increase in cost of the medications during this time period. Because we are a Medicare-certified hospice program, we are reimbursed on a per diem basis. From this money, we must pay for all medical, lab, durable medical, pharmacy, and radiology supplies/equipment related to each individual's terminal illness. By having the CNS mentor the case manager, the decrease in cost can be directly related to the case manager's increased awareness of delivering quality, cost-effective care. For example, a client often has three or four physicians. Frequently, the third doctor does not know what the first doctor has ordered. The case manager coordinates the care to prevent duplication. In hospice, the goal is palliative care, so routine monitoring is rarely done unless it will promote comfort. By having the case manager collaborate closely with the physician, routine monitoring is eliminated.

Another cost-effective measure is utilizing the case manager to coordinate the patient's care, thereby enhancing symptom management. Rarely is it necessary to transfer patients back to the hospital for management of acute care symptoms.

Another example of how integrated care promotes cost effectiveness is illustrated in the following case's cost analysis. The home health department provided care to an end-stage leukemic who received blood transfusions, amphotericin, and lab work, as well as regular nursing assessments. The patient lived 45 miles from the hospital. Had he been hospitalized, the care would have cost $20,066 (see Figure 5). Coordinating home health care with the Medicare skilled intermittent home care agency would have cost $13,736. By going a step further and using integrated care, the cost was $7,056, a substantial increase in savings due to the case manager coordinating and integrating the care.

The case manager was a nurse who resided in the patient's community and who also worked on the unit to which the patient was typically admitted. The nurse coordinated her visits with her unit shifts, which decreased the number of extra trips back and forth to the hospital for medications, blood draw, etc. She integrated the care with the lab and pharmacy departments to facilitate the delivery of nursing care in a timely manner.

We are pleased with the progress we have made at this time in meeting our goals. Integrated care does make a difference. But it is important to remember that anything worthwhile takes persistence.

❑   ❑   ❑

Figure 1
Practice Role of Nurse:
Interface of Role Components

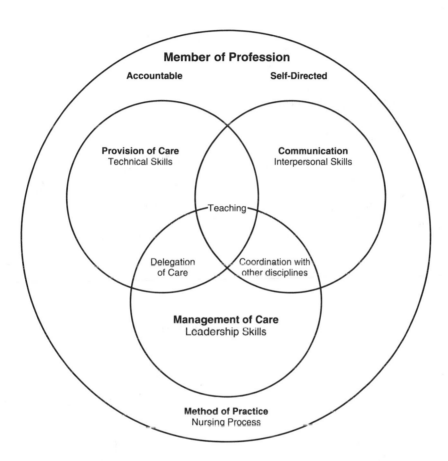

Figure 2
Value of Role Function Characteristics

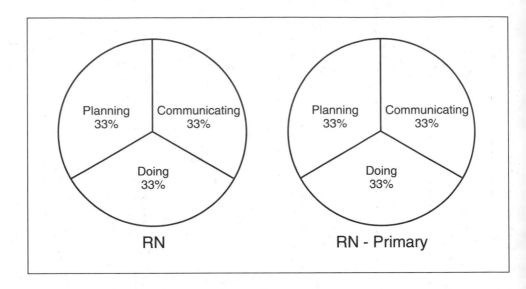

RN

RN - Primary

Figure 3
Time Allocated to Each Role Function

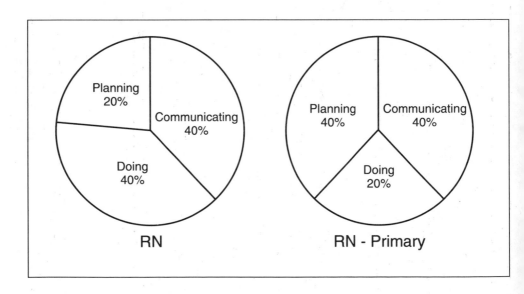

RN

RN - Primary

Figure 4
Hospice Utilization Review

	1988–1989	**1989–1990**
Medical Supplies	1.01/day/pt	.58/day/pt
Lab	2.46/day/pt	.08/day/pt
DME	.53/day/pt	.07/day/pt
Pharmacy	2.95/day	4.31/day
Radiology	.87/day	.40/day
Other Total		50.59—ER
		106.20—Enteral

Figure 5
Cost Analysis of Client Care

Type of Care	**Cost**
Traditional hospital care	$ 20,066
Coordinated home health care	13,736
Savings	$ 6,326
Traditional hospital care	$ 20,066
Integrated home health care	7,056
Savings	$ 13,010

Block Nursing: Practicing Autonomous Professional Nursing in the Community

Marjorie K. Jamieson, M.S., R.N.

She is 82-years-old, has no relatives, lives in the house in which she was born, and receives a social security check of $309 per month. Arthritis prevents her from simple meal preparation because she cannot open a carton of milk or a box of cereal. She must pay for someone to clean her house and provide her personal care from her small income because these services are not eligible for Medicare reimbursement, she does not qualify for Medicaid, and she has no family nearby. To make ends meet, she is gradually selling pieces of her heirloom furniture. She is fiercely independent and does not even want to consider a nursing home if (when) her resources run out.

This may be a familiar story, but the ending has a different twist. Through the efforts of the innovative Block Nurse Program in St. Anthony Park in St. Paul, Minnesota, this elderly lady has been able to remain safely in her home.

Long-term care identifies a broad range of services needed by elderly persons when they can no longer function independently. In the United States, long-term care is usually associated with nursing home care; Americans have institutionalized the "medicalized" care of the elderly. Yet, a study conducted in 1979 by the U.S. General Accounting Office showed that 20–40% of the elderly in

Originally published in 1990, *Nursing & Health Care*, May (11)5: 250-253. Reprinted with permission.

nursing homes would not need to be there if they could get some help at home. In 1989, 25% of Minnesota nursing home residents could remain at home with similar assistance. Despite these findings, the present reimbursement system still does not pay for some of the support services delivered to elderly persons in their homes. Instead, society seems to have chosen the more expensive route (both in terms of cost and dignity) by providing Medicaid reimbursement for nursing home care when elderly persons have exhausted all of their funds.

Formal service providers are a major resource for the elderly. But the formal system represents a complex array of independently functioning public and private agencies. Without a mechanism to coordinate the resources available with the broad-ranging needs of an elderly person, it is difficult for a single agency to provide for the very individual needs of each elderly person living at home. This complex current service delivery system makes it extremely difficult for elderly persons and their families to put together their own package of services. In addition, services that would enable elderly persons to remain at home safely rather than be admitted to a nursing home are generally not eligible for Medicare and Medicaid reimbursement.

Most Americans believe that Medicare pays for nursing home care. However, Medicare pays for less than 2% of the total costs of nursing home care and covers an elderly person for a maximum of 180 days following hospitalization as long as improvement is significant. Once the patient is no longer acutely ill, has no rehabilitation potential, and requires only custodial care, it becomes his or her own responsibility to pay for care. Most elderly persons in nursing homes spend all their savings within six months, thus becoming eligible for Medicaid (also called Medical Assistance or Welfare). To protect themselves against these costs, 70% of Medicare beneficiaries purchase at least one Medicare supplemental insurance policy. However, these policies pay for less than 1% of nursing home care because reimbursement criteria do not include custodial/maintenance care. Cost-effective alternatives to long-term institutionalization are a critical issue for long-term care policy formulation at the federal, state, and local levels.

The Block Nurse Program which began in 1982 in St. Anthony Park, a community in St. Paul, Minnesota, is one alternative that is both a cost-effective and innovative solution to the delivery of health and long-term care services — conceived, implemented, and managed primarily by nurses.

In the St. Anthony Park community of 6,969 residents, of whom 12.5% are aged 65 +, 41.3% of its housing units are owned by the people who live in them. About 55.1% of the residents are college graduates. The poverty level is 7.3%, with 5.2% of all people aged 65 + below the poverty level (1980 census). St. Anthony Park has demonstrated that a community and, more specifically, a neighborhood can play an essential role in providing the coordination and access to services required by the elderly in order to remain at home.

Imagine a model in which:

- A reclusive person who has not left her home for two years because she is incontinent becomes a part of the community again. Her family does not want to repair her washer because "she needs to go into a nursing home and is so stubborn that we are not repairing anything for her." With Block Nurse services, she completes a bladder control program, her family repairs her washer, she has a new wardrobe and hair style, and her family is now involved with their mother, who is active again.
- A Block Nurse, as a neighbor, drops off milk and bread to a shut-in client.
- A clerk in a local dry-cleaning store discusses her elderly neighbor when a Block Nurse drops in to pick up her dry cleaning. She offers to pave the way for a needed assessment.
- A local clergyman discusses the needs of elderly parishioners in his church with the Block Nurse.
- A couple in their eighties, one of whom is confined to a wheelchair and the other to a walker, enjoy each other's company in their home of 49 years with occasional visits by the Block Nurse and support from the Block Companion and Block Volunteer.
- Respite care for a retired college professor's wife is provided. For two years she has remained at home without a break, caring for her chronically ill, disabled husband.
- Nurses ski to client homes during a snowstorm.
- Neighbors stop by to take clients to doctor appointments, concerts, etc.
- Nurses' spouses fix dripping faucets.

- Retired people feel needed because they are Block Volunteers and become vocal proponents of the program.
- A Block Volunteer, trained to deal with loss, addresses the needs of a 70-year-old who has had cataract surgery, lost her driver's license, and can no longer drive her three friends to their weekly shopping and lunch date.

After seven years of providing services to elderly clients, the Block Nurse Program has found that services can be made available based upon the needs of the elderly rather than eligibility for reimbursement. What is required is alternative funding; professional and volunteer community members; and an informal network of family, friends, neighbors, church and civic groups, and service groups such as Boy Scouts and Rotary Clubs. The last two criteria already exist in most communities, and the first — and most critical — is becoming more accessible as the government and third-party payers are becoming more interested in containing their costs. What is most difficult to put in place is a structure that distinguishes this model from more traditional providers.

Answering questions about whether Johnny needs stitches or queries about someone's blood pressure is the fate of any nurse in most neighborhoods. Ida Martinson, PhD, RN, FAAN, knew about this firsthand, having lived in St. Anthony Park for many years. She began creating a vision for a different model for meeting the needs of the elderly, a system whereby younger neighbors — some of whom were nurses — could deliver services to their older neighbors (Jamieson and Campbell, 1987; Jamieson and Martinson, 1983; Martinson et al., 1985; Selby, 1983).

To make this vision practical, two basic tenets of the program are still in effect: 1) clients, paid staff, and volunteers all live within the defined parameters of the community; and 2) existing city, county, and private agencies and resources are used so that no new layers of management are created. The staff, although living in the neighborhood, are all employees of Ramsey County Public Health Nursing Service. This agency provides quality assurance programs, operational mechanisms such as payroll and client charts, and access to third-party payers for those in the program who are eligible.

Rather than convening the directors of other formal service agencies to create a master plan for accessing their services, the nurse determines client need, and prescribes and coordinates those services that are appropriate. Turf issues and the costs of bureaucracy and centralization are therefore minimized. Periodically, the agencies that provide services (such as the Red Cross's provision of transportation) are given data about the services they provide to the program.

The results have been beneficial to the professional nurse as well as the client. The role of the professional nurse has been maximized. The Block Nurse works with the client and family to develop a care plan that is acceptable to them and that meets their needs. In the North End-South Como replication site, because the nurses and home health aides/homemakers are neighbors, they have gotten into homes refused to other service agencies; fear because of vulnerability and suspicion of "welfare" is very real! Building trust over time is a luxury that is too expensive for most programs. As case manager, the nurse is also a gatekeeper to the system so that the "woodworking effect" is less likely to occur. Only the right services at the right time and in the right amount are delivered. This primary Block Nurse is also responsible for those services delivered by the Block Companions (home health aides/homemakers), the trained Block Volunteers, and other volunteers. A program director (also a community resident) functions as liaison between the community and the county nursing service. The program director reports to the board of directors, which is composed of residents of the community.

Indirect time necessary to arrange and coordinate services, plus direct time with clients, are the basis for changes. Indirect time is reduced because many services are available in the community. Only actual time is billed, and there is no minimum for nursing, home health aide, or homemaker time.

The commitment to include everyone 65 and over means that any necessary service is provided, regardless of entitlements or ability of the client to pay. After third-party payers are billed for services for which the clients are eligible, clients are billed based upon their ability to pay.

All nurses have completed a course in gerontics in addition to the requirement that each primary Block Nurse be public health certified. The Block Companions have attended vocational school and are certified as home health aides/homemakers. Block Nurses and Block Companions are paid by the county according to community standards, which puts them among the top 15% in the country. Block Volunteers are trained through a 30-hour course to provide support, peer counseling, and socialization according to the care plan developed by the nurse and the client. These volunteers receive no reimbursement.

The staff component is in frequent contact through the telephone. Orientation and supervision in client homes is continuous because everyone lives as neighbors. Biweekly care conferences include the volunteer coordinator, to whom referrals from the nurses are directed for implementation.

In September 1985, an external evaluation done by Jeanne Campbell, PhD, and Michael Patton, PhD, found that:

- 85% of the Block Nurse Program clients would be forced to enter nursing homes without care.
- The total cost of living with Block Nurse Program care is at least 24% less than the minimum cost of a nursing home *without* nursing services.
- All indicators show that the Block Nurse Program tends to increase and enhance family involvement in the care of elderly relatives.
- Nine dimensions explain the qualitative distinctions between home health care programs and the Block Nurse Program: client-centered programming, coordination and integration of services, community-based staffing, prevention/recovery focus, early intervention, management of chronic illness/ disability, delayed or reduced institutionalization, case mix openness, and fee flexibility.
- Block Nurse Program fees for Block Nurses and Block Companions are lower than for any other program surveyed, yet staff is paid according to community standards.
- The lack of a program policy requiring a minimum number of hours per visit is distinctive of the Block Nurse Program and accounts, in part, for its lower fees.

This evaluation of the pilot in St. Anthony Park suggested that the model needed to be tested for replicability and that an evaluation of the replication and of the nursing practice arrangement and cost savings needed to be done. An "Innovations in State and Local Government" award from Harvard University and the Ford Foundation enabled the writing of proposals for funding a three-year demonstration project.

In January 1988, funding from the Division of Nursing, U.S. Department of Health and Human Services and from the W. K. Kellogg Foundation enabled replication and evaluation to begin in three diverse communities. Highland Park has the largest number of elderly living in their own homes and is the most affluent neighborhood in St. Paul. North End-South Como has the largest number of people below the poverty level in the city. The third community is rural Atwater, Minnesota, a city of about 1,100 residents (the program includes the surrounding farm community).

The average client across all Block Nurse Programs is an 83-year-old female who lives alone and has no support system. Upon admission to the program, a nursing assessment is done to determine the client's ability to perform eight activities of daily living (ADLs). Preliminary data on 129 clients shows that:

- 45% need no help with ADLs (but usually require chronic disease management).
- 39.5% need help with one, two, or three ADLs (some require disease management).
- 8.5% need help with four, five, or six ADLs (some require disease management).
- 7.0% need help with seven or eight ADLs (some require disease management).

Specific ADL needs of the initial 108 clients in one community show that:

- 47% need help bathing.
- 20% need help dressing.
- 19% need help grooming and toileting.
- 13% need help walking.
- 11% need help transferring.
- 10% need help eating.
- 7% need help moving in bed.

In 1989, the average overall cost of Block Nurse Program services in this community was $106 per month per client. Thirteen Block Volunteers have gone through various levels of training to do friendly visits, socialization, and other activities. Thousands of hours have been contributed by the community in planning and implementing the model (this includes monthly meetings of the community board of directors). A similar commitment of volunteer hours occurs at all sites.

Other assessments measure cognition, family function, nursing care complexity, financial status, and other demographic variables. One tool used by nurses and aides provides exhaustive information about a wide range of activities such as who (clients, family, volunteer nurse) defrosts the refrigerator, buys groceries, cuts toenails, shampoos hair, cuts grass, does the laundry, etc.

In three Block Nurse Programs in St. Paul, the following reimbursement sources paid for the costs of the direct services to clients in 1989:

- Veterans Administration 2.1%
- Medicare 4.6%
- Alternative Care Grant (ACG) 6.2%
- County discount 6.2%
- Medicaid 11.3%
- Client fees 25.8%
- Grants 43.8%

During the seven years of the pilot and two years of replication in three other sites, some trends are surfacing, especially in the pilot site:

Community
- Over 80% of the referrals come by word of mouth from the neighborhood.
- A "bottom-up" neighborhood participation endeavor seems more successful and better sustained than a "top-down," superimposed system.
- The community adapts the program to fit its needs without bureaucratic constraints.
- The community has become sensitized to the needs of the elderly and asks for group involvement, such as church youth clubs or individuals concerned about a neighbor.
- The neighborhood furnishes its own informal quality control in the form of contacting direct caregivers or the program director, all of whom are neighbors.

Client/Family
- Families and family surrogates (usually neighbors) have become more involved with their elderly neighbors. Staff report that the ability of the family to meet the needs of clients is enhanced.
- Approximately 15% of the clients have elected to be discharged form nursing homes to Block Nurse care.
- People plan differently for their retirement when they know services will be available at home.

- Of those clients who have died, some have chosen to die at home utilizing Block Nurse care.

Cost Effectiveness
- Health education, prevention, and early intervention have prevented hospitalization for about 25% of the clients.
- Less time is spent managing care, since all staff know the client and client support system.
- By combining home health aide and homemaker functions in one job description, greater efficiency is demonstrated.
- Staff are available during inclement weather or odd hours.
- Although a chart may be formally "closed," staff and volunteers often continue informal client contact; therefore, prevention is addressed. Also, the nurse can build upon the interventions and support that have previously worked.

The replication project is currently demonstrating methods to improve access to nursing services in noninstitutional settings through nursing practice arrangements in communities. The ultimate goals of the Block Nurse Program are to design an appropriate service delivery model for meeting the needs of the elderly and to create a new and more inclusive system for paying for health and long-term care.

❏   ❏   ❏

Excellence for Nursing Practice: Transition Into the Future

Thomas E. Stenvig, M.P.H., R.N., C.N.A.A.

Excellence for Nursing Practice (ENP) is a differentiated nursing practice project involving four facilities of the Aberdeen Area Indian Health Service (IHS), a federal health care agency serving American Indians in North Dakota, South Dakota, Nebraska, and Iowa. Developed as an evaluation research project, the project includes demonstration and evaluation components using a differentiated case management nursing practice model. ENP began in March 1990, with a title chosen by nurses who are themselves participating in the project.

The four project sites are located in the South Dakota communities of Pine Ridge, Rapid City, Rosebud, and Wagner, with each project site serving a population composed primarily of Sioux Indians. With the exception of Rapid City, the four project sites are rural and reservation-based. Each project site includes nurses providing services in both hospitals and public health nursing programs. Hospitals at all four project sites are accredited by JCAHO and the community-based program is accredited by the Community Health Accreditation Program (CHAP). Table 1 summarizes the service population, hospital size, and number of nursing staff participating at each location.

The opinions expressed in this paper are those of the author and do not necessarily reflect the views of the Indian Health Service.

Project Overview

Excellence for Nursing Practice represents a continuing effort to implement differentiated nursing practice in South Dakota that began with the work of the steering committee for the South Dakota Statewide Project for Nursing and Nursing Education in 1986. This group was charged with responsibility for developing a plan for two levels of nursing in the state. Work of the steering committee was influenced by behavioral research in nursing sponsored by the Midwest Alliance in Nursing that began nearly a decade ago to describe and distinguish between the competencies of nurses prepared at the baccalaureate and associate degree levels (Pettengill, 1987). In considering competencies of nurses believed to be consistent with the future needs of the state, the differentiated case management model developed by Primm (1987) was recommended and selected for implementation at four demonstration centers in the state. The work of the steering committee officially concluded in 1988, when a final report was completed that described preliminary findings of the South Dakota demonstration project sites (South, 1988).

The ENP project reflects continued use of the differentiated case management model in South Dakota and is among the first projects nationally to test differentiated competencies in a rural setting in small facilities serving a minority population. Although the model in its original form describes two differentiated nursing roles (case manager and case associate), the practical nurse role has been included in ENP since the agency continues to employ practical nurses who are often individuals from the local community with senior career status. Using the same process applied in the original South Dakota demonstration centers, registered nurses participating in the project were factored into either the case manager or case associate role. Table 2 summarizes these and other key points about the project.

Study Purpose

The overall purpose of the ENP project was to evaluate the effectiveness of the model in the current IHS delivery system, with a focus on the impact of implementation on patient care as well as the satisfaction and professional autonomy of nurses participating in the project. Monitors were therefore needed to measure changes in the quality and effectiveness of nursing care and variations occurring in the practice and professional attitudes of nurses participating in the project.

In addition to these two broad areas, the project was designed to generate information that could be of value in determining agency policy affecting employment practices in the workplace through clarification of roles and responsibilities of nurses with varied educational preparation and competencies. Project results could prove to be of value to administrators, consultants, supervisors, and practicing nurses in making choices about delivery systems and decisions about staffing needs and hiring practices intended to improve patient care to Indian patients. Study findings also would assist in determining educational needs of caregivers and patients and in defining evaluative functions in ongoing quality assurance, risk management, and utilization review activities. Information generated would, therefore, be of value in planning for the future needs of the agency consistent with trends affecting nursing and health care.

The concept of differentiated nursing practice in this project employs the definition developed by the National Commission on Nursing Implementation Project, which stated that "roles and functions of nursing personnel should be based on education, experience, and competence, and nurses should be compensated accordingly" (National Commission on Nursing Implementation Project, 1989). While the ENP project attempts to differentiate nursing roles and functions, it was determined that the project should not be implemented for the purpose of altering the salary structure, and that changes in the compensation structure would be beyond the scope of the current project.

Project Implementation

Project implementation and development of the evaluation plan has been a lengthy and involved process evolving around the work of a technical advisory committee and four separate work groups. Each work group has included consumers, nurses from each project site, and other individuals and consultants with expertise in a particular area.

Staff Development Work Group

This work group met frequently before the project was implemented and focused on the need for staff education, and methods to assess the impact of implementation on nurses participating in the project. Therefore, different measures were suggested related to job satisfaction, professional awareness, recruitment and retention, and similar variables. A total of eight different monitors were developed, including separate validated instruments to measure the professional autonomy and job satisfaction of nurses participating in the project.

Basic understanding about the model and the project were also of concern since the project sites are isolated, rural, and separated by hundreds of miles. None of the project sites have organized staff development departments. Therefore, the implementation plan included development of separate independent study modules to introduce participating nurses to the differentiated practice model, and to familiarize them with care planning and the use of nursing diagnosis in relation to the model. Additionally, many nurses from the project have participated in continuing education and conferences, and several have assisted in development of an educational poster display related to the project. A logo and other materials from earlier work with differentiated nursing practice in the state have been used liberally since the beginning of ENP to provide reinforcement and assist nurses in identification with the project.

Patient Care Outcomes Work Group

Responsibilities of this work group included identification of methods to measure the impact of the model on patient care, and to resolve practice issues at the project sites. A total of 12 different monitors were proposed and are in varying stages of implementation, including separate instruments to measure patient satisfaction in both the hospital and community health settings. The number of nurse-initiated referrals was monitored, and the number of prenatal visits was established as a clinical monitor of concern to all nurses participating in the project.

Documentation of nursing care was monitored through use of a chart audit tool, with audit statements derived from the differentiated job descriptions. This activity served multiple purposes, since individual chart audit statements can be used in quality assurance activities. Risk management and utilization review items have been added to the tool. In addition, individual nurses have become more familiar with differentiated roles simply by performing retrospective chart audits using the statements included in the chart audit tool.

Patient Care Data Work Group

Activities of this work group have focused on coordinating the collection of data for staff development and patient care outcomes work groups. It is implied that data-gathering systems used in the project should be automated whenever possible. This work group's task has been facilitated by the installation of standardized computerized patient care record systems at all project sites during project implementation, thereby increasing the familiarity of all nurses participating in the project with basic computer technology and facilitating data gathering at every level.

Employee-Management Work Group

All nurses participating in ENP have volunteered to be part of the project; their continuing participation is not a condition of employment. A mechanism was needed to alter job expectations while reviewing employee and management rights and responsibilities in the federal employment system. Therefore, the work of this work group has focused on the administrative process for changing job descriptions among project volunteers, and making other adjustments in practice roles and employment status related to the project. In addition to separate job descriptions for the three levels of providers participating in the project, a model performance standard also was developed for optional use by participating staff.

Project Outcomes and Conclusion

Since this project has been in effect less than a full year, conclusions about outcomes are premature at this point. Participating nurses continue to experience indecision about role choices and struggle with fundamental barriers to implementation, including fear of change, resistance to change, lack of knowledge about the model, and difficulty in role conceptualization.

Nevertheless, it is encouraging to note that:

- Hospital nurses serving as case managers are expressing the desire to follow patients when they are discharged home. Public health nurses show interest in continuing as the case manager for hospitalized patients they have previously followed in the community.
- Nurses in general are dissatisfied with existing forms that communicate poorly across settings. Nurses are developing new tools and strategies to provide for continuity of care between providers and across settings.
- A new patient assessment format has been developed as part of the project, focusing on the functional patterns of patients rather than their medical problems. The nursing care plan, not the medical diagnosis, is becoming the basis for nurse-to-nurse communication.
- One nurse has expressed her reaction to the project as "thinking smarter, not harder."

Excellence for Nursing Practice will continue through 1991, when data gathering will conclude and a final report on the project will be developed. Regardless of the findings from each of the evaluation measures selected for use in the project, ENP has already been successful in providing opportunities for IHS nurses to become familiar with new and evolving practice models for nursing, and to participate in program development and research activities. While ease of project implementation has varied greatly from site to site, the commitment and dedication of nurses who have chosen to participate will be a factor in the continued use of various project elements, as well as their willingness to innovate in finding solutions to problems in patient care.

Today's environment and limited resources continue to create a richness of opportunity for those who are willing to look beyond yesterday's answers to the problems of tomorrow.

❏　　❏　　❏

Table 1
Excellence for Nursing Practice Project: Project Site Service Population, Hospital Beds, and Participating Nursing Staff

Location	Service Population* (1990)	Hospital Beds	Participating Nursing Staff		
			Hospital	PHN	LPN
Pine Ridge	18,454	46	12	7	7
Rapid City	5,453	30	14	0	3
Rosebud	9,782	35	13	7	4
Wagner	2,423	10	12	3	0
			Total 51	20	14

*SOURCE: Office of Health Systems Planning, Aberdeen Area Indian Health Service, Aberdeen, South Dakota.

Table 2
Excellence for Nursing Practice Project Summary

The present system as compared to the future:

- Nursing roles and nursing care are ineffectively communicated to others.
- Nurses are considered interchangeable — "a nurse is a nurse is a nurse."
- Nurses believe they are limited in autonomy and accountability.
- Nurses do not use a common language.
- There is insufficient data to demonstrate the effects of nursing care.
- Nursing is often considered a job rather than a profession.

What the project is:

A redefinition of nursing roles for two differentiated levels of RNs at participating IHS project sites in the Aberdeen area, based on the experiences, education, and background of individual nurses.

An explanation of the concept:

- Two role options for registered nurses.
- Support staff for RNs (LPNs, aides, etc.).
- Placing value on the nurse in direct patient care.
- Increased accountability and autonomy in nursing practice.
- Better utilization of present personnel.
- Planning for continuity and quality in patient care.

What is the value of the project?

- Improved patient care.
- Improved recruitment and retention of nurses.
- Increased nurse satisfaction.
- Increased patient satisfaction.
- Increased voice in the decision making of nurses in patient care.
- Cost effectiveness in patient care.
- Improved patient care outcomes.
- Improved compliance with standards of care.
- Development of the model for changes in the federal personnel system.

What is involved?

- Staff education in the use of nursing diagnoses and nursing care plans.
- A change in philosophy that changes nursing roles.
- An opportunity to participate in important professional nursing research.
- Sequential demonstration and evaluation of project components.
- Personal choices in RN role selection.
- Commitment and dedication to improvements in nursing care.
- Data collection to develop an information base for better nursing care.
- Consensus in decision making by nurses about their own practice.

Part IV

Innovation and Technology

Technology and Differentiated Levels of Decision Making

Peggy L. Primm, Ph.D., R.N.

A dvancement of technology and differentiation of nursing practice are only two of the many issues and developments that will affect the structure and process of nursing in the twenty-first century. It is relevant, therefore, to consider how development of technology will affect differentiated nursing practice and/ or whether differentiation of nursing practice will influence the incorporation of technology into nursing practice settings.

This paper will review the original Levels of Functions Model for differentiation of nursing practice and examine the implications of developing technologies for those components of practice.

Development of a framework or model for differentiation of levels of nursing practice began in the late 1970s. Primm sought to define commonly held components of nursing that could be developed into a framework for definition in the preparation and delivery of levels of nursing practice (Primm, 1978). Figures 1 through 5 illustrate the five levels of complexity of decision making that continue to be generic to the definition of differentiated, mutually valued levels of practice. The concept of fully competent, mutually valued levels of practice was germane to the useful definition of increasing complexity and avoidance of "better than" / "less than" valuing statements. Differentiation of practice in the "real world" setting of patient care demands fully competent practice at all times. Thus, practice behaviors and characteristics could not follow the traditional valuing of "less than expected," "average competence," and "exceeding expectations."

Five levels of decision making in an inclusive or Guttmann scale format comprised the original Levels of Functions Model. These five levels of decision-making complexities fully represent competent practice at that level. Each level beyond the first incorporates all the earlier levels within its structure of complexity. Thus, any level incorporates competent completion of the earlier levels as a basis for practice decisions at the most complex level.

Figures 1 through 5 illustrate the complexity of decision making as incorporated into the Client Response Documentation System (CRDS) of differentiated case management. The least complex expectation of anyone providing care for patients is that care is completed within standards of practice. Thus, this level requires definition of standards of practice and places accountability for competent practice at the level of each individual staff nurse or care provider. Further, each aspect of care provided has a concomitant set of patient response data to be collected. In differentiated case management's CRDS system, this data set is specified within the nursing order (see Figure 1). If technology were programmed, taking into account the risk parameters of the patient population, it could possibly identify emerging patient data trends. Because that level of practice incorporates the overall minimum standard that patient care screening needs, negotiations with other labor-related groups would be greatly enhanced.

The second level of complexity (see Figure 2) includes documentation of the specified data to indicate the cares completed. In differentiated case management, the structure of documentation of specified data will result in useful data trends indicating patient response to nursing care.

The third level of complexity of decision making (see Figure 3) is the comparison of the data collected to accepted or published normal parameters of patient response. When a patient's individual response is outside expected parameters of response, the nurse makes a decision to implement protocols to intervene. At this level, the parameters of safety or risk are well defined, as is the protocol to be implemented at the time. Complexity of time line is also a differentiating concept. At the third level, accountability for time management has progressed from task-to-task efficiency to across-the-shift evaluation of data trends.

Figure 4 indicates the increased complexity at level four of the decision-making model. Multiple data sets and data trends are compared to individual knowledge of the patient's responses, and thus create short-term alterations in the client's nursing care.

The fifth level of decision-making complexity (see Figure 5) indicates redesign of the patient's comprehensive nursing plan of care in order to alter his/her response to nursing care. This level of decision making implies independent nursing practice, and thus has the intent, across the length of stay, to resolve nursing diagnoses. The decision that a nursing diagnosis is resolved is based not only on the immediate assessment of patient status, but also on the data trends indicating progress toward and consistent with the mutual goal for the nursing diagnosis. These decisions can only be made if the nurse can count on fully competent care and collection of data by everyone who provides nursing care for the patient (level one). The patient response data must be accurately documented within the data trend patterns relevant to that patient (level two).

Every RN is licensed for practice at levels three and four. The delivery system already in place will structure reporting of these data trends and document the effectiveness of the nursing care implemented in response to trends.

Level five's redesign of nursing care is an ongoing expectation for the nurse planning the care across the hospital's (or other agency's) length of stay (see Figure 5).

With this definition in mind, it is clear that most technologies may assist in data collection, may document those data, and may even notify nursing personnel when data is outside the programmed parameters. At that time, the nurse intervenes to maintain or regain patient response.

Hardware or process technology may thus collect and record discrete data, but the hardware or process technology itself cannot individualize nursing care in reference to multiple, nonstandard data trends. That remains within the role of the nurse monitoring the technology. The incorporation of telemetry equipment into the practice area provides an example. The leads on the equipment collect repetitive discrete data, then program (process technology) those data trends by reports or by screen documentation. Some monitoring systems can be programmed to identify data patterns as outside the expected parameters and to notify nurses of that trend. Perhaps, then, it is possible to program a computer to respond to an identified data trend by altering occlusive pressure on a piggyback bag line by adding a specific medication to the IV line. But is it desirable to do so? Is the addition of specified medication to the IV line the essence of nursing? Does that drug administration activity mirror or replace nursing assessment and intervention? Does the continuing documentation of the data trend comprise assessment of the patient's response to that intervention?

If the role of the nurse is viewed as multiple, self-contained assessments and preplanned interventions, the above example could be accepted as a nursing process. However, the role of the nurse as defined for differentiation of practice incorporates an independent practice component not addressed above. That independent practice incorporates the patient into the planning of nursing care in order to set mutual goals for patient expenditure of resources to resolve the nursing diagnoses.

Do nurses support technology or does technology support nurses?

The setting for nursing practice includes the professional practice culture. If nursing care is defined by the need for data collection, technology may incorporate that aspect of practice, thus freeing nurses for independent nursing practice. If, on the other hand, the technology collects and documents the data, it might free the nurse by data collection.

The concept of technology in nursing and health care can mean many things:

- the sophisticated hardware developed for monitoring and treating patients,
- the process of deriving information from those hardware systems,
- nursing practice actions (protocols) developed to intervene in patient conditions, or
- patterns of care behaviors intended to result in a defined outcome for patients.

Both the intent and resource requirements of incorporating technology into the practice of nursing must be considered when deciding to invest time, space, and nursing efforts in the use of technology.

This paper will provide a model for definition of the practice role of nurses, as well as portions of the conceptual framework for differentiation, by complexity of decision making of levels of nursing practice. The Practice Role of Nurse Model can then be applied to discussions of possible implications of technology development in the future of nursing.

The purpose of this section of the conference is to review the literature and conceptual frameworks regarding the ongoing development and incorporation of technology into the practice settings and educational programs for differentiated nursing practice in the twenty-first century. We further seek to address the implications of the movement to differentiate levels of nursing practice and to incorporate technology in the future. This paper will provide a conceptual framework for differentiation of nursing practice. Further, it will synthesize, from a clinical point of view, the development of technologies currently being developed in clinical settings and challenge nurse executives and educators to take an informed proactive stand in maintenance of nursing resources prior to incorporation of technologies into the daily responsibilities of nurses.

Before incorporating technology into practice settings, most nurse managers must budget for the fiscal commitments of installation and maintenance of technology. In-servicing of staff to work with the technology is also part of the unit budget. These expenses are included in the nursing unit's cost statement addressing whether or not technology supplements, substitutes for, or expands the capability of nursing or other disciplines.

In light of shortages and the high cost of professional nursing resources, nurse managers also must consider the cost/benefit of technology to the nursing staff providing bedside care. It can no longer be assumed that technology provides a benefit of greater accuracy of data or time savings in patient care. Some technologies may be installed to format collaborative practice data already routinely monitored by nurses. Many hospitals are experiencing a time drain on the nursing staff expected to maintain or monitor technologies for other disciplines. Nurse executives must routinely include studies of cost/benefits of data to be made available and nursing time and effort required to initiate, run, monitor, maintain, and bill for the technology. Conservation of resources and a focus on efficiency of care will continue to escalate into the twenty-first century. Thus, nursing administration must include studies of resources required and resources saved or gained in the proposal to incorporate technologies into the daily cares of patients.

The cost of technological hardware is certainly a concern to educators attempting to incorporate these skills into a curriculum. The time required to teach quickly evolving technical skills within an educational program must also be balanced against the need for maintenance of more traditional content.

A common definition of nursing practice is basic to the discussion of the implications of technology for differentiated practice. This paper makes use of the Practice Model of Nursing initially developed by the Kellogg Project and developed from the Levels of Functions that illustrated complexities of decision making (Primm, 1986; Primm, 1987). This concept was further developed by Primm into the Differentiated Nursing Case Management System. This same conceptual framework is useful in structuring differentiated curricula, and is thus proposed as a means of incorporating technologies within the educational programs aimed at preparing nurses for the twenty-first century.

Three major and three minor components make up the role of the nurse within the culture of professional practice. These have been documented through the integrated system of Applied Nursing Diagnosis and Client Response Documentation System (see Figure 6).

The first major component is that of direct care. This refers to all the skills and techniques incorporated into observable nursing practice. One technology or approach to differentiation of practice is to give away "non-nursing cares" to persons such as nursing technicians or nursing assistants. If so many of the common nursing skills are moved to the assistant role, then the nurse lacks direct contact with the patient. How, then, will he/she identify and evaluate the patient's response to nursing care? If a high proportion of the direct care skills are relegated to the technician's role and a process technology is available to standardize nursing response to changes in the patient, when will the patient need a nurse? If the technician decides when a nurse needs to reenter the care process, then nursing has given away the final decisions of the nursing process.

The second major component of nursing practice is communication, including the therapeutic skills that provide a basis for communication with patients. Negotiation skills and communication of client data also fall within this component. Some delivery systems are built on standardization of cares through critical or clinical pathways. If those pathways become a technology, as defined by Jacox, that limit the independent or individualization of practice of nursing to meet patient needs, they may effectively reduce the differentiation of practice.

Where therapeutic communication intersects direct care of the patient, the component of patient teaching is identified. Technology is now available to merge patient diagnostic data with standardized teaching content or plans. This technological approach to the need for patient individualization has the potential to either free nurses from notating this information, or cause them to teach "nice to know" content at the expense of individualization of care.

The third component of nursing is management of nursing and patient resources to meet patients' goals. There are many technologies available to computerize or standardize the scheduling, monitoring of cost, utilization, and projection of future needs. If these components are considered replacements for the nurse manager role, and if case manager staff nurses manage client resources, what will the nurse manager manage?

Where negotiation intersects management of nursing care, the coordination and collaboration of nurses with other disciplines is identified. If maintenance of physiological monitoring mechanisms and recording of discrete data become the role of the nurse, how will nurses have access to data on which to base their collaborative practice decisions? [See Figure 7.]

Finally, the last component of the model intersects management of care with the provision of direct care through delegation of care within nursing. Technologies are growing to provide task lists and standardized time lines. This raises the question of how the nurse will individualize nursing care to meet the clients' nursing needs.

❑   ❑   ❑

Figure 1
Levels of Functions Model: Level One

	Documentation of client response data indicates completion of each nursing order or delegated aspect of care. Data to be collected is specified in each nursing order to the nursing care provided.			
Cares completed and data collected consistent with standards of practice.				

Figure 2
Levels of Functions Model: Level Two

	Data documented indicating completion of each nursing order or delegated aspect of care indicates client response to the nursing care provided.			
Cares completed and data collected consistent with standards of practice.	Data collected while completing cares used to document completion of care.			

Figure 3
Levels of Functions Model: Level Three

	Data sets collected within each shift become the basis of within-shift evaluation of risk or that the client's response remains within normal and expected parameters.			
Cares completed and data collected consistent with standards of practice.	Data collected while completing cares used to document completion of care.	Within-shift data trend compared to accepted parameters of client response.		

Figure 4
Levels of Functions Model: Level Four

Client response data collected during cares and documented across multiple shifts are compared to integrated knowledge of standards and parameters of risk, and individualized expected response as set forth in mutual goals.

Cares completed and data collected consistent with standards of practice.	Data collected while completing cares used to document completion of care.	Within shift data trend compared to accepted parameters of client response.	Multiple data trends evaluated against integrated knowledge and individual parameters of response.	

Figure 5
Levels of Functions Model: Level Five

Based on documented within-shift and across-shifts data, the nursing care plan is redesigned to alter the focal client's progress toward the mutual goals for resolution of nursing diagnoses.

Cares completed and data collected consistent with standards of practice.	Data collected while completing cares used to document completion of care.	Within-shift data trend compared to accepted parameters of client response.	Multiple data trends evaluated against integrated knowledge and individual parameters of response.	Nursing care redesigned to alter the focal client's response to nursing care.

Figure 6
Differentiated Case Management
Model of Nursing

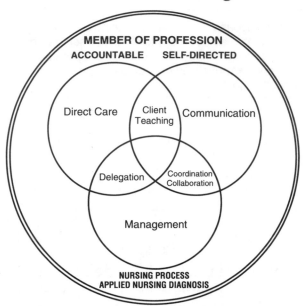

Figure 7
Nurses Supporting Technology
or Technology Supporting Nurses?

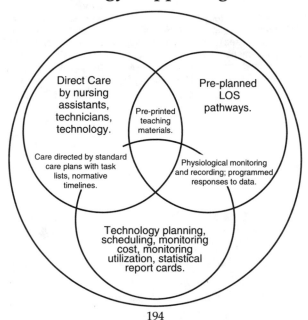

Technology and Differentiated Nursing Practice

Gail A. Harkness, Dr.PH., R.N.

T he challenge to our profession today is to both redesign nursing roles in practice settings, and to also create new nursing care delivery patterns that will move the profession forward in an age of rapidly changing health care. Increasing patient acuity in hospitals, cost containment, and limited resources are being imposed upon a high-tech/high-touch, aging society. The proliferation of sophisticated technological advances in health care, from both pathophysiological and social perspectives, is affecting the type and intensity of nursing care required and the environment in which nursing care is delivered. Within this scenario, there are new opportunities and responsibilities.

Promotion of the differentiation of nursing practice is one method of redesigning nursing roles. It is an attempt by the profession to demonstrate the effectiveness of utilizing nurses according to their education, experience, and competence (American Organization of Nurse Executives, 1990). For too long, nurses have been used interchangeably without regard to their background or preparation. As a result, individuals have not been challenged to reach their potential, and work settings have not utilized their nursing manpower resources in a cost-effective manner.

Classically, the need for change precedes change. Changes in nursing roles, delivery patterns, educational preparation, and licensure for nursing practice are long overdue. However, these changes will not occur unless the need for change, and its effectiveness, are demonstrated in the practice setting. Documentation of the effectiveness of differentiating nursing roles and functions in the practice setting will meet this need. Indeed, one of the primary difficulties in implementing the two categories of nursing practice, as envisioned by the American Nurses Association (1965), is due to the fact that the recommendation preceded the documented need for change in nursing practice.

The differentiation of nursing practice not only addresses the need for clarification of roles, but also the need for change in nursing care delivery patterns. The staff mix of nurses assuming new roles should be identified, and a delivery pattern established that will best accomplish the work to be done. It is feasible that this may vary within every institution, within every unit in a hospital, or within every caseload carried by a community agency. Only when roles are clearly defined within the framework of a flexible, dynamic care delivery system can the challenge of incorporating new technology into nursing practice be met.

Incorporating New Technology into Nursing Practice

Health care technology is already a major component of nursing practice. Technology associated with the pathophysiological condition of the patient primarily centers around mechanical devices and pharmaceuticals. These have recently been labeled technological "hardware." Devices include equipment such as infusion pumps, ostomy bags, defibrillators, arteriolines, and patient monitors. Correspondingly, advances in the procedures used in health care, in the organizational systems in which care is delivered, and in information systems and legal systems are referred to as technological "software" (Pillar, 1990).

Both technological hardware and software have a significant impact upon the patient and the nurse. The patient's pathophysiological condition is often treated by a combination of devices, drugs, or new procedures. Fear, confusion, and physical discomfort may result. Therefore, the type and intensity of nursing care must vary with each individual according to need. The nurse must interface between the patient and the hardware or software, responding appropriately to both. The consequences of making mistakes in life-threatening situations are severe and highly stressful. Often, these decisions must be made in a tense, volatile work environment.

However, technological software is also providing nurses with accurate, time-saving information systems that can individualize nursing diagnoses, create nursing care plans, monitor patient responses at the bedside, prepare workload schedules, calculate acuity indexes, and assist in the decision-making process. Nurses are already piloting hand-held terminals that scan bar-coded labels on both the nurse's badge and patient's wristband, accept vital sign data, and scan the bar-coded labels on intravenous solutions and medications. The information is then transmitted from the terminal to a base unit on the wall, and on to the central database where the information is compared with physician orders, possible drug interactions, and other data. Warning indications appear on a small screen if deviations are found (Center for Devices and Radiological Health, 1989). Advances such as these have easily been accepted into nursing practice, but whether dealing with devices, drugs, procedures, or information processing systems, significant nursing responsibility exists that has not yet been clearly established.

Recognizing the need for clarification and interpretation of nursing practice, Jacox, Pillar, and Redman (1990) have proposed that a classification of nursing technology be created. Their concept is comprehensive, including everything within the legal scope of nursing practice as well as those activities that overlap other professions. Nursing technology associated with devices and drugs would be included, along with biomedical procedures, psychosocial relationships, administrative and organizational arrangements, and health care delivery models. Coordinated with the development of the Nursing Minimum Data Set (Werley and Lang, 1988), this taxonomy would provide the framework for future development of the profession, incorporating new knowledge as it develops.

This taxonomy also would define the varying levels of knowledge and responsibility required of nurses as they interact with technology's hardware and software. It would give credibility to the nurse's role in device management. Nursing input into device design would be encouraged, as would nursing research into the outcomes of device use. Adequate documentation would support nursing's right to reimbursement for care of patients requiring device use. It is only when we have a clear vision of these responsibilities that differentiation of nursing roles regarding technology can be clarified.

But the question remains concernng how advances in technology will affect nursing practice in the future. Not only will varying levels of knowledge and responsibility be required of nurses, but nurses also will be expected to assimilate new knowledge and responsibilities into their decision-making processes. A great deal will depend upon the characteristics of the specific device, drug, procedure, or information system; their use in nursing practice could range from the simple to the complex. Some technologies will expedite the nursing process, while other types, beneficial in the medical treatment of patients, will expand and complicate nursing practice. The latter is particularly true when invasive devices are used. False alarms associated with arrhythmia monitoring (Larsen and Sherer, 1983), high rates of device-related nosocomial infections (Larsen, 1985), and mix-ups in body tubes (Hutchinson, Himes, and Davis, 1987), are just a few of the problems that complicate nursing care at present.

In the areas of decision-making complexity and accountability (Primm, in press), technology will interface at all levels, from competent task performance to redesigning nursing care to improve client response. This can be applied to models for differentiated practice. For instance, a nurse whose responsibilities are primarily to deliver direct care to patients would have several expectations to fulfill: to be competent and accountable in task performance associated with a device; to collect, report, and document data regarding the device; to assess the data against normal standards for risk; and to initiate protocols for risk situations. A nurse functioning as a case manager would evaluate individual responses associated with the device according to multiple standards, and redesign care to alter client outcomes. As nursing roles such as these are differentiated, and a taxonomy of technology that addresses the levels of knowledge that nurses require to interact with new technology develops, the nurse's role in decision making will become clearer.

Challenges for Education, Practice, and Research

The educational implications for the use of advanced technology are challenging. Overall, technology should be considered as a vehicle for enhancing nursing practice, yet it has three distinct applications: as a mechanism for the provision of direct nursing care, as a communicating mechanism, and as a manager of resources.

Technology as a Mechanism for Direct Nursing Care

Technology associated with direct care primarily involves "hardware," such as devices, drugs, and patient monitors. Devices are multiplying rapidly. It is estimated that 5-10% of the medical devices on the market today were unavailable a year ago (Center for Devices and Radiological Health, 1989). Although devices are often considered as tools associated with physician treatment of patients, it is the nurse who assesses the device according to patient outcomes.

In caring for patients with mechanical devices, nurses are obligated to understand the operation of the device, know when to use it, and be capable of interpreting results. The response of the patient, whose condition is often unstable and unpredictable, requires analysis and proper intervention. Appropriate patient adaptation to the device requires the nurse to teach patients its purpose, operation, hazards, and limitations while allaying their fears. We should be aware, however, that devices such as programmable pacemakers are becoming increasingly computerized. As a result, nurses may become more focused on data interpretation and analysis of patient outcomes in order to initiate changes in nursing care. Nurses need to understand their role, responsibility, and authority, and be accountable for the technology they employ (Lindeman, 1989). Obviously, a great deal depends upon appropriate education in the use of technology.

An expanded knowledge base regarding the principles underlying how devices function should become a part of nursing curricula. Lack of knowledge is the primary obstacle to the present integration of new technology into nursing practice. Undergraduate curricula should not only offer the foundations of physics, biochemistry, pathophysiology, and other sciences, but should also provide practical experience with medical devices. Nursing faculty should be accountable, both for teaching students how to apply scientific principles to the use of devices, and for remaining informed about their use. Interactive computerized learning programs, videotapes, and samples of devices should be available in learning laboratories. Examinations for achievement, licensure, and certification should include assessment skills associated with devices.

Abbey and Shepherd (1989) have developed a device education model intended for undergraduate, graduate, in-service, and continuing education. It is based on four levels of complexity:

1) Operational Procedures

   Clearly state the purpose of the device, followed by
   a general description of how the device accomplishes
   that purpose.

2) Fundamentals of Procedures

   Focus on the relationships between the parts of the
   device, methods for using the equipment, its effect on the
   patient, and the desired outcome. This implies understanding of the mechanisms by which mechanical devices
   interact with the patient.

3) Science and Technology

   Include the basic scientific principles, such as principles
   of physics, associated with design characteristics.

4) Systems Principles

   Provide an interactive paradigm showing the relationships between the device, nurse, patient, facility,
   and environment. This includes the ability to interpret
   the patient's cues that indicate his/her need to use,
   adjust, or discontinue use of the device.

This model clearly presents the essential knowledge and skills
associated with bioinstrumentation. From this model, criteria can be
developed for evaluating competent, safe nursing practice. Clinical
agencies should make this information (plus other educational
materials about devices) accessible in a learning resource center. To
ensure that device information is available to all nurses, the Abbey
and Shepherd model should be incorporated into the development
of a taxonomy of nursing technology, establishing a national device
information center for nursing.

In addressing the educational implications for technology as a
direct care mechanism, nursing's responsibility for research in the
field cannot be overlooked. Although innovative devices are developed by other professionals, they often become integral components of nursing practice. Nurses must be involved in the design,
development, use, clinical testing, and evaluation of these products.
The management of device-generated data, and the analysis of
device use on patients, families, and nursing staff, are very much
within the realm of nursing. Nurses at the University of Arizona
Health Science Center have designed a unique way to develop and
maintain competence in device use (Clochesy, 1987) by initiating a
task force style of introducing and supporting the use of new tech-

nology. Each task force is individually appointed, and includes an engineer, a clinical nurse specialist, and staff nurses. A variety of educational methods are used to keep nurses up-to-date on equipment, and learning resources are readily available.

Technology as a Communicator

Technology's ability to communicate is based on its software, especially information systems or computers. The potential for this technology is limited only by human ingenuity. We already have computerized nursing diagnosis, bedside charting, and bar-coded data entry and monitoring. The potential use of artificial intelligence offers exciting new possibilities for future use. Computers also can be therapeutic communicators. Patient monitors have the potential to transmit data to other computer systems for analysis. At present, however, the usefulness of patient monitors is limited by the development of sensor technology (Brimm, 1987). Finally, computers can be significant teaching tools. Interactive computer systems have proven to be excellent educational tools for patients, nurses, and students.

The educational implications require all faculty and undergraduate and graduate students to be computer-literate, with a foundation in computer knowledge that will allow adaptation to new computer technology in the future. Faculty and students should interact with computerized systems in clinical facilities. Similarly, continuing education staff in clinical facilities should be accountable for assuring that all nurses are competent users of information systems. Nurse educators also should assume the responsibility of developing interactive computer programs that address the learning needs of both patients and staff regarding the use of innovative technology.

Technology as a Manager of Resources

Another use of software is as a planner, resource allocator, and monitor of efficiency. A dynamic, sophisticated system with seven tools to help managers obtain high productivity from their staff has been developed at Piedmont Hospital in Atlanta, Georgia (Silva and Aderholdt, 1989). Actual workload is measured and productivity is monitored through an automated Kardex and care plan. The result is a reliable determination of each patient's requirement for care and the associated nursing workload. The next logical step is computer-based assignments for patient care based on nursing skill level. The educational implications for this type of technology resemble those of technology as a communicator.

While it is exciting to ponder the present and future technological advances that will affect the evolution of nursing practice, they raise some issues of concern. Karl Marx and Max Weber warned of alienation in the domain of work (Coser, 1977). As labor becomes more complex, the worker becomes increasingly alienated from the work product, losing all sense of belonging. Frustrated comments such as, "I didn't study nursing to nurse machines," indicate alienation. The trend toward participative and shared governance is an attempt to address this issue. In spite of stress and burnout, nurses may continue to practice the science of nursing, but the art of nursing may have been lost.

The depersonalization of care associated with advancing technology is disturbing. According to Naisbett (1984), every technological advance must be accompanied by a counterbalancing human response (high-tech/high-touch). Health care technology allows decreased human interaction, often creating barriers to human touch. In spite of technological advances, we need to preserve the essence of nursing — the comforting, caring presence and touch of the nurse (Henderson, 1985).

❑   ❑   ❑

The Relevance of Health Care Technology Assessment to Nursing

Barbara Barth Frink, Ph.D., R.N.

I n the past few decades, one of the greatest impacts on the quality and delivery of health care has been the interaction between technological innovation and a cost reimbursement payment system (Aaron and Schwartz, 1985; Garrison and Wilensky, 1986; Light, 1986; Roe, 1985). The health care policy shift to a prospective payment system changed the demand for information about the development, use, assessment, and evaluation of health care technology to providers and managers of health care (Finley, Young, and Morris, 1985).

Health care technology assessment is a form of policy research. In its broadest definition, it examines the consequences to patients and society of the use of medical devices and systems which would include health services research. A narrower interpretation is the evaluation of specific medical technologies and their long-term effect on society (Institute of Medicine, 1985; Steering Committee on Future Health Scenarios, 1987).

Nursing is both a consumer and provider of health care technology. Therefore, it participates in the process of technology assessment as it applies to nursing practice, organization, and delivery. In addition, nursing uses medical practice technologies in clinical

The author would like to thank J. Sanford Schwartz, M.D., Executive Director, Leonard Davis Institute of Health Economics, The Wharton School of the University of Pennsylvania, for review of this paper.

work with patients and families, and thus has a role in evaluating technologies that may be used by several disciplines.

Relevance

Multiple federal agencies are involved in health care technology assessment (Institute of Medicine, 1985). Until late 1989, health care technology assessment was sponsored and conducted by the National Center for Health Services Research and Health Care Technology Assessment (1985). Through the Omnibus Budget Reconciliation Act of 1989, the center has become the Agency for Health Care Policy and Research (AHCPR), which is responsible for health care technology assessment. Nursing is active in many aspects of the new agency's program (Lang, 1990). Another role of this new agency is to support studies on the outcomes of health care services and procedures used to prevent, diagnose, treat, and manage illness and disability (Agency for Health Care Policy and Research, 1990).

The National Center for Nursing Research (NCNR) at the National Institutes of Health (NIH) has established several priorities that support the health care technology assessment framework, such as technology dependence across the lifespan, information systems, and nursing resources and the quality of patient care. In 1988, NCNR, the American Nurses Association (ANA), and representatives from other nursing organizations participated in a conference titled, "Nursing and Technology: Moving into the Twenty-first Century," which focused on educational needs for nurses and interrelationships with other disciplines in both the public and private sectors (U.S. Department of Health and Human Services, 1989). Nursing organizations, including ANA, the American Organization of Nurse Executives, and the American Academy of Nursing, have developed goals and priorities that support the implementation and evaluation of organizational care delivery systems, including differentiated practice and comprehensive payment systems.

Nurse researchers, executives, managers, and expert clinicians have had the opportunity to add to the nursing knowledge base in the critical area of health care technology assessment. This opportunity is important for several reasons. First, evaluation of the effect of nursing information systems and nursing care delivery systems, including differentiated practice, on quality of care and patient outcomes is critical to the economic and clinical justification of nursing

204

services. Second, nursing must be able to document through research that clinical nursing interventions contribute to positive patient and/or family outcomes. Third, nursing cost methodologies must be evaluated from both payer and patient perspectives. Nursing is the major health care provider delivering both episodic and continuous patient care. There is potential for patients to be ill served from both clinical and economic perspectives if nursing does not evaluate the effect of its delivery and system technologies on processes and outcomes of care.

Health Care and Nursing Technologies

Health care technology is defined as the "drugs, devices, medical and surgical procedures used in providing health services, and the organizational and supportive systems through which health care is delivered" (National Center for Health Services Research, 1986). Based on this definition, a proposed definition of nursing technology is the devices and nursing care interventions used in providing nursing services, and the organization and supportive systems through which nursing care is delivered (Frink, 1985).

Certain aspects of technology used by nursing are shared with other disciplines, yet some are unique to nursing. Devices and interventions used by nursing are the more "tangible" and shared technologies, while nursing care delivery systems and organizational systems may be unique to nursing. This raises the issue of the health care technology assessment paradigm. The current literature is primarily focused on individual disciplines. Although I strongly advocate the appropriateness of nursing's involvement in the technology assessment process, I also believe we are remiss if we fail to consider collaborative research with other disciplines and the promotion of a patient- centered paradigm of health care technology assessment. Examples of nursing technologies used in the management of nursing care delivery and clinical practice in a tertiary care setting are presented in Table 1.

Nursing executives, managers, and clinicians plan, purchase, evaluate, and use health care and nursing technologies. However, until recently, little systematic effort has been made to identify or classify nursing technologies or to educate nursing leaders as to the applicability of technology assessment to research and evaluation of current nursing practices. In a review of nursing cost-effective analysis studies, Fagin and Jacobsen (1985) identified studies that examined organization of nursing services, tested nursing interventions, examined substitution of nurses for other providers, and tested alternative models of practice. They concluded that the weakest area was the study of organization of nursing services. Based on the evidence thus far, no conclusions about cost-effectiveness of different organizational patterns could be made. They recommended more stringent study designs, with emphasis on control of variables and the use of the most sophisticated designs for determination of cost-effectiveness analysis.

In Pillar, Jacox, and Redman's (1990) article on technology assessment, they defined the assessment methods of randomized clinical trials, cost-benefit analyses, and consensus methods. They acknowledged that nursing is only peripherally involved in technology research, and called for greater participation by nurse researchers. They concluded by suggesting some policy implications for nursing. In a second article on technology assessment in nursing, Jacox, Pillar, and Redman (1990) described the current conflict in the discipline over defining nursing's unique contribution to health care, while acknowledging the overlap with other disciplines in both practice roles and the use of technologies. The authors proposed that an appropriate taxonomy would classify nursing technologies within the domain of nursing as well as those domains that cross disciplines. They specified guidelines for the development of this taxonomy, one of which was to identify the complexity of the technology. The concept of complexity of care forms one of the major links between nursing technology and differentiated practice. What, then, is the relationship between the concept of differentiated practice and the complexity of health care technologies used in patient care?

The Process of Health Care Technology Assessment

Several descriptions of the components of the health care technology assessment process already exist. Terms frequently used to describe the process include, "feasibility," "efficacy," "effectiveness," "economic appraisal," "benefits," "risks," "costs," and "ethics" (Jennett, 1986; Riis, 1988). In 1986, Berwick presented a detailed review of the components that define the technology and the population, and examined alternative technologies in the context of neonatal intensive care technology. The review presented herein is based on the work of Berwick (1986), utilizing examples from nursing technology in tertiary care.

Defining the Technology

Clearly defining the technology to be studied is an obvious starting point in a systematic assessment. It is often difficult, however, to distinguish the boundaries between technologies.

For example, the simultaneous implementation of a new nursing patient classification system and the automation of that system is a likely occurrence. When conducting a study to determine the accuracy or reliability of the nursing patient classification system, the study outcomes related to classification would need to be clearly distinguished from the possible effects of the automation.

A second aspect of defining the technology is that of clearly defining the context in which it is studied. Is the study conducted in a controlled experimental situation, or in the "real world"? Terms used to distinguish between these two contexts are efficacy and effectiveness. The performance of a technology in experimental conditions is efficacy; performance under real world conditions is described as effectiveness. The effectiveness of a technology is almost always less than its efficacy.

The context in which a technology is assessed may have implications for interpretations related to policy — for example, the context of risk influences the policy for screening technologies. Kiely and Meister (1987) applied standards of technology assessment in a literature analysis on tests used in prenatal screening for neural tube defects. They distinguished the assessment issues of multistage testing in individual patient screening from issues of multistage testing in mass screening for neural tube defects. They identified several gaps in the literature related to assessment of multistage testing for mass screening protocols and discussed the implications of policy-mandated screening.

Defining the Population

Once the technology to be assessed is defined, it is necessary to specify the population in which the technology is to be studied. As many relevant variables as possible should be collected on the population of study, with particular attention paid to variables that may affect the outcomes under study. For example, a nursing patient classification instrument developed and validated in one setting may not be valid in another. Another example is that of identifying problems resulting from the transfer of equipment technology from the acute pediatric setting to home care (Feetham, 1986).

Alternative Technologies

Technology assessment almost always involves the measurement of the technology against some gold standard, baseline data, or a specific alternative technology. The effectiveness of a technology is assessed in the real world as marginal effectiveness (Berwick, 1986). That is, the incremental change brought about by this technology is opposed to that of an established technology.

For example, in studies evaluating the effectiveness of primary care nursing, the alternative technology was team nursing (Betz, 1981; Felton, 1975; Giovanetti, 1980; Jones, 1975; Shukla, 1981). In a review of cost-effectiveness studies in nursing, Fagin and Jacobsen (1985) reported that in each of the evaluation studies on primary nursing, there was no adequate evidence of equivalence of the experimental or surveyed nursing unit with the team nursing unit. Giovanetti (1986) supported this finding in a review of research evaluating primary nursing. She reported that nursing does not generally demonstrate the efficacy of a concept before implementation. Implications are that nursing has implemented new technologies that have greatly affected nursing practice (such as primary nursing) without demonstrating either efficacy or effectiveness.

One of the deficits of the discipline has been the lack of a standardized clinical data set for use in research, quality assurance, and evaluation. This has influenced the evaluation of nursing technologies against baseline data. Efforts to identify a minimum data set for nursing began in the 1960s, which led to the identification of a nursing minimum data set in 1985 (Werley and Lang, 1988). McCloskey (1990) proposed that standard variables be identified and controlled in nursing administration research; Cleland (1990) described data sets for projecting costs of differentiated practice. These efforts should enhance nursing's ability to evaluate technologies using baseline data.

Continuum of Technology Assessment

Every health care technology can be described by the stage of its diffusion. There are four stages on the continuum that describe the diffusion of a technology: emergent, new, established, and obsolete (Goodman, 1985). The design and methods of health care technology assessment are influenced by the stage of the diffusion.

Methods of Analysis

Depending on the nature of the assessment, both quantitative and qualitative methods are used in health care technology assessment. Each method has identified strengths and weaknesses. Quantitative methods, such as experimental and quasi-experimental studies, provide evaluative information for technology assessment that support generalization. Quantitative measurement techniques, such as receiver operating characteristic (ROC) curve analysis, Bayesian analysis, and sensitivity analysis, can be used to evaluate validity of study findings. Qualitative methods, such as consensus techniques, clinical expert judgment, and Delphi techniques, are also used in technology assessment. Literature syntheses may include both qualitative analyses and measurement techniques. Modeling techniques, such as decision analysis, decision matrices, cost-benefit analysis, cost-effectiveness analysis, and risk analysis, are all useful with regard to evaluating the effectiveness of a technology (Fagin and Jacobsen, 1985; Doubilet et al., 1985; McNeil and Pauker, 1984; Nutt, 1984; Weinstein and Fineberg, 1980).

Models provide a perspective on the future while dealing with the uncertainty of the present. They provide explication of the variables or values that may produce substantial effects in real life (Institute of Medicine, 1985). Advantages of models are that they permit identification of issues arising from a technology before application occurs, they force rationality on decision processes surrounding the technology, and they allow for testing the technology under changing conditions. Disadvantages are that models are usually developed based on aggregate data and may not be applicable to the individual clinical situation. They are helpful only to the degree that they reflect truth of the real world.

Decision matrices, the ROC curve, and Bayesian analysis are appropriately used when the efficacy of a diagnostic technology is being evaluated (Centor and Schwartz, 1985; McNeil, Keeler, and Adelstein, 1975; Swets et al., 1979). Other methods appropriate for use with emergent technologies are randomized controlled clinical trials, epidemiologic methods of cohort and case studies, and simulation modeling (Fetter et al., 1989; Fox, 1986; Goodman, 1985).

Group judgment, expert judgment, and literature syntheses are most often used with established technologies (Goodman, 1985). Nurse executives and managers may be directly involved in nursing technology assessments and the use of these methods. Minimally, they should be familiar with the techniques in order to evaluate the results of technology assessments made by interdisciplinary groups in clinical and academic settings.

Conclusions and Recommendations

Control over the environment in which nursing is practiced must include informed decision making about the nursing technology the profession purchases, designs, implements, and uses. Choices need to be made regarding the technology employed by another discipline which has a direct impact on nursing regarding resource allocation and practice patterns. The restructuring of nursing organizational arrangements and delivery patterns must be accompanied by prospective and retrospective studies that focus on the effects, costs, and risks of the delivery of care compared to established patterns. As nursing develops comprehensive payment systems for services, issues of economic incentives and professional choices regarding technologies become much more critical, as has been demonstrated in medical studies (Glaser, 1986; Luft, 1986).

Health care technology assessment provides a framework in which to guide the development of programs of nursing research that would address these critical issues. It also provides a systematic method for executives and clinicians to evaluate the stage of a health care technology and the appropriate questions to raise about the technology and its potential effect on groups of patients and society. Nurses may have a unique view of the effect of technology on patients, which should be considered in interdisciplinary collaborative research on health care technology assessment.

Suggested objectives for nursing with regard to technology assessment are:

- To identify technologies that are uniquely developed and used by nursing.
- To establish priorities for the evaluation of those technologies.

- To identify the existence of a unique nursing perspective on the effects of health care technology on patient and society outcomes.
- To define a nursing role for contributing to interdisciplinary health care technology assessment.
- To take an active part in forums where policy formation and research interact.

Health care technology assessment, rich with quantitative and qualitative investigative methods, should enhance the research programs of nursing while contributing to the evaluation of health care policy for both groups of patients and for society.

❏   ❏   ❏

Table 1
Examples of Nursing Technology in Tertiary Care

Management of Nursing Operations	Management of Clinical Practice
• Staffing and scheduling systems	• Clinical protocols
• Management information systems	• Practice patterns
• Patient classification systems	• Resources allocation
• Nursing financial systems	• Therapeutic devices
• Nursing delivery systems	• Monitoring devices

The Role of Professional Organizations in Establishing Standards of Practice and Guidelines

Joanne M. Disch, Ph.D., R.N.

Introduction

Over the past 15 years, specialty nursing organizations have actively participated in the development of standards for specialty practice. The American Nurses Association (ANA) has also invested much time and effort in the development of standards, often in conjunction with the specialty nursing organizations. Standards serve as a framework for guiding and evaluating nursing practice. Collaboration on their development and implementation is, obviously, desirable.

However, there are distinct responsibilities on the part of specialty nursing organizations and ANA in setting standards. This paper will review the responsibilities of specialty nursing organizations in establishing and promoting standards of practice and guidelines. An overview of several related specialty nursing organization projects which are currently underway will be highlighted. Finally, a few issues of concern will be raised regarding the current status and future prospects.

Specialty Organizations

Specialty nursing organizations have come a long way over the past 50 years. Early pioneers in this effort were the American College of Nurse Midwives and the Association of Operating Room Nurses. In the 1970s, many new organizations flourished. The history of specialty nursing organizations is fascinating, but certainly beyond the scope of this paper. Fortunately, researchers such as Joan Lynaugh at the University of Pennsylvania and others are tackling the topic and their efforts will yield data soon.

Currently, it is estimated that specialty organizations number more than 225,000 nurses as members, and represent between 75 and 100 special interests. Many nurses belong to more than one organization. Some organizations, however, while representing specialty interests, lack a formal structure.

Furthermore, definitions as to what constitutes a specialty nursing organization vary. Groups such as the National Intravenous Therapy Association admit non-nurse members. Certain groups which are comprised solely of nurses, such as the American Organization of Nurse Executives, do not primarily address clinical practice issues; yet some nurses would — and do — argue that the practice of management is a legitimate, specialized practice role in the broad sense. Finally, organizations such as Sigma Theta Tau are comprised of nurses, but have a very specific purpose which is not principally practice-oriented.

For the purpose of this paper, specialty nursing organizations are defined as those organizations which are comprised primarily of professional nurses, have as a primary mission the advancement of nursing practice, and address a body of knowledge and skill in a defined area of clinical practice. While it would seem that these limiting characteristics would result in groups of very narrow scope and small size, that has not always been the case. Some groups are very small, with only a few hundred members; others are quite large, like the American Association of Critical-Care Nurses, with more than 68,000 members.

For the most part, the mission of all specialty nursing organizations is to improve and advance the nursing practice of a particular group of practitioners. The expected beneficiaries of the organization's activities are certainly its members, although patients and their families are also implicitly expected to benefit.

Because of the emphasis on nursing practice which is so integral to the mission of specialty nursing organizations, they have assumed several responsibilities related to the scope of specialty practice — i.e., standards for competency in the specialty area and certification of competency. The responsibilities outlined below are those related to the establishment of standards and practice guidelines for differentiated practice.

Responsibilities

One of the primary responsibilities of specialty nursing organizations is to define specialty practice. From the definition evolves the scope of practice, standards of practice, and all other documents and activities of the specialty group. These definitions may change, as in the case of perioperative nursing. This specialty originated decades ago within the confines of the operating room and was called operating room nursing. Today, it encompasses a wide variety of settings and extends throughout many institutions, from preadmission through discharge.

The names of organizations also change. For instance, the American Association of Industrial Nurses has become the American Association of Occupational Health Nurses. The American Association of Cardiovascular Nurses was given its current name (American Association of Critical-Care Nurses) when the association's need for a broader scope was realized. [This also explains the hyphenation of "critical-care" in the name of the organization so that it would continue to fit with the acronym, AACN.]

A second major responsibility of specialty nursing organizations is to establish appropriate standards. The right and responsibility to develop standards is a critical activity, for standards define the specialty practice base. They form a cornerstone for specialty practice; shortly after incorporation, specialty nursing organizations usually develop a set of standards for nursing practice in their particular area. As mentioned earlier, many of these standards have been developed in close collaboration with ANA. In this way, they are congruent with and expand upon the generic standards of professional nursing under which all nurses practice.

In a similar vein, specialty nursing organizations are responsible for developing appropriate practice guidelines. The specialized knowledge of the practitioners is particularly helpful here. Activity in this arena will become increasingly important, especially as initiatives such as those of the Agency for Health Care Policy and Research are advanced.

Through printed materials, continuing education sessions, national meetings, and numerous other mechanisms, specialty nursing organizations disseminate information about standards and guidelines to practitioners. A major thrust of specialty nursing organizations is not only to develop standards, but also to educate their members about standards and practice guidelines and assist in implementing standards for the improvement of nursing practice. Additionally, specialty nursing organizations educate other constituencies about the existence, role, and benefits of standards — e.g., legislative bodies, lawyers, administrators, and the public.

A fifth responsibility which specialty nursing organizations have undertaken is the development of measures for judging the competency of practitioners in particular areas of practice. Once standards have been developed (whether for structure, process, or outcome purposes), a means for evaluating their attainment must be established. Through affiliated or independent certification programs, competence in the area of specialty practice can thus be reflected.

Specialty nursing organizations also conduct and fund research and clinical trials. This responsibility is consistent with the trend among all nursing groups today to support the utilization of research for the purposes of establishing a more scientific basis for nursing practice. The focus of study and funding for specialty nursing organizations is predominantly clinical practice, although some organizations do fund studies and conduct projects on related topics, such as the health care environment, ethics, and the nursing shortage.

One responsibility that has not previously been well-executed, but which promises to demand much attention, is that of developing a nursing data base. Specialty nursing organizations are generating rich data bases which will eventually contribute to a greater understanding of nurses, nursing practice, patient care outcomes, and health care issues.

Finally, a critical responsibility of the specialty nursing organizations in the development of standards and practice guidelines is to collaborate with ANA in the development of a framework which accurately represents the entire spectrum of nursing practice — a practice we all share, yet which differs from patient group to patient group. Ongoing dialogue and debate must occur so that all perspectives are represented.

The responsibilities listed above have generated a few observations:

- While most organizations have tackled *some* of these responsibilities, few have aggressively addressed them all. As individual nursing organizations evolve from infancy to maturity, they progress through organizational stages, limited at times by the resources available to them. Over time, most of the organizations strive to address all responsibilities.
- The responsibilities are shared; responsibilities of specialty nursing organizations often overlap with ANA and with each other. This requires a win-win or both/and approach to issue identification and problem resolution.

Current Programs and Initiatives

Specialty nursing organizations have aggressively pursued the development of programs and initiatives to execute their responsibilities. Their efforts are represented in a wide variety of outcomes, some of which are highlighted below.

As mentioned earlier, most groups develop a set of standards shortly after the organization is incorporated. These are often in the form of process standards, similar to ANA's *Standards of Nursing Practice* (American Nurses Association, 1973). But some groups have developed additional structure and/or outcome standards. The Oncology Nursing Society is an example of an association which developed outcome standards early in its evolution. The American Association of Critical-Care Nurses (AACN) recently published *Outcome Standards for Nursing Care of the Critically Ill* as an addition to the second edition of its *Standards for Nursing Care of the Critically Ill*.

In conjunction with the emphasis on differentiated practice, a few specialty nursing organizations have developed competency statements for differentiated practice in their particular areas. For example, in 1989, AACN published *Competence Statements for Differentiated Nursing Practice in Critical Care*, differentiating practice for the professional and associate nurse. In addition, the Oncology Nursing Society recently finished its competency statements for advanced practice in oncology nursing.

AACN and some other specialty nursing organizations have undertaken role delineation studies. Using the Delphi technique or other exhaustive survey methodologies, the purpose of these efforts is to identify critical elements of nursing practice, and to provide a basis for direction and validation of the certifying examination. In this way, the knowledge, skills, and abilities necessary for practice with a particular patient population can be identified.

The conduct and utilization of research has received increasing attention by specialty nursing organizations over the past 10 years. Today, many organizations fund studies; provide research fellowships and awards; select distinguished scholars or researchers; and share methods and findings of research studies at local, national, and international meetings. Added to these activities, AACN is sponsoring three additional projects which promise exciting results:

1) The Demonstration Unit Project, an effort funded by AACN for the past three years, which has evaluated changes in patient care outcomes over time at a site in which core AACN values and programs have been integrated.

2) The National Study Group on Suctioning, a project involving a group of senior researchers, each interested in complementary aspects of suctioning protocols, which received support money from AACN so that proposals for national funding and continuation could be developed.

3) The Thunder Project, a multihospital clinical trial being conducted through the auspices of AACN to investigate the impact of heparin in the maintenance of arterial lines and to promote clinical research (the title was suggested by a project planner who wanted the study to "stir up a little thunder in clinical settings").

Not included in this brief overview of specialty nursing organization efforts related to the development and dissemination of standards, but certainly noteworthy, are numerous other activities and projects supported by these nursing organizations to reach nurses. Comprising a major portion of specialty nursing organization efforts, these activities include the publication of journals, books, and monographs; the creation of audiovisuals and congresses, courses offered through continuing education, and symposia; collaboration with other health care providers and stakeholders in interdisciplinary projects; and the development of public service announcements which communicate nursing's responsibilities to the broader public.

Issues

Specialist Practice versus Specialty Practice

In *Nursing: A Social Policy Statement* (American Nurses Association, 1980), a specialist is defined as a nurse who meets two primary criteria:

1) an earned graduate degree (master's degree or doctorate) that represents study of scientific knowledge and supervised advanced clinical practice related to a particular area within the scope of nursing; and
2) eligibility requirements for certification through the professional society or completion of the certification process.

Many specialists belong to specialty nursing organizations; however, many do not. Conversely, the membership of most specialty organizations includes a majority of non-master's-prepared clinicians. Responsibility for the setting of practice standards must somehow be shared between the members of the relevant specialty organization and specialists in the particular field.

Role of Specialty Organizations in the Certification Process

The relationship between specialty organizations and their complementary certifying bodies is reflected by a diverse, sometimes confusing, array of structures, philosophies, and arrangements. Hopes for a national credentialing center or process stem from the belief that coordination of this issue is crucial. This situation is not unique to nursing, and certainly is not solely an issue for specialty nursing organizations, but it serves as an excellent example of the inevitable push-pull between a national, professional organization and groups with narrower, yet more defined goals and purposes. Whereas the 1980s focused on the need for collaboration between ANA and specialty nursing organizations in the development of standards, collaboration in the 1990s will be needed to resolve the credentialing issue for nursing. Hopefully, the past 10 years have taught us strategies that will serve us well in the future.

Synergism Between ANA and the Specialty Organizations

Over the past several years, impressive strides have been made in resolving disagreements and forging helpful alliances between ANA and the specialty nursing organizations. Total consensus is not the order of the day, yet what has emerged is a more realistic integration of the different roles of these organizations. Ongoing attention and efforts to understand and support the different contributions to be made by each nursing organization must be a priority for all.

Summary

Working both individually and collectively in developing and implementing standards for nursing practice, specialty nursing organizations and ANA have progressed well. A great deal has been learned in the process, and a conference such as this one speaks to the commitment and effort of many nursing leaders. Tasks for the 1990s include developing practice guidelines and forging a common agenda for certification issues. While there is certainly much that remains to be done, a good foundation has been established.

❑   ❑   ❑

Differentiated Practice:
The Competency Model

Caryle G. Hussey Wolahan, Ed.D., R.N.

Introduction

E ducational preparation for nursing practice has been an issue for the profession for many decades. History indicates that discussions in the early part of the twentieth century frequently focused on what type of education was needed to prepare a professional practitioner. These discussions continued throughout the following decades, becoming a major issue during the last 25 to 30 years.

Entry, as it has become known, has been of particular interest since 1965 when the American Nurses Association published *Educational Preparation for Nurse Practitioners and Assistants to Nurses: A Position Paper*, which called for the education of all those who are licensed to practice nursing to take place in institutions of higher education. Specifically, this position paper recommended that 1) minimum preparation for beginning professional nursing practice be baccalaureate education in nursing, and 2) minimum preparation for beginning technical practice be associate degree education in nursing (American Nurses Association, 1965).

The American Nurses Association's position on entry created considerable debate and study within the nursing community.

The outcomes of this competency model have been modified from the original outcomes which were copyrighted by and are reprinted with permission from Donna Peters, Ph.D., R.N., F.A.A.N.; and Susan Lange, M.S., R.N.; © 1979.

Some states took action to implement such a plan. The New York State Nurses Association was one of the most outspoken and visible groups to do so. Many other states began to look at the issue, although at a more relaxed pace. In 1974, the New York State Nurses Association passed a resolution requiring the bachelor's in nursing degree as a condition for registered nurse licensure by the year 1985. The "1985 Proposal," as it came to be known, brought the issue of educational preparation for nursing practice to the forefront, where it has remained to this date (New York State Nurses Association, 1985). In addition, the 1985 issue made nursing educators and nursing service administrators more cognizant of the competencies, skills, and knowledge base needed for delivery of nursing care in the complex health care delivery systems both in the United States and worldwide. Competencies and differentiated practice became issues demanding examination and action.

In 1978, the ANA House of Delegates reiterated support of its 1965 position by formally adopting a "Resolution on Identification and Titling of Establishment of Two Categories of Nursing Practice" (American Nurses Association, 1978). This resolution called for the identification and titling of two categories of nursing practice by 1980, stipulating that by 1985 minimum preparation for entry into professional nursing practice would be satisfied by the baccalaureate in nursing. The resolution also called for ANA to work with other nursing organizations to define two categories of nursing practice, and to identify national guidelines of implementation with a report to the 1980 ANA House of Delegates. North Dakota is the only state to date that has been able to formally define two categories of nursing practice; all other states continue to move toward this goal.

Entry Issue in New Jersey

New Jersey began to identify and implement two categories of nursing practice shortly after the 1965 ANA position was adopted. The New Jersey State Nurses Association Board of Directors appointed a committee on nursing education in January 1967, which was charged with developing a "blueprint for nursing education in New Jersey based on orderly transition" (New Jersey State Nurses Association, 1967). This committee presented its blueprint to the nursing community in 1968, titled *Nursing Education in Transition: A Plan for Action in New Jersey* (New Jersey State Nurses Association,

1968). However, it was not enthusiastically received, although it was well developed and included recommendations, timetables, and statistical data.

During the next 10 years, the New Jersey State Nurses Association did little work on the isue of two categories of nursing practice. From 1978 to 1982, its membership gave the New Jersey State Nurses association varied and often conflicting directions; however, by 1982, the membership voted to establish two categories of nurses and to form a task force to plan the timely implementation of the position (New Jersey State Nurses Association, 1982).

The task force, led by Drs. Caryle G. Hussey Wolahan, Donna Peters, and Theresa Valiga, began its work in 1983 by examining a number of documents related to the issues of levels of practice and competencies. The task force believed that before nurses could be expected to practice differently, be licensed differently, and be educated differently, the differences or distinctions separating the professional nurse from the associate nurse needed to be clearly defined in a manner that was understandable and meaningful. Work by a 1978-1979 New Jersey State Nurses Association committee on utilization was most helpful to the task force in this regard.

This committee had combined the ANA *Standards of Nursing Practice* (American Nurses Association, 1973) with the nature of the setting in which care was delivered to provide a framework for defining the competencies of the associate and the professional nurse (see Appendix 1). The task force used this work as its basis to develop the Competency Model, a practice-based model.

ANA Standards

The debate surrounding the entry into practice issue, when focused solely on the education aspect, is meaningless if not translated into the practice setting. Since nursing practice in all settings needs to be guided by some standard, and since ANA has clarified such standards, it was obvious to the task force that these standards should be used as part of the framework in developing two categories of nursing practice.

An assumption was made that all nurses would be familiar with the standards of practice and, therefore, would hold in common certain expectations of nursing practice that would serve as a basis for the model. Those using the model would not need to learn a new language. The *Standards of Nursing Practice* are so closely related to the nursing process that they have become virtually second nature to most practicing nurses (American Nurses Association, 1980).

The Practice Setting

As nurses providing care in various settings implement the ANA *Standards of Nursing Practice*, they are moving toward different goals and different outcomes. By articulating these outcomes, greater understanding can be achieved about who can best meet the identified goals. The practice setting, however, is difficult to define since it can be anywhere that nurses practice: acute care, community health, schools, businesses, independent practices, long-term care, and many other settings. For the purpose of the model, the New Jersey State Nurses Association task force decided to incorporate the terms "distributive" and "episodic" as used by Jerome Lysaught (1970). The task force believed these terms provided enough flexibility to include all settings in which nursing is practiced.

The role of the associate nurse in the distributive care setting and the role of the professional nurse in the episodic care setting can be clarified. The question of appropriate roles in these two settings often arises when the issue of two categories of nursing practice is raised. Therefore, defining the nature of the practice setting helps us achieve a greater understanding of client outcomes and specific nursing roles.

Competencies

During the past 15–20 years, a great deal of effort has been directed toward specifying the distinct competencies of the associate (or technical) nurse and the professional nurse. The National League for Nursing (NLN) organized numerous committees and task groups to identify these differences and has published many documents regarding competencies and/or characteristics (National League for Nursing, 1987; National League for Nursing, 1989). Currently, NLN is reviewing its work on competencies to determine if what exists is still applicable to the 1990s and, looking even further ahead, to the beginning of the twenty-first century.

Many nursing faculty, particularly those in "ladder programs," debated the differences between the graduates of the associate degree and baccalaureate programs. Some faculty groups accepted the NLN documents without refinement; other faculty groups modified existing statements of competencies to suit their own needs and remain consistent with their own stated beliefs. Still other faculty groups developed totally new statements of competencies. In addition to NLN and nursing faculties, secondary groups were formed or refocused to study the issue of competency levels, including, state nurses associations, state education departments, independent research groups sponsored by the federal government and private funding agencies, the National Commission on Nursing Implementation Project, and ANA.

The 1979 ANA Task Force on Entry into Practice Competency Work Group was established to delineate entry level competencies for the two categories of nurses who will enter nursing in the future. The group addressed competencies of nurses in the roles of:

- provider of client care,
- manager of client care,
- client teacher,
- communicator,
- investigator, and
- participant in the discipline of nursing.

This work group specified that:

Differentiation of the two categories should take into account the nature and amount of knowledge which can be incorporated into the respective curricula of each type, and from this, differences in focus of care, in the kinds of settings in which care is given, in practice roles and in accountability, can be derived (Commission on Nursing Education, 1978).

The New Jersey State Nurses Association task force believed it was essential to differentiate the competencies of the associate nurse and the professional nurse. To do so, they developed the Competency Model, which incorporates practice standards and practice settings, making the model practice-based. Without such a distinction, the expectation of nurses in practice, the focus of new licensing exams, and the legal descriptions of nursing in new nursing practice acts cannot be clarified.

The Competency Model

The Competency Model interrelates 1) the eight ANA standards of nursing practice, 2) the nature of the setting in which nursing care is delivered (i.e., distributive or episodic), 3) client outcomes, and 4) specific activities or competencies of the associate nurse and the professional nurse. This model has been shared with many groups and nursing leaders throughout New Jersey, has been redefined based on input from nurses in educational and practice settings, and has been validated for content.

Despite the extensive work related to differences in responsibilities and competencies between nurses prepared in baccalaureate programs and those prepared in associate degree programs, most health care institutions that employ nurses have not incorporated such distinctions in job expectations for staff nurses. These institutions continue the traditional practice of having all registered nurses function in the same manner and with the same degree of responsibility, regardless of their educational preparation; thus perpetuating the stereotype that "a nurse is a nurse is a nurse."

Given 1) the increased support for two distinct levels of nursing practice, 2) the progress made in articulating the distinctions between these two levels of practice (see Appendix 2), 3) the lack of utilization of such a model in the delivery of nursing services, and 4) the lack of documentation regarding how such a delivery system works in practice settings, the time has come to implement and evaluate such a nursing care delivery system. Based on the Competency Model presented herein, such a demonstration project has been developed, but funds for implementation have yet to be obtained (see Appendix 3).

It is the belief of the members of the task force who developed this Competency Model and its related demonstration project that differentiating practice based on 1) the ANA *Standards of Nursing Practice*, 2) the nature of the setting in which nursing care is delivered, 3) client outcomes, and 4) specific activities or competencies of the associate (technical) nurse and the professional nurse are the best means by which nursing practice can move into the twenty-first century.

❏   ❏   ❏

Appendix 1

American Nurses Association's Standards of Nursing Practice

Standard 1 — The collection of data about the health status of the client/patient is systematic and continuous. The data are accessible, communicated and recorded.

	SPECIFIC NURSING OUTCOMES*		NURSE COMPETENCIES TO ACHIEVE OUTCOMES	
	DISTRIBUTIVE CARE SETTING	EPISODIC CARE SETTING	ASSOCIATE NURSE	PROFESSIONAL NURSE
PRIMARY CARE FOCUS	An accessible, systematic assessment of the client system's health status with identified potential risk factors is documented.	An accessible, systematic data base, including the biopsychosocial aspects of the client system and the suprasystem influencing and/or affecting the client, is documented.	Collects data from the client system and other health care personnel using established tools. Focuses data collection on the client system's presenting problem(s).	Integrates data from the client system to which the client system is linked (e.g., work, church, neighborhood). Focuses data collection on the client system's past and presenting problem(s) and their potential for an enhanced level of health.
SECONDARY CARE FOCUS	An accessible, systematic assessment of the client system's health status and level of adaptation is documented.	An accessible, systematic assessment of the client system's initial compromised health status and the progression of that status is documented.	Communicates data to the professional nurse and on the client system's record. Contributes to the nursing data base and the identification of the client system's immediate nursing care needs on a continuous/ongoing basis. Obtains data through interview, observation, and written records.	Obtains data through health assessment interview, written records, literature search (e.g., research findings), case studies, and research methods. Modifies existing data collection tools or designs data collection tools to be appropriate to the individual client system's situation.
TERTIARY CARE FOCUS	An accessible, systematic and periodic assessment of the client system's modified health status is documented.	An accessible, systematic and periodic assessment of the client system's health status is documented.		

*The nature of Standards 1-4 necessitates that these be *nursing* outcomes, not client outcomes.

Appendix 1 — cont'd

Standard 1 (Cont'd)

	SPECIFIC NURSING OUTCOMES		NURSE COMPETENCIES TO ACHIEVE OUTCOMES	
	DISTRIBUTIVE CARE SETTING	EPISODIC CARE SETTING	ASSOCIATE NURSE	PROFESSIONAL NURSE
PRIMARY CARE FOCUS				Utilizes data collected about the client system's health status to formulate an individualized plan of nursing care.
SECONDARY CARE FOCUS				Communicates data collected to the client system, the nursing team, other health team personnel, and on the client system's record.
TERTIARY CARE FOCUS				

Appendix 1 — cont'd

Standard 2 — Nursing diagnoses are derived from health status data.

	SPECIFIC NURSING OUTCOMES		NURSE COMPETENCIES TO ACHIEVE OUTCOMES	
	DISTRIBUTIVE CARE SETTING	**EPISODIC CARE SETTING**	**ASSOCIATE NURSE**	**PROFESSIONAL NURSE**
PRIMARY CARE FOCUS	The client system's identified potential health risks are reflected by a documented nursing diagnosis.	The client system's risks or potential health risks are reflected by documented nursing diagnoses.	Contributes to the formulation of nursing diagnoses by identifying the client system's needs and problems, based on standard protocols and accepted lists of nursing diagnoses.	Includes the problem and its etiology in formulating individualized nursing diagnoses based on a synthesis of knowledge from nursing, the physical and behavioral sciences, and the humanities.
SECONDARY CARE FOCUS	The client system's identified health problems and adaptation to those health problems are reflected by a documented nursing diagnosis.	The client system's changing health problems are reflected by documented nursing diagnoses.		Analyzes the health status and health potential of the client system in establishing individualized nursing diagnoses.
TERTIARY CARE FOCUS	The client system's modified health status is reflected by a documented nursing diagnosis.	The client system's diminished or altered level of functioning is reflected by documented nursing diagnoses.		Contributes to the body of nursing knowledge by formulating and refining nursing diagnoses which may or may not be on standardized lists.

Appendix 1 — cont'd

Standard 3 — The plan of nursing care includes goals derived from the nursing diagnoses.

	SPECIFIC NURSING OUTCOMES		NURSE COMPETENCIES TO ACHIEVE OUTCOMES	
	DISTRIBUTIVE CARE SETTING	**EPISODIC CARE SETTING**	**ASSOCIATE NURSE**	**PROFESSIONAL NURSE**
PRIMARY CARE FOCUS	The client system's documented goals reflect a plan for minimizing or eliminating identified potential health risks.	The client system's documented goals reflect a plan for minimizing or eliminating defined health risks.	Collaborates with the professional nurse to establish client system goals for each nursing diagnosis. Contributes to the updating and refinement of client system goals based on continuous/ongoing data collection.	Collaborates with the client system, the nursing team, and other health care personnel to formulate short-term and long-range client system goals for each nursing diagnosis. States goals in measureable client system behaviors with assigned time periods for achievement of each goal.
SECONDARY CARE FOCUS	The client system's documented goals reflect a plan for reducing identified health problems.	The client system's documented goals reflect a plan for reducing defined health problems.		
TERTIARY CARE FOCUS	The client system's documented goals reflect a plan for altering the client's compromised health status.	The client system's documented goals reflect a plan for altering the client's compromised level of functioning.		

Appendix 1 — cont'd

Standard 4 — The plan of nursing care includes the priorities and the prescribed nursing approaches or measures to achieve the goals derived from the nursing diagnoses.

	SPECIFIC NURSING OUTCOMES		NURSE COMPETENCIES TO ACHIEVE OUTCOMES	
	DISTRIBUTIVE CARE SETTING	EPISODIC CARE SETTING	ASSOCIATE NURSE	PROFESSIONAL NURSE
PRIMARY CARE FOCUS	The development of the client system's problems is prevented through prioritized nursing interventions.	The client system's defined health risks are reduced or eliminated through prioritized nursing interventions.	Formulates nursing interventions for each client system goal based on established protocols. Implements the plan of nursing care based on knowledge of established nursing practices/protocols.	Utilizes current nursing theory as a basis for designing nursing care and nursing practice/decisions. Collaborates with the client system in identifying priorities of care.
SECONDARY CARE FOCUS	Restoration of the client system to prior health status and/or maintenance of the client system's optimal health status is achieved through prioritized nursing interventions.	The client system's defined health problems are resolved through prioritized nursing interventions.		Utilizes multifaceted approaches in meeting the client system's individual needs and achieving the short-term and long-range goals derived from the nursing diagnoses. Formulates nursing interventions for the accomplishment of each client system goal.
TERTIARY CARE FOCUS	The client system's optimal level of health and independence are maintained through prioritized nursing interventions.	Modification of the client system's altered level of functioning and/or maximization of the client system's health potential are achieved through prioritized nursing interventions.		Bases proposed nursing interventions on nursing research findings. Documents an individualized plan of nursing care for the client system. Interprets the plan of nursing care to all members of the health care team.

231

Appendix 1 — cont'd

Standard 5 — Nursing actions provide for client/patient participation and health promotion.

	SPECIFIC NURSING OUTCOMES		NURSE COMPETENCIES TO ACHIEVE OUTCOMES	
	DISTRIBUTIVE CARE SETTING	EPISODIC CARE SETTING	ASSOCIATE NURSE	PROFESSIONAL NURSE
PRIMARY CARE FOCUS	The client system identifies available community resources for health promotion.	The client system identifies its general health status.	Involves the client system in his/her own care according to the specified plan of nursing care.	Assesses the client system's level of ability to participate in his/her own care.
SECONDARY CARE FOCUS	The client system utilizes appropriate community health resources to monitor changes in health status.	The client system participates in the development and implementation of health care.	Carries out individual teaching plans prescribed by the professional nurse in collaboration with the client system to maintain or improve his/her present state of health.	Consults with the client system prior to formulating short-term and long-range goals and prior to planning nursing care.
TERTIARY CARE FOCUS	The client system maintains current health status by utilizing appropriate community health resources.	The client system participates in health restoration modalities and actively complies with the health care regime.	Collaborates with the client system in his/her attempts to participate in his/her own care. Communicates to the professional nurse and in the client system's record the progress of the client system in participating in his/her own care.	Designs teaching plans in collaboration with the client system that help the client system promote, maintain and restore his/her health. Keeps the client system informed of the progress of his/her health status, or refers him/her to appropriate sources for assistance. Acts as a consultant to the client system as he/she attempts to care for self as much as possible. Teaches the client system strategies for health promotion, maintenance, and restoration.

Appendix 1 — cont'd

Standard 5 (Cont'd)

SPECIFIC NURSING OUTCOMES			NURSE COMPETENCIES TO ACHIEVE OUTCOMES	
	DISTRIBUTIVE CARE SETTING	EPISODIC CARE SETTING	ASSOCIATE NURSE	PROFESSIONAL NURSE
PRIMARY CARE FOCUS				Communicates to the client system, the nursing team, other health team personnel, and on the client system's record the progress of the client system in participating in and managing his/her own care.
SECONDARY CARE FOCUS				
TERTIARY CARE FOCUS				

Standard 6 — Nursing actions assist the client/patient to maximize his health capabilities.

	SPECIFIC NURSING OUTCOMES		NURSE COMPETENCIES TO ACHIEVE OUTCOMES	
	DISTRIBUTIVE CARE SETTING	EPISODIC CARE SETTING	ASSOCIATE NURSE	PROFESSIONAL NURSE
PRIMARY CARE FOCUS	The client system demonstrates a knowledge of healthful behaviors and maintains a safe environment.	The client system identifies optimal health status.	Focuses on the strengths of the client system when providing nursing care.	Guides the client system, the nursing team, and other health team personnel in focusing on the client system when providing care.
SECONDARY CARE FOCUS	The client system integrates health information and data to maintain health status.	The client system progresses to an improved level of health.	Supports the client system's decisions that maximize his/her health capabilities.	Assists the client system in making decisions that would maximize his/her health capabilities.
TERTIARY CARE FOCUS	The client system manages health problems through utilization of appropriate nursing interventions.	The client system complies with the health care regime.	Carries out prescribed individual teaching plans to help the client system stay in the best possible state of health.	Collaborates with the client system in making decisions that would maximize his/her health capabilities.

234

Appendix 1 — cont'd

Standard 7 — The client's/patient's progress or lack of progress toward goal achievement is determined by the client/patient and the nurse.

| SPECIFIC NURSING OUTCOMES | | NURSE COMPETENCIES TO ACHIEVE OUTCOMES | |
DISTRIBUTIVE CARE SETTING	EPISODIC CARE SETTING	ASSOCIATE NURSE	PROFESSIONAL NURSE
PRIMARY CARE FOCUS — The client system demonstrates a degree of achievement toward elimination of identified potential health risks.	The client system demonstrates a degree of achievement toward elimination of identified and/or potential health risks.	Uses criteria established with the professional nurse to evaluate the effectiveness of nursing interventions.	Designs evaluation strategies to determine client system progress toward short-term and long-range goals.
SECONDARY CARE FOCUS — The client system demonstrates a degree of achievement toward elimination of identified health problems.	The client system demonstrates a degree of achievement toward elimination of identified health problems.	Gathers data for the evaluation of nursing care. Participates in the evaluation of goal achievement by communicating to the professional nurse and on the client system's record observations made regarding the client system's progress.	Plans for the involvement of the client system in evaluating his/her progress toward goal achievement. Determines how data obtained from an ongoing evaluation of the client system's progress toward goal achievement will be utilized.
TERTIARY CARE FOCUS — The client system manages his/her health care problems.	The client system manages his/her health care problems.		Coordinates the data and persons involved in the evaluation process. Communicates to the client system, the nursing team, other health team personnel, and on the client system's record the client system's progress toward achievement of short-term and long-range goals.

235

Appendix 1 — cont'd

Standard 8 — The client's/patient's progress or lack of progress toward goal achievement directs reassessment, reordering of priorities, new goal setting, and revision of the plan of nursing care.

	SPECIFIC NURSING OUTCOMES		NURSE COMPETENCIES TO ACHIEVE OUTCOMES	
	DISTRIBUTIVE CARE SETTING	EPISODIC CARE SETTING	ASSOCIATE NURSE	PROFESSIONAL NURSE
PRIMARY CARE FOCUS	The client system's degree of progress toward elimination of identified potential health risks determines the community's future health needs.	The client system's progress toward elimination of actual and/or potential health risks determines the future health needs.	Contributes to the revision of the plan of nursing care as needed by collecting data regarding the client system's progress toward goal achievement.	Plans for the involvement of the client system in designing an approach to the ongoing evaluation and revision (as necessary) of the plan of nursing care.
SECONDARY CARE FOCUS	The client system's degree of progress toward elimination of identified health problems determines the revision and implementation of the plan of care.	The client system's degree of progress toward elimination of identified health problems determines the revision and implementation of the plan of care.		Collaborates with the client system to reorder priorities, set new goals, and revise the plan of nursing care based on the data collected regarding the client system's progress toward the achievement of short-term and long-range goals.
TERTIARY CARE FOCUS	The client system's degree of progress in managing health problems determines the revision and implementation of the plan of care.	The client system's degree of progress in managing health problems determines the revision and implementation of the plan of care.		Communicates the revised plan of nursing care to the client system, the nursing team, other health team personnel, and in the client system's record.

Appendix 2
Summary of Differences in Levels of Practice

VARIABLE	ASSOCIATE NURSE	PROFESSIONAL NURSE
Care Setting	• Secondary	• Primary • Secondary • Tertiary
Problems Addressed	• Common • Well-defined • Psysiolog-Illness-Focused	• Screening • Psychosocial • Networking in health care system • New
Client Population	• Individuals in the system with prescribed regimens	• Groups/families/communities as whole or as individuals entering the system
Setting/Context	• Institutions • Structured • In the mainstream	• Developing or nonexistent/role • Unstructured
Interventions Used	• Common • Predictable • Recurrent • Established protocols	• New • Untried • Speculative
Characteristics	• Semi-independent • Informed follower • Data gather • Decision maker (on a limited scope) • Member of nursing team	• Independent • Self-directed • Risk taker • Critiquer • Predictor • Analyzer • Decision maker (on a broad scope) • Developed member of broader health care team
Nursing Process	• Assess with guidance • Have input to the plan • Carry out care • Have input to evaluation—teacher	• Perform total assessment plan care • Carry out care • Evaluate—outlines teaching plan and teaches
Focus of Concern	• Quality of care in *own* practice and setting • Identification of problem areas in nursing practice	• Quality of health care in general contributes to nursing science • Investigate nursing problems

Appendix 3
Two Levels of Nursing Practice: A Demonstration Project

Abstract

This proposal sets forth a demonstration project designed to ascertain the advantages and problems associated with the provision of nursing care according to a new care delivery structure. The new model calls for all nursing care to be delivered by graduates of associate degree and baccalaureate nursing programs, each of whom assumes responsibility commensurate with his or her educational preparation. The basis for this care delivery structure is the Competency Model developed by the New Jersey State Nurses Association, which is based on the American Nurses Association's *Standards of Nursing Practice.*

The existing nursing care structure fails to utilize nurses according to the competencies for which they were educated. Thus, utilizing nurses prepared at the associate level rather than those professionally prepared at the baccalaureate level for patient care that requires complex decision-making skills and judgment may jeopardize rapid recovery free of complications. Such mismanagement could result in longer hospital stays involving additional costly services and supplies. Misutilization or under-utilization of nurses also is likely to contribute to their role dissatisfaction and the subsequent loss of qualified nurses from the profession.

The proposed demonstration project spans a 30-month period of time and includes 1) the establishment of a demonstration medicalsurgical unit in an acute care facility in New Jersey; 2) the full implementation of a care delivery model on that unit 24 hours-a-day, seven days-a-week for a minimum of 18 months; 3) the ongoing and final evaluation of the advantages and problems associated with the demonstration unit care delivery model; and 4) the preparation of a written report about the project.

Appendix 4
Definitions

Associate Nurse	That nurse prepared in an associate degree nursing program.
Client System	A term that can refer to the client, the client's family, and/or the client's significant other(s).
Competency	A cognitive, psychomotor, and/or affective ability derived from the present and evolving roles of nursing in the health care system that implies integration of performance behavior.
Distributive Care	That area of concentration in nursing practice which emphasizes prevention of disease and maintenance of health and is largely directed toward continuous care of persons not confined to health care institutions.
Episodic Care	That area of concentration in nursing practice which emphasizes the curative and restorative aspect of nursing and which usually involves patients with diagnosed disease, either acute or chronic.
Primary Care Focus	Includes generalized health promotion as well as specific protection against disease. Is comprised of 1) health promotion: activities directed toward *sustaining* or *increasing* the level of well-being, self-actualization, and personal fulfillment of a given individual or group; and 2) primary prevention: activities directed toward *decreasing* the probability of encountering illness, including active protection of the body against unnecessary stressors.
Professional	That nurse prepared in a baccalaureate nursing program.
Secondary Care Focus	An emphasis on early diagnosis and prompt intervention to halt the pathologic process, thereby shortening its duration and severity and enabling the individual to regain normal functions at the earliest possible point.
Structured Setting	A practice setting in which definite lines of communication and patterns of organization exist, collaboration and supervision are readily available, roles and functions are relatively constant, and care is adapted to the needs of the individual.
Tertiary Care Focus	An emphasis on a defect or disability that is fixed, stabilized, or irreversible. Rehabilitation, the goal of tertiary prevention, involves halting the disease process itself — it is the restoration of the individual to an optimum level of functioning within the constraints of the disability.
Unstructured Setting	A practice setting in which collaboration and supervision are less available, there is greater opportunity to practice independently, roles and functions vary, and care is adapted to the environment as well as to the individual. In such settings, consumers have more control over their health care and their environment. There are more variables to be managed.

Part V

Projecting the Costs
of Differentiated Practice

A Differentiated Pay Structure Model for Nursing

Virginia Cleland, Ph.D, F.A.A.N.

The Problem

I t was well documented by Aiken (1987), Inglehart (1987), and
Buerhaus (1987) that constraints on increases in nurses' salaries
in response to the greatly increased demand for nurses directly
resulted in a shortage of nurses. The managers of nurse compensation, faced with prospective salary limitations, prevented a normal market response to the greatly expanded demand for nurses in
new roles both outside and within hospitals. This had an economically predictable effect. Salary controls decreased the number of
nurses willing to work for the wages and working conditions which
hospitals offered.

While improvements in entry-level salaries have supposedly
eased the shortage, the American Hospital Association's most recent
survey (April 1989 data) showed a 12.66% vacancy rate, the highest
since 1986 (Study Sees RNs Still Gripped by Pay Compression,
1990). It is obvious that simply raising entry-level salaries is a costly
and inadequate approach to the problem.

Equating Nurses' Preparation

While the pay level of nurses has been examined in many
professional and trade surveys, limitations placed on nursing's pay

structure — that is, the relationship of nursing positions — has been just as harmful. A common institutional goal was to avoid increased salary costs associated with baccalaureate-prepared nurses. This policy initially worked well to limit nursing costs, but now it is increasing costs. In San Francisco, an associate nurse without any nursing experience can begin at $43,000. In no other occupation is the associate-degree graduate compensated at this level.

This costly practice can be corrected by redefining job descriptions and practice expectations according to the level of preparation. A draftsman is not paid the same as an architect; an associate engineer is not paid the same as a professional engineer; a laboratory technician is not paid the same salary as a medical technologist. In 1983, the National Commission on Nursing recommended that, "Salaries and benefits for nurses should be commensurate with their level of responsibility, preparation, experience, and performance" (National Commission on Nursing, 1983). This recommendation was reiterated in the *Final Report* of the Secretary's Commission on Nursing (1988).

Licensure as a registered nurse is a minimal standard to protect the public welfare. It is only one prerequisite for employment in any particular nursing position. Licensure of nurses provides the citizenry of a state with considerable protection, but it is inappropriate to use licensure to achieve professional goals. Medical staffs evaluate the training and skills of physicians currently licensed in the state and desiring to practice in a particular setting. Likewise, nursing staffs can evaluate the education and practice competencies of nurses licensed by the state and desiring to practice in a particular facility.

Growth of Part-Time Nursing

Nursing's splendid record of over 80% labor force participation (Schoen and Schoen, 1985; Division of Nursing, Health Resources and Services Administration, 1988) is offset by the excess use of part-time employment. In a small study of part-time nursing in five counties in western Michigan, Cleland found that only 50.7% of the nurses who worked part-time had children under 18 years of age. Another random survey in California of 115 part-time nurses found that only 32% had any children under 18 years and only 24% had children under five years of age (Cleland, Quinn, and Eggert, 1988).

The stereotype of the part-time nurse with young toddlers is simply not true. In truth, most nurses work part-time to avoid the pressures of working unwanted hours. Prescott (1986) clearly documented that agency nurses providing supplemental nursing services are the same nurses formerly employed in hospital positions.

If staff nurses use part-time employment to control work schedules, it is necessary to examine shift differentials. In contrast to the practice of American hospitals paying $1 to $2 per hour for shift differentials (Mattera, 1987), hospitals in the Netherlands pay a 20% differential on Monday–Friday evenings; a 30% differential on Saturday days and evenings; a 40% differential on Monday–Saturday nights; and, finally, a 45% differential on Sundays, holidays, Christmas Eve, and New Year's Eve (Department of Social Services and Labor, 1984). Shift differentials in American hospitals simply have not been adequate.

Clinical Ladders and Salary Compression

Another longstanding employment problem in hospital nursing has been the lack of recognition of experience and performance levels in the nursing pay structure. This includes experience gained in both previous employment and in the present setting. It is rare to find a hospital where the expert nurse is paid more for her expertise than the beginner when both are new hires for the same position. When pay differences do occur, they are more likely to be based on longevity. Instead of receiving a higher salary, a capable nurse is expected to support and offset limitations in the services of the incompetent. The proficient nurse may be assigned to evenings or nights because another nurse is not able to handle the responsibilities. Nurses in a tight job market are sometimes discharged for insubordination, but rarely for incompetence.

In the American Hospital Association's nursing personnel survey of March 1981, several questions were devoted to determining the position levels and salary differentials for clinical (nonmanagement) positions (Beyers et al., 1983). In a 20% national random sample of about 1,200 hospitals (59.9% response rate), data indicated that 48.2% of hospitals had one clinical level and no promotion plan; 22.5% had two levels; 17% had three levels; and 12.3% had more than three levels. Criteria for differentiating levels included experience, level of responsibility, clinical activities, and education

(American Nurses Association, 1984). With two levels, the RN achieving the higher level could anticipate a maximum increase of $.68 per hour; with four levels, the maximum increase was $2.27 (or $.75 per hour per level). One can conclude, therefore, that in most hospitals, economic incentives for climbing a clinical ladder have been minimal.

In a survey conducted by Hay Management Consultants (Study Sees RNs Still Gripped by Pay Compression, 1990) of 370 hospitals employing nearly 90,000 registered nurses, particular attention was directed at the four levels of nursing personnel. The survey defined level 1 as the novice or RN recently returned to practice; level 2 as a fully competent staff nurse; level 3 as a nurse practitioner and/or nurse clinician; and level 4 as a clinical nurse specialist. Hay Management Consultants reported that shortage pressures had driven level 1 salaries to a new high of $27,800; level 2 nurses were earning $29,500; level 3 nurses were earning $32,000; and level 4 nurses were earning $32,500. These data indicate that recent pressures on nursing salaries have had no effect on the traditional compression and, in fact, may have made it worse.

The Rationale for Pay Structure Changes

Goals

The Differentiated Pay Structure Model has been developed to achieve several goals:

- to make professional nursing a more attractive career choice in order to maintain an adequate supply of nurses (recruitment),
- to increase the average weekly hours worked by the individual nurse (productivity),
- to separate the major roles and employment expectations for professional and associate nurses employed in hospitals (staff mix), and
- to maintain budget neutrality (cost management).

Pay level is a market issue and varies by region of the country. To resolve the problem relating to pay structure, the relationships between nursing positions must first be clarified. This is a problem relating to pay structure.

The Work Force of Nursing

The categorization of nurses can most easily be portrayed with a diagram of concentric circles [see Figure 1] (Cleland, 1978). If the model is viewed in cross section, it forms a cone with the profession at the top. The nursing profession (center space) is composed of registered nurses possessing a baccalaureate or higher degree with a major in nursing. The academic emphasis is stressed because the actual nursing degrees may have different names, but upper division nursing knowledge is essential in order to be a professional. Professional nurses would include most members of job categories such as practitioners, clinical nurse specialists, educators, researchers, consultants, administrators, etc. A large number of them would have master's or doctoral degrees.

The occupation of nursing (center and middle spaces) includes all professional nurses plus registered nurses prepared in associate degree and diploma programs, as well as licensed practical nurses (LPNs or LVNs).

The work force of nursing (all three spaces) includes professional nurses, associate nurses, and licensed practical nurses, plus assistive personnel who are not registered and who are most commonly trained on the job by the institutions employing them, such as nurse assistants, technicians, and orderlies. Unit clerks and other clerical personnel are not part of the work force of nursing since they do not provide direct care to clients or patients, although they are essential employees of nursing departments.

The outer border of the diagram is indicated by a broken, semipermeable line to indicate that individuals are able to move rather freely in and out of nursing employment at the assistive level. The other two circles are drawn with continuous lines because licensure and professional regulations have defined these groups.

Nursing's educational model, based on approximately two, four, six, or eight years of education, requires additional formal education to move to the next level (see Table 1). It must be made be clear that each educational route prepares the nursing student for a different level of nursing practice. With practice level and salary distinctions, it will be possible for individual nurses to select the most cost-effective route by which to pursue his or her own career goals and to add advanced educational preparation as appropriate.

Pay Structure of Hospital Nurses

The employment models used for nursing in many health service institutions violate important principles upon which salaries should be based. The end result is that nurses' salaries show great compression at the clinical levels, creating little economic incentive for the development of advanced skills and competencies (Lewis, 1984; Mattera, 1987; New Salary Wars Promise Solid Gains This Year, 1988). Yet it is nurses with advanced skills whom institutions find in particularly short supply.

Wage and salary administration within nursing departments needs to be modified to provide individual nurses with sufficient economic incentive to invest in their own preparation. Such investment involves both direct costs of advanced schooling and the expenses of income lost while one is in school. The common practice of grouping all clinically practicing nurses into the same job description denigrates the professional practice of nursing — the essential service of providing patient care. Such employment practices have had a negative affect on nursing education in colleges and universities. Also, high school advisors frequently direct students to community college nursing programs as being the most cost-effective. Ultimately, the negative image leads to recruitment problems.

Differentiated Pay Structure Model

The Differentiated Pay Structure (DPS) Model is composed of six factors, described in the order in which they appear in the model. Following the description of each factor is the algebraic formula that applies to that particular factor. Each factor is treated as an independent variable, with the nurse's ultimate salary being the dependent variable — thus becoming linear equations in the DPS model. The effect is one of compounding instead of treating the variables as being simply additive.

Generic Model Formulae
Y = Dependent variable:
     Hourly wage.
a = Point where the line intersects the X axis:
     Existing hourly wage of new hire, without
     experience, in a staff nurse position.
b = Slope of the line:
     Increase in pay level brought about by each of the
     independent variables.
X = Independent variables:
     Education (E), Position (P), Performance (PF),
     Differentials (D), Longevity (L).

DPS Model $= Y = a + b_1E + b_2P + b_3PL + b_4PT + b_5D + b_6L$

Education Factor (E)

Description. Education is defined as credits and degrees recognized by institutions of higher education. In this model, the BSN degree (which has been designated by the American Nurses Association as the entry level for professional nursing) is used as the benchmark position (see Table 2). It is easily compared with baccalaureate-prepared nurses employed at other institutions and baccalaureate-prepared persons in other occupations/professions. There are two educational levels above this one (MSN and DNS/PhD) and three levels below it (namely, associate degree/diploma, LPN, and nursing assistants). LPNs have traditionally been paid about 30% below the staff nurse position. This model drops the level to 40% because the BSN is used as the benchmark position. Nursing assistants, who are defined by the health industry, are included because the model includes the total work force of nursing.

The three categories below the BSN level are protected by the Fair Labor Standards Act and occupants would be entitled to time-and-a-half for overtime. Overtime pay (and time clocks) would be discontinued for professional level personnel. These latter employees would be salaried and exempt from the Fair Labor Standards Act. Professional nurses could receive compensatory time for working overtime.

Formulae
$Y = a + b_1 E$
     or
$Y = a + (a \cdot E) = a_1$

Position Factor (P)

Description. The second major factor, that of position, reflects the activities collected within a job description (see Table 3). Position includes all the functional areas of nursing — practice, teaching, administration, research, and evaluation. Faced with a head nurse position vacancy, nursing management could appoint an associate nurse, a baccalaureate-prepared nurse, or a master's-prepared nurse. Depending on the level of preparation of the appointee, the position would be developed appropriate to that skill level.

This implements the phrase "salary commensurate with preparation," seen so often in advertisements. This method is more fair for both the institution and the nurse, as there is acknowledgement of true expectations. Institutions may try to save money in making the appointment, but there should be no false expectations of professional nursing performance from associate nurses (i.e., expecting a BSN nurse to have the advanced social interaction/management skills of an MSN graduate). Revising the job description to accurately reflect the appointment does not violate Title VII of the Civil Rights Act or the Equal Pay Act.

For nurses engaged in clinical practice, there are three possible job series, beginning with the two series of general clinical practice — namely, staff nurses with associate degree/diploma preparation, and clinical nurses with a baccalaureate degree. Nurses in advanced clinical practice possess the master's degree. Thus, an institution could have staff nurse, clinical nurse, and clinical nurse specialist series.

Many hospitals provide only basic care; therefore, there is no advanced clinical practice. Basic care consists of carrying out physicians' directives, as well as assisting patients with activities of daily living. If there are no professional nurses planning and providing care, there is no professional care and no advanced clinical practice. In such instances, third-party payers should share in the institution's reduced costs.

Formula

$$Y = a_1 + (a^1 \cdot P) = a_2$$

Performance Level (PL)

To each position is added a performance level (see Figure 2). This should not be confused with traditional employment steps where the worker advances a step each year and then, after six or seven steps, reaches the maximum pay level, except for across-the-board increases.

To conceptualize the performance level, one may refer to the work of Benner (1984), who has defined performance stages as "Novice, Beginner, Competent, Proficient, and Expert." These five stages are developmental in nature and evolve from the seven domains of practice described by Benner.

In the DPS model, use of titles for the levels of development is avoided. Instead, there is provision for appointments to staff nurse 1 through 5, clinical nurse 1 through 5, and clinical nurse specialist 1 through 5:

Level 1
- Probationary period — defined by the institution, but generally extends for six months. Applicable to new hires at any level of employment. Probationary status has legal implications regarding job rights.

Level 2
- This would commonly describe the completion of the first year of employment, but this level can be extended as appropriate. New transfers to a clinical service would initially be employed at Level 2.
- Per diem staff are employed at this level.

Level 3
- Most commonly, nurses would be at this level for a minimum of three years. This level can become a permanent level of performance.
- Part-time nurses cannot progress beyond this level.

Level 4
- A nurse would not be considered for level 4 with less than four years of clinical experience, two years in the specialty, and two years with the present employer.
- Full-time employee.
- Certification in the area of specialty as offered by ANA or recognized by ANA.
- Successful management and peer review.

Level 5
- This level is defined by the nurses who have achieved level 4 in the institution using an outside consultant for assistance. The final criteria and standards will be approved by

the nurse administrator of the clinical area and by the chief nurse in the institution.

A nurse manager can advance nurses from levels 1 to 2. Following consultation with nurses at level 3 and above, the nurse manager may advance a nurse to level 3. To achieve levels 4 and 5, a formal peer review process, including portfolio review, is required.

The use of the three series and five levels enables the nursing department to reward staff appropriately for individual levels of performance. Money saved in levels 1 and 2 positions by the employer can be used to reward levels 4 and 5 nurses. Level 1, at 20% below position level, protects the institution economically from the high cost incurred in preparing new graduates for practice positions. If the individual practitioner must absorb the cost of being employed at levels 1 and 2, that nurse will want to demonstrate competence at level 3 as quickly as possible; and, if achievement of that goal is delayed unduly, the nurse will bring pressure on the school of nursing for its inadequate preparation for the expected role. Levels 1 and 2 are deterrents to unproductive job hopping. With each job change, the nurse is again returned to levels 1 and 2 temporarily.

Formula
$$Y = a_2 + (a_2 \cdot PF) = a_3$$

Part-Time Factor (PT)

Description. The fourth factor is an adjustment for part-time employment. The presence of part-time positions is essential to hospital nursing departments, as well as to some nurses. However, the practice has been abused by both management and staff. Nursing appears to be the only field of employment where it is common practice to prorate a full-time salary into per diem wages.

In determining pay rates for part-time employment, one must recognize that part-time nurses do not assume equivalent responsibilities for the unit as a whole. They add to communication and quality control problems, increasing the cost of recruitment, orientation, staff development, and termination; and they decrease the productivity of nursing, both within the institution and throughout nursing as a whole. However, part-time nurses also enable the full-time staff to work more flexible hours, and they save the institution money through unpaid employee benefits. Smeltzer (1990) has reported a compensation plan which awards nurses a 20% increase in the hourly rate for all hours worked beyond a 24-hour minimum.

For the part-time nurse in any position, the model calls for a 20% salary cut, with the remaining 80% salary and 100% employee benefits prorated across five days. This 20% savings for the institution contributes to the hidden costs of excess employees on the payroll. In addition, there is a 1% penalty for each hour less than 40 worked in a one-week period. This penalty reflects that fact that a nurse who works eight hours-per-week is less valuable than the nurse who works 32 hours-per-week. In this model, it is suggested that institutions allot no more than 30% of their full-time positions to part-time nurses.

Formulae

$$Y = a_3 + (a_3 \cdot PT) = a_4$$
$$(a_3) - ((a_3 \cdot .8) \cdot (.01 (40 - \# \text{ hrs worked}))) = a_4$$

Differentials Factor (D)

Description. Shift differentials make up the fifth factor. Hospitals will not solve their staffing problems until they pay a market price for the hours worked outside the Monday through Friday daytime hours. A manager can no longer convince a staff member with arguments such as, "you know you must share the unpleasant hours" or, "you knew when you elected to become a nurse that patients are sick 24 hours-a-day." Society is accustomed to paying higher prices for services outside normal daytime business hours; hospital work is no different. Every nursing job can be dispersed among the available work force if the price is right. Staff nurses on the day shift are overpaid if they do not rotate shifts, for shift work is assumed in the position. Day shift assignments cannot be used to reward longevity because they create an impossible recruitment barrier. Nurses have been so relatively inexpensive and undervalued that other departments routinely ask nursing to take on many of their tasks after 5:00 p.m.

In the DPS model, shift differentials (see Table 4) are shown as 15% for evenings, 10% for weekends, 20% for nights, and −15% for day shifts. Shift differentials are not applied to nonshift employees. In addition, there is a provision for a 5% differential for the relief charge nurse. Percentages are adjusted to achieve the goal of volunteerism. Hospitals have preferred to use an hourly bonus for shift differentials, but percentage of base rate is a more fair way, facilitated by computerization of payroll files.

Formulae

$$Y = a_4 \cdot D_1 \cdot \# \text{ hrs}_{\text{Days}}) + (a_4 \cdot D_2 \cdot \# \text{ hrs }_{\text{PMs}}) +$$
$$(a_4 \cdot D_3 \cdot \# \text{ hrs }_{\text{Nocs}}) + (a_4 \cdot D_4 \cdot \# \text{ hrs WE}) +$$
$$(a_4 \cdot D_5 \cdot \# \text{ hrs }_{\text{RC}}) = a_5$$

Longevity Factor (L)

Description. Longevity rewards, the sixth and final factor, are paid as a bonus and not added to the base rate of pay (see Table 5). Awards of sizeable sums are expected to keep workers who might otherwise resign on a whim. In contrast to bonuses, annual salary increases are costly and buy the institution little in employee longevity. Edward Lawler III (1990) has called these annual increments "annuities," for they are paid each year to the employee. Since bonuses are special awards for particularly loyal service, they are appropriate only for full-time employees (and only after informing those employees there is an expected minimum of six months' service after receiving such bonus awards).

The armed forces have had extensive experience with enlistment bonuses and found them to be generally effective. The military varies the bonus according to the anticipated need for the worker's particular skill category. Such a mechanism of variable bonuses is not recommended for use within the nursing division, but an institution might consider this tactic in recruitment of nurses.

In this model, the nurse is paid a 10% bonus on employment anniversary dates at two, four, and six years, and a 20% bonus at 10, 15, and 20 years. This is budgeted at 5% of payroll per year, minus the money saved based on projected turnover rates for that level of tenure.

Formula

$$L \text{ bonus } = a_3 \cdot \underline{\hspace{1cm}} \%$$

Projected Effects

In summary, the Differentiated Pay Structure Model can be expected to produce savings with some variables and increased costs with others.

Possible Cost Savings

- Reducing orientation costs paid through salary control until employees reach productivity.
- Eliminating across-the-board increases, except for cost-of-living adjustments.
- Limiting longevity bonus pay to reflect one-time payments which are not added to base pay.
- Eliminating overtime pay for professional nurses.
- Reducing staff development costs (CEU allowances, CPR and ACLS training) by delegating more responsibility to the individual nurse.
- Eliminating the practice of overpaying the underprepared.
- Reducing costs of excess turnover by employing nurses who volunteer for evening, night, and weekend work.
- Reducing the cost of day shift employment.

Possible Cost Increases

- Increasing differentials for evening, night, and weekend work.
- Adding payment to reflect educational level (possibly offset by salaries held steady for the lesser-prepared).
- Adding longevity bonus payments (offset by eliminating annual increases).
- Adding professional nurse salaried positions (but eliminating overtime pay).

Implementation

Although the components of the model can be implemented individually, this is not recommended. The total model provides areas where money can be saved to offset added costs in others. Also, the total model provides gains and losses for each category of nurse and the potential for more widespread acceptance. It is the total model which promotes economic rewards for nurses who a) are better educated, b) assume greater responsibility, c) engage in full-time employment, and d) achieve advanced performance levels. These are the same achievements rewarded in other fields.

Testing of the Differentiated Pay Structure Model is taking place with funding from the Agency for Health Care Policy and Research (formerly the National Center for Health Services Research). Stage I utilizes computer simulations of the personnel data bases of two local hospitals to demonstrate that with a phased-in period of implementation, the inequities in nursing's pay structure can be corrected in a manner that is budget-neutral to the institution. When the inequities have been corrected, institutions can adjust staff mix and pay level as appropriate to that particular health service market. Stage II of the research will involve actual implementation of the model in selected medical centers across the United States to determine whether changes in pay structure produce the projected behavior changes in nurses.

❑　　　❑　　　❑

Figure 1
A Model of the Three Components
of the Work Force of Nursing

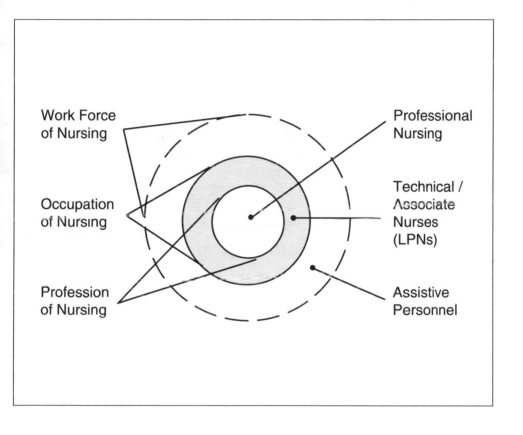

Figure 2
Performance Stages

−20%	−10%	00%	+10%	+20%
1 ———	2 ———	3 ———	4 ———	5

Table 1
Educational Model

Years	Level	Degree
2	Technical Nursing	AD or ADN
4	Professional Nursing	BSN, BS, BN
6	Advanced Specialization	MSN, MS, MN
8	Research Competence	PhD, DNS

Table 2
Education Factor

+30%	DNS/PhD
+20%	MSN
00%	BSN (benchmark position)
−20%	Associate Degree/Diploma
−40%	LPN/LVN
−60%	Nursing Assistant

Table 3
Position Factor

+50%	Director: Clinical Service, Staff Development, Research, or Quality Assurance
+40%	Unit Manager/Head Nurse
+30%	Consultant: Practice, QA, Staff Development
+20%	Case Manager, Assistant Unit Manager, Nurse Practitioner
+10%	Preceptor, Charge Nurse, Infection Control Technician
00%	Clinical Practice

Table 4
Differentials

Evenings	=	+15%
Nights	=	+20%
Weekends	=	+10%
Days	=	−15%
Relief Charge	=	5%

Table 5
Longevity Bonus

After 2 years ... +10% of base salary
4 years ... +10%
6 years ... +10%
10 years ... +20%
15 years ... +20% (and every 5 years thereafter)

Computer Simulation of Projected Costs of the Differentiated Pay Structure Model

Michael Moore, M.S., R.N.

Overview of the Simulation Process

As Virginia Cleland points out in the paper preceding this one, the ideas behind the Differentiated Pay Structure Model are relatively straightforward. My part in this research project was to turn the model's concepts into a software program. The goal of this program was to make the requisite analysis to find a budget- neutral solution. The program also had to allow easy addition, deletion, and changing of the model variables. A personal goal of mine was to make the software as generic and simple to use as possible.

While this analysis of costs could, in theory, be done by hand, the use of a computer makes the process realistic, and speeds and simplifies the repetitions of factor adjustments used to find a budget-neutral solution. The computer also allowed us to use actual demographic data from hospitals that participated in the study, and to group this data by the individual, unit, division, and department.

While we might have relied on hypothetical staff data, real demographics seemed important to use for the credibility of the results. It is important to remember that our results and figures so far are relevant only to the particular hospitals studied in the San Francisco Bay area. Some adjustment to the base rate and model factors would have to occur when other areas of the country are studied.

Table 1 illustrates the steps forming the process of the analysis. So far, we have completed the first four steps. Although the first two steps (collection of staff and unit data) could be completed simultaneously, we found that the design of the computer data base and program had to follow, even though we were unsure of what data would be available and what assumptions and compromises to make. As it turned out, most of the necessary data was available, although it came from multiple sources within the hospital and much of it had to be entered into our data base manually.

Once we had constructed the data base and knew what was missing, we could make assumptions about what could be randomly assigned and what could be inferred. The next step was to see how the model, in its original state, would change the salary cost of this group of nurses. We then adjusted the model factors to come up with a budget-neutral solution.

Our next objective will be projecting these results to determine the cost of staffing — comparing what was actually spent and what would have been spent under the model. Finally, we will evaluate the impact of the new job descriptions and model costs over time, using linear programming to determine the optimal configuration of staff.

While we anticipated data collection to be relatively straightforward, there were some unanticipated barriers to be overcome. The data elements we gathered are listed in Table 2. The information needed was simple; however, we found from this research project and from selling scheduling software to other clients that this information is typically scattered throughout most hospitals, with several departments possessing a piece or two, but with no central collection facility for all relevant staff data. Generally, human resources may have the first seven or eight elements, while nursing may have the last four. We have often found, though, that when there is overlap, the data conflicts. The data in each department may or may not be stored electronically. In the case of the first hospital we studied, critical elements were not stored on a computer, so employee personnel files had to be searched manually, with nurse managers completing the data forms.

This situation pointed out the hidden costs to an organization of territoriality in information storage. The data is usually redundant, often inaccurate or conflicting between departments, and when it is stored manually, it is, for all practical purposes, inaccessible. This situation affects not only those of us wanting to do research, but the organization itself when timely information is needed for decision making.

I would like to suggest that the most efficient possible information system would involve networked data sharing between personnel and all the other departments in a hospital, with each user taking responsibility for keeping his/her information current. Hopefully, this method will someday become a reality in hospitals.

Other data collection issues revolved around the concern for confidentiality of staff information. While we collected staff names, they were used only for validation and additional data collection. Once the data we needed was collected, the names were removed from our files. Another problem surfaced when, in one hospital, data collection had to be suspended until labor negotiations were completed. There was even some fear that discussion of a differentiated pay structure might complicate the collective bargaining process.

Not all data were available for each staff member, so any missing elements — such as education or competency — were randomly assigned, based either on frequencies in groups of the same position and unit or on assumptions made in the original model.

The Differentiated Pay Structure Model, represented in a linear equation, is used to calculate the costs of the model (see Figure 1). The dependent variable is Y, the staff hourly wage. This wage relates only to direct pay, and does not include any benefits or other indirect costs.

Once the hourly wage is determined for each employee, it is then converted into an annual wage and aggregated at the unit, divisional, and departmental levels.

The variable a represents a base salary figure, which is adjusted based on the factors in the model, and from which the final study salaries are derived. Originally, we had planned to use a starting salary for a new graduate; however, this resulted in a severe pay cut for most staff. As the average staff nurse tenure was eight years, the variable a was changed to $39,000 — which reflects the average pay for a day shift staff nurse. We could have achieved budget neutrality by keeping a low baseline salary and varying the adjustment factors more, but this caused excessive wage spread among staff.

The variable b is the slope of the line, and represents the change in pay level brought about by the independent variables. As originally conceived, the effect of the independent variables (education, position, etc.) is additive — i.e., the effect of each factor is compounded on the previous factors. Therefore, the impact of the independent variables diminishes as one moves from left to right in the equation.

This compounding of factors also increased salary variability and decreased wage compression. Coding the software so as to be user selectable for compounding versus straight addition added more flexibility. If compounding is selected, the education factor, being the first applied, has the greatest impact on the final salary.

For the purposes of the study, we decided that nursing assistants, nursing technicians, and LVNs/LPNs should be excluded from the calculations. While their costs are included in the final totals, they are not directly affected by the Differentiated Pay Structure Model, and essentially pass through the cost calculations unchanged.

In the next variable, staff positions, the adjustment factors were designed to reflect certain positions that are not associated with shift or weekend differentials. Given a decrease in day shift differential (essentially a negative differential), the pay loss would need to be offset.

A competency or performance level for each staff member was assigned based on certain assumptions — that novices and beginners would make up about 15% of the total, and that the remaining 85% would be divided into 50% competent, 30% skilled, and 20% expert. The novice and beginner levels were assigned based on hire dates. We arbitrarily chose one year's experience as the end date for the beginner/novice group. Using that criteria, the actual percentage was about 17½%. For the rest of the staff, we needed to have data on their performance evaluation level as a guide to assigning competence levels. However, since this was not available to us, we randomly assigned their competence in proportions of 50%/30%/20%, using a computer program.

The part-time differential is noteworthy because the effect of the formula we used is progressive and linear, as the FTE levels decline. This means that hourly rates continue to decrease with FTE decreases. Roughly, that means that if a full-time nurse was earning $20 per hour, a .7 nurse would earn $18 per hour, and a .4 nurse would earn $16 per hour. The slope of this decrease is selectable with the software.

The important feature of the shift differentials variable is the decrease in pay for day shift work. The assumption here is that the day rate is too high relative to other shifts. Differentials of 15% and 25%, for evenings and nights respectively, are designed to create a volunteer work force for these shifts. [Australian hospitals, we have learned, pay 50% and 75% differentials on the weekends. Not surprisingly, they have little trouble staffing weekends.] The weekend differential in the model here is a more modest 10%. All differentials are additive, so that weekend nights would get a 35% increase.

Finally, longevity bonuses are given in lieu of automatic pay increases, and are to be phased in rather than immediately prorated on implementation. For the purposes of analysis, the software can be configured to either include or exclude the effects of the longevity bonuses on the final cost.

The next step was to design the software to analyze the data. Most people are familiar with spread sheets for data analysis, but this is not always the best choice. The reasons for choosing a spread sheet over a data base are that it is easy to create the data tables and formulas, and easy to modify formulas and visualize the relationships between model elements. No complex programming is generally required.

Conversion of existing organization data is simpler using a data base than a spread sheet, and data is more easily exported back to the organization's main data base. It also is simpler to make global changes or replacements in the data. The size of the staff data base is virtually unlimited, which makes it very easy to project the global effects of changing any value or factor of the model. If new model elements are needed, they can be easily added. Lastly, a data base system allows more flexible reporting.

Actually, we ended up using a hybrid approach. We did initial simulations on a spread sheet to see if the numbers we were projecting were reasonable, and then we created a data base system to do the bulk of the analysis.

An overview of the data base system design appears in Figure 2. As illustrated therein, there is a central staff data base that is connected to six other small data bases — education, position, competency, shift differential, weekend differential, and longevity bonus. What this connection means is that if a staff member has a BSN degree, then the education data base is automatically positioned at the entry for BSN, and will return the value of the factor associated with that degree. What each of these small data bases does is modify the value of the base salary until, at the end of the analysis, the final model cost for that person has been derived. The advantage to this approach are that it allows addition, change, or deletion of any of the possible values in one of the small data bases without reprogramming. This is especially important to the position and differential data bases. For instance, if a hospital had a 12-hour day shift starting at 11:00 a.m., the software could easily add that shift and designate it as either a day or evening shift. This design also allows additional model factors to be easily added. For instance, a factor for certification could be included quite simply (provided the certification information existed in the staff data base).

Once the data has been gathered, the design completed, and the software coded, the process of running simulations is relatively straightforward. I varied the baseline salary first, trying to achieve a total cost similar to the current cost, and then adjusted the model factors to keep the cost of a benchmark nurse (that is, a BSN-prepared, full-time, competency-level nurse) at the current rate. It was important to keep a reasonable spread in salary levels. Rather than wage compression, the model tended to create large divergences of pay rates. In practice, this involves changing a factor and seeing the effect on the total cost, as well as on individual nurses.

Ultimately, by adjusting the base salary, differentials, and some of the education factors, I was able to derive a budget-neutral solution for the nursing department as a whole. The budgets for individual units varied widely, based on the composition of their staffs. Not surprisingly, nursing administration costs increased, as did units with highly skilled, long-term staff, while costs in the general units tended to drop.

While the model equation is linear, linear programming techniques cannot always be applied to find the best answers. Typically, linear programming seeks out the optimal answer to a problem. The commercial software we used looks for the most efficient scheduling of nurses (meaning least cost) by reducing as much as possible the variance between supply and demand. This is a well-defined linear programming problem.

On the other hand, trying to apply linear programming to the Differentiated Pay Structure Model is a bit like going to the grocery store with $100 and trying to determine the "best" allocation of that money. To one person it might mean spending it on nutritious foods, while to another it might mean spending it all on frozen pizzas and cookies. There really is no "best" answer, as reaching such a conclusion involves making a value judgement.

I made the numbers balance by increasing the weekend differential, decreasing the day shift penalty, and raising the AA/ADN and diploma rates slightly. How the model will actually be implemented, however, depends entirely on the values of the organization's leadership.

The next step of this project is to take all the financial data for a study period (in this case, June 1990), and use the newly adjusted factors to calculate the cost of staffing for that actual period. As the model includes provisions for some staff on salary, overtime for this group will have to be adjusted and converted to some type of compensatory time.

We will then make projections of costs at two and four years past the study date, taking into account compensation trends and the market and labor distribution effects of implementing the differential pay structure model. By using the newly defined job descriptions, staffing will be predicted and costs analyzed as compared to the cost of traditional staffing and job roles. Finally, the cost of schedules will be analyzed with linear programming, and the optimal full-time/part-time mix with regard to cost will be determined.

❑   ❑   ❑

Table 1
Computer Simulation Steps

- Collect data on individual staff
- Collect data on unit hours and costs
- Design and set up data bases and software
- Vary model factors to achieve budget neutrality within the staff data base
- Calculate the cost of unit staffing with the new pay rates
- Compare the study cost with the actual cost for the target period
- Run linear programming optimization to determine optimal skill and FTE mix

Table 2
Data Collection: Staff Information

- Name
- Employee number
- Position
- Unit
- Hourly pay rate
- Hire date
- Hired FTE
- Pay step
- Performance level
- Hired shift (and rotation if applicable)
- Weekend frequency
- Highest nursing degree

Figure 1
DPS Model

$$Y = a + b_1E + b_2P + b_3PL + b_4PT + b_5D + b_6L$$

Y = Dependent variable: hourly wage
a = Intercept of the line on the X axis
b = Slope of the line
E = Education factor
P = Position factor
PL = Performance level
PT = Part-time factor
D = Shift differential
L = Longevity bonus

Figure 2
DPS Data Base Model

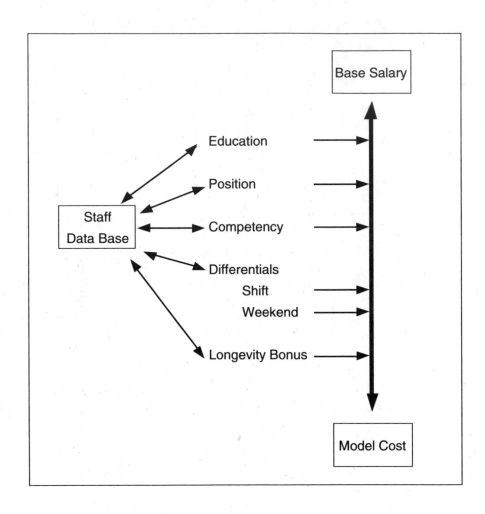

Persuading the CEO/CFO to Try Differentiated Practice

Janet Barron, M.S., R.N.

I t is exciting to realize that nursing can now develop and implement pay structures which reward professional and organizational values. Dr. Cleland's Differentiated Pay Structure Model is a mechanism to reward desired professional behaviors, an alternative to rewarding nurses for just showing up.

PolyOptimum is pleased to be working with Dr. Cleland on this project, because it corresponds with our corporate philosophy that a health care institution should make decisions in keeping with its organizational culture and values. Not everyone would agree on the emphasis that should be placed on each factor. Some may believe that working nights is more difficult than working weekends and should be compensated accordingly. Others may feel that precepting new staff is a part of every professional's role, and should therefore be included in the basic salary package without additional compensation. When opportunities for advanced education in the community are limited, competency level may be more heavily valued than educational preparation.

One of the beauties of Dr. Cleland's model and its use of computer simulation is that factors can be weighted and adjusted to meet the organization's philosophy, goals, and values while maintaining budget neutrality. A small rural hospital may draw on a very different professional work force than a large urban teaching hospital. It is quite possible to compensate the behaviors that offer the greatest benefit to the organization and its patients. Rewarding desired professional behaviors is possible, even in the cost-constrained world in which we live.

My role focuses on convincing the CEO and CFO that compensating differentiated practice and maintaining budget neutrality are achievable even in a unionized setting. Some might doubt that CEOs and CFOs will readily embrace the idea of compensating RNs for different roles, yet almost any hospital in this country today utilizes dramatically varying levels of pay based on differences in practice. The RN who is planning the care may not be the one who is generously rewarded; instead, the greater reward may be given to the nurse who is following someone else's plan. Similarly, the nurse who is managing and directing the care for several patients may not be rewarded as well as the nurse who is simply following orders. The RN who assumes greater roles or responsibilities may not receive the greatest compensation; instead, it may be the nurse who shuns additional responsibilities and simply wants to put in his/her eight hours of work. Most hospitals are setting different practice expectations and compensating one group significantly more than others. *Registry nursing* means compensating nurse applicants who merely show up with a license in hand — they do not have to do much; all we ask is that they get through the next shift.

While CFOs may not like it, they have tolerated the current differentiated practice compensation model for years. The issue, then, is how to convert to a model that rewards professional behaviors instead of mediocre practice. Selling CEOs and CFOs on this new approach requires looking at the issues from their perspectives. The CEO and CFO need to achieve a bottom line that is acceptable to the board or governing body. Top management jobs may be on the line if financial performance is not achieved. It will no longer suffice to legitimately justify cost overruns; only results matter when jobs are in jeopardy. Top level executives will scrutinize any change that has financial consequences. Therefore, achieving consensus on a dramatic shift in compensation requires some serious measures.

The current federal administration has made it clear that it intends to limit health care expenditures. As a result, we are witnessing a shift from a health care environment that is service-driven to one that is resource-driven. In a service-driven mode, the organization identifies the service it wants to deliver and asks, "What are the resources I need to deliver this service?" In a resource-driven mode, the organization looks at its resources and asks, "What service can I afford to deliver?"

This is not far from the ideal environment in which to promote increases in compensation. Yet, it is possible because CEOs and CFOs are committed to improving the bottom line.

Given our reimbursement mechanisms, we may not control the amount of money that nursing has to spend to deliver care, but we may be able to control how the money is spent. We may choose to reward the professional behaviors we want to see, while paying less for the worker who functions as little more than a pair of hands.

To ensure the financial viability of the organization, leaders must control costs. It is tempting to argue that if the existing wage compression were eliminated and professional behaviors were adequately compensated, nursing positions would be filled and registry staff would no longer be needed. That approach is probably unrealistic. All too often, nursing leaders have pushed for higher salaries that never resulted in any noticeable reduction in registry use. For example, a hard fought increase in the differential for nights may result in night staff cutting back one night a week.

A dramatic shift must take place before an organization can hope to sell differentiated practice in a cost-constrained environment. Nursing has to let go of hours as a measure of staffing productivity. We must learn to manage the cost per patient day and allow the hours to free float.

On the surface, it appears that the typical CFO has an undying loyalty to the hour as the universal indicator of health care labor productivity. After all, those hours grow into full-time equivalents (FTEs) that can be easily counted and tracked. CEOs and CFOs are often measured and compared by their organization's FTEs per occupied bed. In fact, hours are nothing more than a surrogate for the true measure of productivity — cost. If cost, then, is the critical factor, why have institutions focused so strongly on the hours of care delivered?

Until recently, it was not possible to accurately measure and report cost on a daily basis. The actual cost of care was determined by payroll or finance two weeks or two months after the care was given and the cost incurred. It was hard to measure cost, but hours were a different story. Any institution could count staff bodies and hold managers accountable for the hours of care they delivered. Even without computers, nearly any hospital could measure the hours in every unit and compare one unit with another.

As long as the skill mix remained constant and the cost of a nursing hour of care fell within a narrow range, the cost per patient day served as an adequate estimate of cost; that is no longer the case. Now the cost of a nursing hour of care may vary greatly from an in-house nursing assistant to a registry RN on overtime. One hourly rate could be ten times another, and yet we still count the hours and hope the budget will fall into place.

When the financial picture looked bleak, institutions cut back on hours. Reducing hours, however, did not always result in reduced labor costs — overtime and expensive registry staff ate up any potential savings. When faced with a limit of five people for the next shift, staff fought for the highest level of professional staff possible, thwarting efforts to change skill mix. Until nursing relinquishes hours and focuses on the cost of staffing decisions, we will be hard pressed to control labor expenditures, and even less likely to gain widespread acceptance of compensating differentiated practice.

While there is early evidence that differentiated practice may result in reduced costs or lengths of stay, the success in other institutions may not be enough to convince a dubious CFO to revamp the entire compensation structure. Nursing administrators can increase the chance for success in their institutions by incorporating a cost-per-patient-day approach to staffing, scheduling, and productivity monitoring. First, nursing administrators will have to take the initiative and demand, "Give me X amount of dollars per orthopedic patient and I will provide nursing care within that limit. If I choose to spend more of those dollars on overtime and registry, then I will' accept fewer people. If, on the other hand, I choose to spend the dollars on different levels of practice, then I will do so within the dollar limit." Nursing administrators will then have to follow through on this agreement.

To put a cost-per-patient-day system in place, annual budget figures must be translated into cost-per-patient-day targets. Managers need to have data available to plan their staffing guidelines, with consideration for the cost of each alternative. Staff need to be sensitized to the cost implications of their requests for more help. They may elect to use two unlicensed staff instead of the registry or overtime RN. This requires the flexibility to adjust the way care is delivered on a daily basis according to available staff, exposure to modes of delivery, and the knowledge and skill to work within each mode.

Managers, supervisors, and staff need to know the impact of their staffing choices in real dollars prior to finalizing their decisions. Additionally, they need to see each day's results so they can adjust in time to make their goals; and they need the freedom to exceed their target on a particular day/shift as long as they keep within their year-to-date figures. Given their firsthand knowledge of the patients' needs and the staffing options with their associated costs, managers and staff can make financially sound decisions while delivering their desired level of care.

CEOs and CFOs will support the concept of compensating for differentiated practice if nursing can demonstrate its ability to provide care within the budgeted cost per patient day. The first step we need to take as a profession is to abandon body counts and allocate our nursing resources according to the level of value for the price paid.

❑   ❑   ❑

Part VI

Outcome and Evaluation of Differentiated Practice Models

Implementing Differentiated Practice as Part of a Professional Practice Model

Doris Milton, Ph.D., R.N.
Joyce Verran, Ph.D., F.A.A.N.
Carolyn Murdaugh, Ph.D., F.A.A.N.
Rose Gerber, Ph.D., R.N.

T his paper presents the issues of implementing differentiated practice as part of an integrated professional practice model entitled Differentiated Group Professional Practice. "Differentiated Group Professional Practice in Nursing" is a five-year research project cooperative agreement jointly funded by the National Center for Nursing Research and the Division of Nursing.

The project's purpose is to test the effectiveness of a unit-based professional practice model on nurse satisfaction, nurse resources, quality of care, and fiscal outcomes. The implementation of a model that includes components of professional practice as supported by previous research is hypothesized to result in increased measures of professional environment and nurse satisfaction with practice. Increased satisfaction should increase nurse retention and decrease turnover, which, in turn, should increase quality of care outcomes while decreasing or maintaining fiscal resources needed.

The authors are co-principal investigators on a research project cooperative agreement award, "Differentiated Group Professional Practice in Nursing," funded by the National Center for Nursing Research, NIH and the Division of Nursing, Bureau of Health Professions, Health Resources and Services Administration, 1988-1993 (#UO1 NR02153).

Specifically, we are collecting data related to professional practice (indexed by group cohesion, organizational commitment, autonomy, and control over nursing practice), nurse work satisfaction, nurse resources (indexed by vacancy, retention, and turnover measures), patient outcomes (indexed by patient satisfaction, complications, and nursing process documentation), and fiscal outcomes (indexed by operating costs, personnel and supplemental agency costs, costs per patient day, and overtime costs).

The Differentiated Group Professional Practice Model is being implemented in four hospitals in Arizona — a tertiary medical center in a metropolitan urban area, a community hospital in an urban area, and two community hospitals of varying sizes in different rural settings. Data to test the research model are being collected at these facilities and also at comparison sites.

The integrated Differentiated Group Professional Practice Model has three major components: group governance, differentiated care delivery, and shared values in a culture of excellence. Group governance incorporates four subcomponents to create a participatory nursing group practice at the unit level: participative unit management, shared decision making through staff bylaws, peer review, and a professional salary structure. Participative unit management provides a structure in which staff and managers jointly make decisions that affect nursing care delivery and the management of the unit. Bylaws are developed through group consensus and are intended to guide the actions of the nurses in the group practice. Peer review provides a framework for the evaluation of a nurse's credentials and performance by colleagues. A professional salary structure is used to compensate professionals for the entire job performed, rather than for specific tasks within the job, as in hourly wage structures.

Differentiated care delivery includes three subcomponents: differentiated RN practice, the use of nurse extenders, and primary case management. Differentiated RN practice provides for two RN staff roles based on an individualized assessment of knowledge and skill base. Position descriptions reflect the competencies expected of future graduates from ADN and BSN nursing education programs. Nurse extenders are assistive personnel who have been trained to perform clinical and nonclinical skills under the direction of an RN. Primary case management provides a framework for describing, monitoring, and tracking patient care and outcomes during a stay on one or more hospital units.

Shared values in a culture of excellence include three subcomponents: quality of care, support for creativity and intrapreneurship, and internal and external recognition. Shared values involve the adoption of homogeneous attitudes and beliefs by individuals throughout an organization. One of the values most consistent with excellence is the quality of care or service that is provided. Support for intrapreneurship is necessary to foster creativity and innovation on the part of staff who develop and test alternate strategies for improving care. Both formal and informal recognition programs reward those who demonstrate commitment to the values consistent with a culture of excellence.

In this integrated professional practice model, RNs are expected to participate in managing their unit, to share in making decisions that affect their practice, to participate in peer review, and to be compensated in accordance with a professional salary structure. They perform nursing functions commensurate with their knowledge and skills, have assistive personnel to perform non-nursing tasks related to patient care and unit operations, and participate in a case management system to monitor patient progress. Behaviors that reflect the value of quality care are supported; creativity and intrapreneurship are facilitated; and efforts are recognized both internally and externally.

Certain issues have arisen as we implemented this integrated professional practice model with differentiated practice as a subcomponent. We believe that these issues differ from those that occur when only differentiated practice is initiated. They may reflect conditions that could occur in facilities that also share aspects of a professional practice. These issues will be addressed in relation to each of the three components: group governance, differentiated care delivery, and shared values in a culture of excellence; some overlapping of the components is inevitable. In order to present the issues in an organizational fashion, I artificially separated components of a model that is wholly integrated. I will also discuss how the issues have been resolved in our demonstration sites. In many cases, these points of resolution are in transition, as is our model of differentiated practice.

Also, for ease of presentation, I will refer to the two differentiated RN staff roles as "baccalaureate degree-type" and "associate degree-type." In the future, it is our intent to base placement in the two RN roles solely on formal education. However, in this transition period, not all RNs in the baccalaureate degree-type role have baccalaureate degrees — some have associate degrees or diplomas, and some RNs in the associate degree-type role have diplomas.

The four issues that have evolved in implementing the first model component, group governance, have been:

1) creating avenues for participation in unit management and decision making,
2) identifying who is a peer,
3) reconciling differentiated roles with clinical ladder programs, and
4) analyzing the fit between salary structure and role descriptions.

The first issue concerns the degree to which RNs in the two different roles participate in unit management and decision making. Should RNs in both roles have an equal voice in all decisions related to unit management and patient care? If not, how will their roles in decision making differ without devaluing one or both of the roles? Also, discussions have taken place regarding how much assistive personnel should participate in decisions that affect both the care they provide patients and the management of the unit.

The type of participation that RNs in both staff roles have in decision making and unit management can affect the position descriptions for the two roles, as well as the changes in patient assignment methods after differentiation. In our experimental sites, we have found that since many shared decisions related to unit management concerns may violate longstanding traditions, changes are more easily accepted if RNs in both roles have an equal voice in those decisions.

The implementation of peer review — a component of group governance — has led to interesting discussions at each site about who is a peer. When a clinical ladder program is in place, is a peer an RN at the same clinical ladder level? Does that peer also need to be in the same differentiated role type? Should the clinical ladder program be redesigned so that the requirements for progression would include a broader scope of practice, thereby incorporating both roles? Or should two distinct clinical advancement programs be in place — one for RNs in the baccalaureate degree-type role and one for RNs in the associate degree-type role? Would two separate ladders help define beginning to advanced levels of expertise in both roles?

At this point, we are finding that the clinical ladder programs in our facilities have levels that generally correspond to each scope of practice, although there is some overlap between levels. Also, the existing clinical ladder programs are taking the beginning step toward establishing a pay differential for RNs in both role types.

The fourth issue related to the implementation of the group governance component is that of the fit between salary structure and the two different role descriptions. Most professional salary structures propose compensating all RNs on an annual salary basis. Yet, if nurses prepared with an associate degree are more focused on providing care during a specified time period, should they be paid on an hourly wage or an annual salary basis? Also, separate clinical advancement programs for RNs in the two roles may necessitate increasing the annual salary for advancement in the baccalaureate degree-type role and increasing the hourly wage for advancement the associate degree-type role. We have not yet resolved this issue at any of our sites.

The two major issues in implementing differentiated care delivery have been:

1) performing non-nursing tasks when assistive personnel are not present; and,
2) in case management, separating the nurses' roles from the case manager role.

The first issue has centered on the performance of non-nursing tasks when there are insufficient assistive personnel to perform these tasks or until assistive personnel are employed. Which of the two RN positions then becomes responsible for the performance of non-nursing tasks? Should baccalaureate degree-type RNs and associate degree-type RNs divide the non-nursing tasks, or should the associate degree-type nurse perform these tasks? At most of our demonstration sites, RNs in both roles presently perform non-nursing tasks when assistive personnel are unavailable.

The second issue in this model component has been that of how to distinguish the RN roles in the case management of patients from the RN baccalaureate degree-type role. This confusion occurs primarily because the leadership needed in case management matches the profiles of the RN in the baccalaureate degree-type role. Secondly, we called this role "case manager." It seems clear that, in order to be responsible for case management of patients and their families, an RN would need the scope of knowledge and skill associated with the baccalaureate degree-type role. What is not clear is how the RN in the baccalaureate degree-type role, without primary accountability for the case management of a specific patient, still manages *not* to function as an associate degree-type RN. That is, the baccalaureate degree-type RN still uses his/her full scope of knowledge and skill, and cannot arbitrarily begin to function within a narrower scope of knowledge.

A great deal of staff development is needed to reinforce the need for the RN in the baccalaureate degree-type role to demonstrate leadership at all times, whether acting as the case manager of a patient or not. This educational process is ongoing and constant in all sites.

The third component of this integrated model involves shared values in a culture of excellence. The three major issues related to implementing this component are:

1) identifying the contributions of both roles to quality of care,
2) distinguishing differentiated types of creativity, and
3) fostering mutual valuing of roles versus equality of roles.

Emphasis on the quality of care provided to patients and their families is the most critical of these values. Providing quality care requires the best possible match between patient/family care needs and the appropriate differentiated RN role type. For that match to be optimized, the current method of using RNs in both roles interchangeably needs to change. For patients and families to receive quality care, the contributions of nurses in both roles are important. With RNs functioning to the optimal extent of their capabilities in both roles, patients and families receive the fullest possible scope of nursing care.

The second issue is that of distinguishing and fostering differentiated types of creativity and innovation. Strategies for fostering creativity may differ for RNs in the two roles, since their attitudes and performance expectations differ. Associate degree-type nurses, for example, are creative in devising more efficient ways of completing a plan of care during their shift and methods to individualize a standardized plan of care. Baccalaureate degree-type nurses tend to be creative in developing plans of care to increase the efficiency of resource use during the patient's hospital stay and in modifying a plan of care for a patient with complex family dynamics.

The third issue in this component centers on fostering mutual valuing of roles versus equality of roles. Problems in valuing the contributions of all RNs to quality care arise when "mutually valued" is interpreted as being synonymous with "equal value." Contributions by individual RNs are not the same because of their differing knowledge and skill base. Both roles, however, are of value and are viewed as complementing each other.

When developing formal and informal recognition mechanisms, the focus needs to be on ways in which both the baccalaureate degree-type nurse and the associate degree-type nurse can be recognized. In our experience, mechanisms other than those we now have for rewarding nurses — especially external recognition mechanisms — are greatly needed. Because of their differing mind-sets, the contributions of the nurses in the two roles differ, yet most of the current reward mechanisms (such as clinical ladder programs and professional or specialty association awards) are more likely to recognize the baccalaureate degree-type RN. Although we have not developed concrete solutions to this dilemma, we need to begin by refining internal recognition mechanisms (such as clinical ladder programs) to ensure that the contributions to patient care of the associate degree-type nurse are recognized.

Implementing an integrated professional practice model has presented some interesting challenges to all of us involved with this project. We are excited to have this opportunity to influence redesign in diverse acute care practice settings, and are confident that by the end of our project our outcome data will demonstrate that this type of change is effective. As Barry and Gibbons (1990) recently wrote, "Changing circumstances have become so compelling that it is no longer a question of *whether* familiar systems need redesigning, but rather *how soon* and *by what means* a different system will take the place of the existing one."

Since we are at the beginning of the third year of our five-year project, I look forward to a future opportunity to report on the success of this innovative nursing care delivery model.

❏   ❏   ❏

Affecting Patient Outcomes Through Innovative Nursing Practice Models

Patricia Moritz, Ph.D., R.N.

Abstract

T his paper will discuss the development and evaluation of innovative practice models, their relationship to differentiated practice, and their potential impact on the changing health care system.

The increasing need to differentiate nurses by their knowledge and clinical competence has been recognized, and responses are being implemented and evaluated. "Quality" and "outcomes of patient care" have become buzzwords within the overall health care system. To respond to this changing emphasis, nursing must be able to demonstrate the impact of care provided by its practitioners through measures of outcomes of patient care. Putting innovative practice models in place that facilitate the ability to provide high quality care, autonomy and independence in practice, participative and collaborative clinical and administrative decision making, and group governance is important. It is necessary to evaluate the models in terms of specific quality and outcome measures that reflect nursing practice. The means to do this is further explored herein.

Introduction

Change, uncertainty, and quality have characterized the health care delivery system for some time, particularly since the onset of the current prospective payment system. Change and quality also have become benchmarks in nursing practice, as hospitals and their nursing departments are being restructured. Similarly, as nursing science has expanded, deepened and strengthened nursing practice, nursing homes are preparing to implement new Medicare regulations designed to improve the quality of life of residents. With the restructuring and reorganizing of the environments in which patient care is delivered, innovative models of nursing practice have been called for, and some models have emerged for evaluation. Several National Center for Nursing Research (NCNR) initiatives have investigated innovative practice models in both hospital and community-based practice, which will be discussed below.

This paper will focus on differentiating nursing practice for the improvement of patient care, using innovative nursing practice models for the strengthening of nursing practice and strategies for evaluating the impact of nursing practice on patient outcomes.

Differentiating Nursing Practice for Improved Patient Care

In the effort to establish a better interpretation of the professional practice of nurses, differentiated practice has been one type of nursing care delivery that has drawn considerable interest and is currently being implemented in a variety of clinical settings. Differentiated practice, particularly with a case management component, is one of the nursing delivery methods that has emerged from primary nursing, and one whose impact on patient care is ready for evaluation. Since the time of Mildred Montag and the development of associate degree education in nursing and of nurses practicing from the perspective of a continuum (Montag, 1980), there have been attempts (albeit unsuccessful ones) to differentiate the roles and functions among nurses with diverse levels of educational preparation and competence.

Nurses do practice within an interdisciplinary framework in all clinical settings, and the relationships among the disciplines vary according to the setting. Thus, it is a complex undertaking to explain the variation in patient outcomes considering the impact of practitioners from the clinical disciplines across settings. For example, in community-based practice, there is considerable independence in practice with limited interdependence on others. However, within acute care settings, interdependence among all the disciplines is common. Moreover, nurses who practice in hospitals also practice collaboratively within a group of clinical nurses, whereas nurses in community-based practice usually do not practice within a group. This aspect of group professional practice is one of the unique features of hospital nursing practice. Community-based practice, both in public health and home care, entails much more isolation from colleagues during caregiving.

Naylor (1990) has indicated that, from a care delivery perspective, there are advantages to maintaining the generalist approach to nurse staffing because all nurses have the same license to practice, regardless of educational preparation. Employers, therefore, would have a larger pool to draw on for assignment across clinical units. Some have argued that certain settings, such as rural areas, take a generalist rather than a restrictive approach to staffing (Fuszard et al., 1990). Other settings, because of the specialized nature of their services, require nurses with specialized clinical knowledge and competence. Recent work on critical thinking — especially that of Tanner (1987), del Bueno (1990), and Benner (1984) — in describing the advancement of clinical nurses from novice to expert, demonstrates a rationale for differentiating among nurses in clinical practice, particularly in different levels of clinical competency.

Such differentiation can lead to identification of nurses with specialized knowledge and competence, achieved through continued career development and/or advanced education. Primm (1987) noted that within the role of the nurse there are differentiated levels of functions which result in collaborative, interdependent, and complementary parameters of practice that are consistent with the educational preparation of the practitioner. Within the differentiated practice model, the ADN- and BSN-prepared nurses are further differentiated by the competencies they should exhibit in clinical practice situations.

The provision of direct care, communication, and management competencies have come from a consensus favoring their identification and have been pilot tested (Primm, 1987). Delineating the competencies for each level of educational preparation, coupled with defining the educational content that would support this kind of differentiation, achieves a better fit with how employers define position requirements and practice expectations. In clinical practice settings, nurses are compensated for the work they do based on position functions and requirements, the competencies that they bring, and the quality of care they provide. Differentiating the level of the clinical work required from different categories of nursing personnel produces an appropriate fit among patient needs and requirements, and nursing competencies and compensation.

The need to differentiate nurses by their knowledge and clinical competence is increasing, and efforts have been made to determine the feasibility of implementing such an approach within nursing delivery settings. At the same time, the concerns of those managing and paying for health care have changed to focus more directly on issues of quality and effectiveness in clinical practice, requiring an examination of the outcomes of care delivery. In describing the tenets of accountable practice, Zander (1985) notes that professional practice is enhanced by changing the locus of accountability for outcomes of patient care. She describes the following tenets:

- The product of nursing service is not nursing care, but rather the outcomes of care — more specifically, the expected results of nursing interventions.
- The nurse as a manager of a caseload of patients uses a systematic production method, called the nursing process, by which outcomes are produced.
- The responsibility of nursing administration is to maintain and improve the production process so that the nurses' work in actualizing patient outcomes is attainable and satisfying.

Strengthening Nursing Practice Through Innovative Practice Models

Over the years, national commissions, task forces, and other groups have examined issues related to the growth and stability of nursing. A variety of groups have suggested numerous solutions to the recurrent nurse shortages, most of which were not implemented (Moritz, Hinshaw, and Heinrich, 1989). Suggestions for modifying nursing practice itself began in 1973, when the National Commission for the Study of Nursing and Nursing Education (commonly called the "Lysaught Commission") made recommendations for nursing practice that included:

- reexamination of nursing practice to decrease non-nursing functions and increase the time clinical nurses have for direct patient care,
- establishment of a Joint Practice Commission to increase dialogue and clarify the roles of physicians and nurses, and
- the creation of nursing as a full partner in shaping health policy.

Ten years later, while examining the adequacy of the numbers of nurses nationwide, the National Commission on Nursing (1983) and the Institute of Medicine of the National Academy of Sciences (1983) echoed these recommendations and called for a substantial reorganization of clinical nursing and the environments in which it is practiced.

More recently, the U.S. Department of Health and Human Services Secretary's Commission on Nursing (1988), which determined that the current nursing shortage reflects a demand rather than a decline in the number of nurses, also echoed these recommendations by indicating a need for change in how nursing practice is structured, how interdisciplinary professional relationships should be modified, how management should support nursing practice, and increased involvement by nurses in governance groups. As long ago as 1923, a concern for "time wasted in non-nursing duties," an essential component of the demand issue, was expressed in the landmark Goldmark Report. It was this report's recommendations that lay the foundation for professional nursing practice as it is known today (Goldmark, 1923).

In another study of the nursing shortages of the early 1980s, Murphy (1989) concluded that there were common recommendations related to nursing practice, including:

- Nursing should be involved in policy development and all levels of decision making.
- Interdisciplinary collaboration should be fostered.
- Allocation and management of resources should be nursing's responsibility.
- Nurses should be involved in decision making about patient care, management, and governance of the organization.

- Nurses should design, implement, and evaluate changing organizational structures and care delivery methods.
- Salaries and benefits should be commensurate with the level of responsibility; career advancement should be promoted.

The findings and recommendations from the various groups that have studied nursing and its recurrent shortages over the years have demonstrated a remarkable degree of congruence, most recently highlighted in the results from the State of the Science Conference on Nursing Resources and the Delivery of Patient Care held in 1988. This conference (National Center for Nursing Research, 1989) noted that the time had come to examine what was known about nurse shortages, to explore the effect of the available nursing resources on patient care delivery, and to evaluate the costs and benefits of bringing about the necessary changes. The conference findings noted that:

- The shortages exist in part because of the problems associated with substituting nurses for other workers.
- Patient care can be expected to suffer when nurses are unable to care for patients due to time spent in substitution activities.
- The availability of appropriate support staff and systems enable nurses to focus on their clinical responsibilities and facilitate quality patient care.

The conference findings also indicated that interdisciplinary collaboration between nurses and physicians has a positive effect on outcomes and needs to be encouraged. The level of competency among clinicians was also found to have a positive effect on outcomes.

The Magnet Hospital Study (McClure et al., 1983) described working environments which were successful in attracting nurses to practice there. Kramer and Schmalenberg (1988), in a recent examination of a selected group of these magnet hospitals, reconfirmed the approaches to nursing care delivery and to the nurses employed in them that directly affect the retention and quality of care delivered. The hospital environments where nurses were successfully recruited and retained, and which were described at the State of the Science Conference (Kramer, 1988), share a profile that includes:

- a high ratio of RNs;
- well-prepared clinical and managerial staffs;

- self-governance with considerable involvement in decision making;
- limited use of new graduates;
- little or no floating;
- salaries rather than wages, with flexible benefits;
- flexible or self-scheduling; and
- flat decentralized administrative structure.

In these environments, nurses were valued as professional colleagues who contributed to the quality of care delivery and made a unique contribution to care outcomes through their professional nursing practice.

The Innovative Nursing Practice Models research program of the NCNR was designed to build on these findings and recommendations. The program's goals were to stimulate change in the hospital practice environments so that innovative practice models could flourish, and to facilitate the movement of what was known from research outcomes into practice through a coordinated study effort. The studies in this program were designed to take into account the environment in which nursing practice is carried out, the environment that enables professional practice, the means to measure change in patient care delivery and the quality of patient outcomes, the compensation packages offered, and the actual and perceived roles of nurses who practice in hospitals. In other words, the program was designed to support and evaluate practice models that achieved the following:

- Restructured nursing practice and the environments in which nursing practice occurs so that nurses could practice at the highest level of their professional competence.
- Directly linked nursing practice, both clinical and managerial, to measures of quality and effectiveness of outcomes.
- Changed compensation to reflect position requirements, clinical competence requirements, and quality of care provided (Moritz, Hinshaw, and Heinrich, 1989).

The overall stimulus for initiating and evaluating these practice models was what I have come to describe as the "desired near future" of nurses in clinical practice. Included are:

- Autonomy and independence in practice.
- Clinical environments that foster quality patient care.

- Compensation and benefits appropriate to the complexity of the work.
- Work environments that foster competent clinical practice, including management structures and processes that facilitate innovation.
- Career advancement and professional recognition.

Three models (in Arizona, New York, and Baltimore) are currently being implemented and evaluated — two are to be discussed in this paper. The Arizona and New York studies are companion research demonstration projects, stimulated by an NCNR request for grant applications.

The Group Professional Practice Model, implemented in Arizona with seven participating hospitals, demonstrates certain components of differentiated practice, group governance, and cultural change. The restructuring of the hospital environment is at the unit level and is designed to enable group practice, decentralized decision making, and peer review. At each implementation site, committees have been formed to ensure ownership. A professional salary structure is planned as a component of shared governance, with a recognition program that will reward innovation and quality performance. The model's impact will be evaluated through both patient and cost outcomes. Examples of patient outcomes include infections, complications, length of stay, and patient satisfaction.

The Enhanced Professional Practice Model being implemented in New York incorporates staff nurse control over practice and resources at the unit level, increased participation in decision making, flexible work hours, interdisciplinary care and discharge planning that facilitates continuity of care through follow up at home, and a salary and benefit program that compensates according to level of responsibility and professional development. The model capitalizes on the capability and leadership of the existing nursing staffs to determine the best means for providing nursing care. It does not attempt to implement a single strategy across all hospitals. With the model components and the staff education strategies planned, it is anticipated that the individual nursing staffs will move toward a competency-based nursing practice that will be unique to each setting.

These two studies share unique features as well as commonalities. It is the commonalities in the models that allow examination of findings across the studies. Among these commonalities are: evaluation of the effect of changes on quality of care, patient outcomes (such as length of stay, infection rates, and patient satisfaction), and costs incurred through the implementation of competency-based practice strategies; staff nurse control over practice; increased participation in clinical and administrative decision making; control over scheduling; and compensation based on salary rather than wages.

The third model being studied was established to determine the effectiveness of the Professional Practice for Nursing Model at the Johns Hopkins Hospital in Baltimore. This model has been implemented on some of the hospital units over several years and will continue to be implemented during the study. The model consists of formal contract negotiation by a nurse and the hospital, in which the nurse agrees to provide 24-hour nursing care to patients on a particular unit in exchange for self-management and a salary. The nursing unit staff is organized to function as a cohesive whole through self-governance. Patient and cost outcomes are being evaluated, including such indicators as continuity of care, patient satisfaction, nurse satisfaction, and group cohesion.

A new NCNR effort in the area of innovative practice models is being implemented as a result of our recent collaborative effort with two other federal agencies to stimulate studies that include demonstration and evaluation of community-based nursing practice models targeted to minority populations. Three studies are being funded: two by the combined efforts of the NCNR and the Division of Nursing, and one by the new Agency for Health Care Policy and Research.

Nursing's Impact on Patient Outcomes

After several years of tight cost controls through the implementation of the Prospective Payment System for Medicare, policy makers have begun to question the quality, appropriateness, and effectiveness of the health care that is being provided in hospitals, nursing homes, and through formal home health care services. Quality of care and patient outcomes have recently become of great interest. As the nursing shortage continues, there is a growing focus on the impact of nursing practice on patient outcomes, and a growing recognition that variance in the patient outcomes cannot be explained by examining physician practice alone. Although the independent functions in each health profession are not questioned, the interdependent relationships among them are now being appreciated, and evaluative structures are being implemented. In order to respond to this changing emphasis, nursing needs to demonstrate the impact of care provided by its practitioners by measuring outcomes of patient care that reflect nursing practice.

Nursing has a long history of involvement in patient outcomes. A seminal work in this area was the Roberts and Hudson (1964) monograph, *How to Study Patient Progress.* The first chapter raises the question, "Why study patient progress?" The authors point out that such information assists in assessing patient needs, reviewing agency policies and programs, and evaluating an agency's care delivery and staff performance. An earlier text on the economics of nursing (Committee on the Grading of Nursing Schools, 1934) also asks the question, "are patients satisfied?", and discusses how to assess the patient situation so as to answer the question.

Horn and Swain (1977), using Orem's conceptual model, developed criteria measures or outcomes that could be applied across several populations. They also developed the reliability and validity for a large number of items. At approximately the same time, Haussman and Hegyvary (1976) were writing their series of monographs on monitoring the quality of nursing care. More recent work has focused on the development of instruments for measuring client outcomes (Strickland and Waltz, 1988), on measures for home care outcomes (Rinke, 1987), on a classification of outcome measures relevant to nursing care (Marek, 1988), and on a synthesis of nursing literature to develop a classification of patient outcomes (Lang and Marek, 1990). These works provided a starting point from which to examine outcome measures that reflect nursing practice. The NCNR has begun to assess the readiness of nursing researchers and others within nursing to undertake this effort.

When the NCNR was organized, no other federal agency had a specific patient care research mission. In December 1989, the Agency for Health Care Policy and Research (AHCPR) came into being with a mandate to implement a Medical Treatment Effectiveness Program that has both a research and a practice guideline development component. The purpose of this program is to improve effectiveness and appropriateness of health care services through better understanding of the effects of health practices on patient outcomes. In spite of its name, this program is focused on health care provided by all practitioners (Agency for Health Care Policy and Research, 1990a).

Through the National Nursing Advisory Group, this agency has sought assistance in describing the potential nursing components of patient outcomes, specifically for practice guideline development. As a result of this group's work, the term "clinical condition" is used instead of a specific diagnostic term. A clinical condition is defined as a patient problem that can be a nursing diagnosis, a medical diagnosis, a diagnosis made and treated by another health care provider (such as a social worker), or a combination of diagnoses (Agency for Health Care Policy and Research, 1990b). This approach has opened the doors to clinical conditions that relate more directly to nursing than to medicine. It also has facilitated conditions more specifically focused on medical practice. Development of specific practice guidelines is now underway.

Seven panels have been implemented, three of which have nurse scientists as chairs or co-chairs. Examples of those panels with nursing leaders include: pain management; urinary incontinence in the adult; and prediction, prevention, and early treatment of pressure sores in adults. The companion Medical Effectiveness Research Program has the goal of improving the effectiveness and appropriateness of clinical practice by developing, evaluating, and disseminating scientific information regarding the effects of presently used health care services and procedures for patients' survival, health status, functional capacity, and quality of life (Agency for Health Care Policy and Research, 1990a). Currently funded research focused on patient outcomes includes assessment of back pain, total knee replacement, acute myocardial infarction, stroke prevention, and drug-related hospitalizations among older people.

To assess whether there is a unique nursing research perspective that could complement this AHCPR effort, the NCNR convened a small group of nurse scientists in May 1990 to review the current status of research on quality and effectiveness of nursing practice, and on patient outcomes; and to assist in determining an approach for a patient care initiative in the area of patient outcomes research. The goals of this planning group were to:

- articulate the scientific issues,
- examine the content for a research focus,
- assess the relevance of existing resources and methodologies for nursing practice-focused outcomes research, and
- recommend strategies for an NCNR patient outcomes research initiative.

The group adopted the concepts provided in a background paper by Dr. Sue Hegyvary (1991), in which she noted, "In concept, patient care outcomes are the end results of treatments." She also proposed the idea that outcomes are defined indicators that reflect the results of clinical practice, most particularly the implementation of nursing interventions in response to a nursing assessment.

The planning group participants strongly supported direct NCNR involvement in patient outcomes research, emphasizing the importance of collaborative activities with AHCPR, other federal agencies, and private sector groups. A framework for developing an NCNR Patient Outcomes Research Program was developed. It included activities for:

- assessing the current state of outcomes research related to nursing practice for the purpose of identifying fertile areas for short-term and long-term emphases;
- supporting an organized program of patient outcomes research based on the emphases identified when outcomes are assessed; and
- supporting research training for new investigators, as well as for those at mid-career who are either interested in adding this area of inquiry to their research or who need training in the measurement issues relevant to this area of research.

The definition of patient outcomes measures has been shifting and broadening from the traditional base of mortality, morbidity, and disability to include quality of life, length of stay, health status, and patient satisfaction. The planning group expressed the need for the identification of nursing-sensitive outcome measures. From my perspective, there are two major approaches to be considered.

One approach is to focus on organization studies by examining structures and processes using variables that could show the effect of nursing practice on patient outcomes at the aggregate level. This can mean, for example, examining decision-making structures and staffing patterns for nurses in intensive care units and their effect on certain outcomes, such as medication errors, length of stay, or even mortality.

The second emphasis is a more clinical one, focusing on validating and comparing nursing interventions to determine their effectiveness and appropriateness for a specific clinical condition. This could include examining the linkages between nursing assessment, nursing intervention, and outcomes for two behavioral interventions for presurgical anxiety. Regarding this more clinical focus on patient outcomes inherent in nursing research, there is considerable work to be done in determining the best measures to reflect the outcomes of practice.

At this time, the NCNR staff are planning a conference to assess the state of the science on patient outcomes research related to clinical nursing practice. AHCPR is also planning a broad-based conference to examine the current status of outcomes research. We anticipate holding the NCNR conference after this broader review has been completed so that duplication does not occur. For the NCNR conference, there are many issues to be identified and explored, as well as aspects of nursing inquiry to be considered as they relate to a successful practice outcome initiative within nursing science.

In summary, I have reviewed the development and evaluation of innovative practice models and the emerging strategies for the evaluation of the impact of nursing practice on patient outcomes as a backdrop for the discussions of the innovative practice models being currently implemented and evaluated in Arizona and New York.

❑   ❑   ❑

Evaluating the Impact of Enhanced Professional Practice on Patient Outcome

Gail L. Ingersoll, Ed.D., R.N., presenter
Sheila A. Ryan, Ph.D., R.N., F.A.A.N., co-investigator
Alison W. Schultz, M.S., R.N., co-investigator

An Enhanced Professional Practice Model of Nursing Care Delivery is being implemented in three hospitals in New York. The intent of the model is to create an environment in which professional nurses can practice according to their educational and experiential preparation. Five conceptual components of the model have been defined:

1) control over practice,
2) continuing education responsive to staff nurse need,
3) continuity of care delivery,
4) collaborative practice, and
5) professional compensation package reflective of education and experience.

Preparation of this paper was supported by Cooperative Agreement Award Number U01 NR 02156 from the National Center for Nursing Research, National Institutes of Health and the Division of Nursing, Health Resources and Services Administration. Its contents are solely the responsibility of the authors and do not necessarily represent official views of the awarding agencies.

Background

Studies of nurse retention and satisfaction have been directed toward surveying staff nurses and administrators to determine the environmental and personal variables affecting nurses' decisions to stay or leave the work setting. Limited attention has been paid to the effect of these variables on patient care delivery. Even less has been directed toward evaluating programs in which the factors are implemented to determine whether they actually make a difference in nursing practice and patient care delivery.

Studies of nurse retention and turnover have identified several factors that contribute to dissatisfaction and movement of nurses from one position to another. The most stable across- studies factor is age, with younger nurses more likely than older ones to change jobs within two years of hire (Donovan, 1980; Lowery and Jacobsen, 1984; McCloskey, 1974; Seybolt, Pavett, and Walker, 1978; Simpson, 1985; Slavett et al., 1979; Weisman, Alexander, and Chase, 1980). Additional personal characteristics include lack of autonomy (Deets and Froebe, 1984; McCloskey and McBain, 1987; Mottaz, 1988; Seybolt, Pavett, and Walker, 1978; Simpson, 1985; Weisman, Alexander and Chase, 1980), limited education (Donovan, 1980; Froebe, Deets, and Knox, 1983; McCloskey and McBain, 1987; Seybolt, Pavett, and Walker, 1978; Wandelt, Pierce, and Widdowsen, 1981), career advancement opportunity (Cronin-Stubbs, 1977; Everly and Falcione, 1976; McCloskey, 1974; McCloskey and McBain, 1987; Wandelt, Pierce, and Widdowsen, 1981), lack of achievement and recognition (Cronin-Stubbs, 1977; Deets and Froebe, 1984; Donovan, 1980; Froebe, Deets, and Knox, 1983; McCloskey, 1974; McCloskey and McBain, 1987; Seybolt, Pavett, and Walker, 1978; Simpson, 1985), interpersonal relationships (Cronin-Stubbs, 1977; Everly and Falcione, 1976; Froebe, Deets, and Knox, 1983; Godfrey, 1978; Wandelt, Pierce, and Widdowsen, 1981), and locus of control (Weisman, Alexander, and Chase, 1980).

A variable labeled "intent to leave" has been identified as a strong predictor of staff turnover in two studies (McCloskey and McBain, 1987; Weisman, Alexander, and Chase, 1981). This "intent," however, is a second-stage outcome of precipitating factors that have prompted consideration of alternate employment options.

Environmental factors predictive of nurse dissatisfaction and turnover are pay (Deets and Froebe, 1984; Donovan, 1980; Everly and Falcione, 1976; Froebe, Deets, and Knox, 1983; Mottaz, 1988;

Seybolt, Pavett, and Walker, 1978; Wandelt, Pierce, and Widdow-sen, 1981); type of organizational structure, whether primary, team, or functional nursing (Froebe, Deets and Knox, 1983); and daily work assignment (Hinshaw, Smeltzer, and Atwood, 1987; Weisman, Alexander, and Chase, 1981). Leadership responsiveness also appears as an important contributor to staff satisfaction (Everly and Falcione, 1976; Godfrey, 1978; McCloskey and McBain, 1987; Mottaz, 1988; Wandelt, Pierce, and Widdowsen, 1981; Weisman, Alexander, and Chase, 1981) and perceived autonomy (Alexander, Weisman, and Chase, 1982).

In studies of quality of care delivery, similar structural and attitu-dinal variables have been reported to be associated with quality of care. Haussmann, Hegyvary, and Newman (1976) studied contex-tual variables, which they describe as those pertaining to hospital characteristics, and unit staff attitudinal variables to determine the influence of these factors on patient outcome. The investigators found that no single variable was associated with nursing care qual-ity. Unit staff attitudes were less likely to influence outcome than were staff mix on the unit, number of patients, volume of care required, and type of unit organizational structure. Higher-quality units, however, did have more favorable unit staff attitudes. Staff reported they had better quality leadership and were more satisfied with their jobs. Unfortunately, the two-month period of data collec-tion was too short to allow for prediction of whether or not these attitudes positively affect nursing retention.

The study most often cited for its description of factors that enhance staff nurse retention is the Magnet Hospitals Study, con-ducted in 1981-82 by the American Academy of Nursing Task Force on Nursing Practice in Hospitals (McClure et al., 1983). The investi-gators surveyed staff and leadership at the magnet hospitals and identified several conditions perceived to be desirable for nursing practice.

Principal among the factors were management style; an organi-zational structure that facilitated professional practice, personnel policies, and programs that were equal to or superior to those of other hospitals; and the presence of professional models of practice that allowed for accountability, autonomy, and direct monitoring of care delivery. Staff nurses reported being able to practice the kind of nursing they believed to be essential to high-quality patient care. Moreover, they perceived themselves to be contributing to the overall health and well-being of their communities through their associations with the magnet hospitals.

As an outcome of this study, the investigators made several recommendations for improving practice in hospitals. These included attendance to both personal and professional needs of staff nurses, developing organizational goals reflective of the values of all members of the system, assurance of congruence between leadership and staff nurses' role expectations, and allowance for staff nurse participation in the control and direction of nursing practice. A systematic method for implementing and evaluating these recommendations has yet to be developed and tested. Consequently, the potential impact of the study has yet to be fully realized.

The Enhanced Professional Practice Model combines positive retention factors identified in previous research. The intent is to test the effect of this comprehensive model on nurse satisfaction, retention, quality of care, and cost in a 720-bed urban medical center, a 120-bed community hospital, and a 62-bed rural hospital.

Description of the Model

Expectancy theory has served as the framework for the model's development. According to expectancy theory, nurses perform better and are less dissatisfied with their work environment when they identify a direct link between their work efforts and high level performance (Seybolt, 1979). This framework was selected since inability to meet personal care delivery standards was cited as a major contributor to turnover in a recent study of nurse satisfaction.

The model focuses on the organizational factors that can be modified to facilitate staff nurse control over practice. These include participation in decision making (Alexander, Weisman, and Chase, 1982), adequate training for the demands of the job (Bailey, Steffen, and Grout, 1980), adequate support services to eliminate the need for completion of non-nursing tasks (Kent and Warner, n.d.; Witzel and Sovie, 1987), adequate staffing mix to meet the needs of the patient population (Hinshaw, Smeltzer, and Atwood, 1987; Kent and Warner, n.d.; Weisman, Alexander, and Chase, 1981), support for professional development (Cronin-Stubbs, 1977; Everly and Falcione, 1976; McCloskey, 1974; McCloskey and McBain, 1987; Simpson, 1985), and a compensation package that is appropriate for the educational and work demands of the position (Deets and

Froebe, 1984; Donovan, 1980; McCloskey and McBain, 1987; Mottaz, 1988; Seybolt, Pavett, and Walker, 1978; Wandelt, Pierce, and Widdowsen, 1981).

Evaluation of Effect

Quantitative and qualitative data are being collected to determine the impact of the model's implementation on nurse satisfaction and retention, and on quality of care and cost. Structure, process, and outcome indicators are being used to monitor change in practice behavior and effect on care delivery. The evaluation plan is a comprehensive one that uses multiple approaches to monitor changes directly attributable to the model, as well as to activities external to the project. Since the study is taking place in hospitals that are dynamic in their own approaches to improving work environments for nurses, clearly identifying the effect of the Enhanced Professional Practice Model is a challenge.

Nevertheless, we have instituted several measures to monitor the effect of the model implementation. Data are being collected from units in which the model is being implemented, as well as from units comparable in terms of staffing and patient mix, annual staff nurse attrition rates, and organizational environment. Medical center units have been matched with other units within the same institution. Community and rural units have been matched with units in hospitals located in similar locales and offering comparable patient support services.

Base-line data suggest experimental and comparison units are similar for all demographic factors, with the exception of usual shifts worked. Differences between the medical center, community hospital, and rural hospital are measured as to age (with younger nurses being employed by the medical center), marital status (with single employees being most evident in the medical center), basic RN preparation (with the medical center having a greater proportion of BSN staff), and usual shift worked (see Table 1).

We are measuring the outcome of the project by monitoring staff nurse turnover, professional advancement activities, quality of care delivery, and cost to the institution. Included in the patient outcome assessment is satisfaction with hospital experience, morbidity, mortality, length of hospital stay, and need for unplanned readmission within seven to 30 days of discharge.

Cost of care delivery is being determined according to nursing care cost per patient day. Cost of implementing the model is being determined through ongoing process evaluation. This process evaluation segment has been an important addition to the project and is providing us with considerable data about the work required to institute a major innovation in an existing work environment. It includes observation of staff nurse interaction with patients and coworkers, monitoring of implementation planning meetings, document review, and focus group sessions. We also are interviewing chief nurse and chief executive officers and physicians to remain informed about what occurrences within the hospitals could influence the outcome of the project. In addition, we have identified three key sources who are interviewed every six months concerning local, state, and national health care activities.

Quantitative and qualitative methods are being used to measure the effect of the model on variables of interest. Quantitative methods include the use of multiple questionnaires and review of existing documents and data bases. Qualitative methods include nonparticipant observation, structured and unstructured interview, focus groups, document analysis, and review of project participant logs. Qualitative data collection was added during the first year of the project to:

- describe the culture of the experimental and comparison units and how they change over time;
- provide a context for interpretation of the quantitative data;
- describe the process of model implementation in the experimental units; and
- identify the individual, unit, and organizational response to the model and its implementation.

To monitor progression toward and final achievement of intervention outcome, the project team identified a series of one-year, two-year, and three-year benchmark indicators for each component of the model. To do so, we worked backwards from our expectation of a positive result at the end of the project. We envisioned the first year of the implementation as involving assessment and planning; the second as focusing on implementation, evaluation, and refinement; and the third as being a time of stabilization and demonstration of a verifiable short-term effect. For each component, we devised a working definition and identified assumptions about why

306

the component was integral to enhanced professional practice and what was intended by including this component in the overall plan. We also determined how each indicator would be measured — whether through qualitative or quantitative means, or a combination of both.

An example of a benchmark indicator for one element of the model component "control over practice" relates to staff nurses' perception of ability to manage patient care delivery and the environment in which care is delivered. By the end of the first year, indication of attainment of that outcome would be staff nurses' identification of what control over practice means to them and how measures can be implemented on their unit so that it is achieved. The project team is measuring this indicator through monitoring meeting minutes, reviewing documents, and holding focus group sessions. By the end of the second year, implementation of changes identified by staff nurses should be evident. Nonparticipant field observation and focus group methods are used to measure extent of attainment. By end of the third year, control over practice is demonstrated by nurse behavior and response to formal questioning. Focus groups, nonparticipant observation, and questionnaire response will be used to evaluate effect.

This ability to control practice is hypothesized to be an important contributor to nurse satisfaction and quality of care. As one staff nurse noted during an initial focus group session, "It does not matter how many rungs you put on some professional career ladder if you still make me call the supervisor at night before I can contact a physician about a patient problem." Not allowing nurses to complete the full cycle in the patient care delivery process thwarts professional responsibility and sets up unnecessary barriers to quality patient care.

Issues Associated with Measuring Effect

Because this project involves implementing and measuring a major innovation in diverse hospitals, a number of issues have arisen associated with both the demonstration and the research aspects of the project:

- identifying appropriate methods for measuring direct and indirect effect of the intervention,

- clearly distinguishing between the demonstration component and the research component of the project when team members are discussing both,
- communicating with numerous individuals at sites removed away from project headquarters,
- working with hospitals with varying degrees of experience in implementing innovative care delivery approaches,
- motivating key personnel at sites,
- collecting comparable data from five hospitals in which availability of existing information differs significantly,
- using persuasion rather than legitimate power to ensure that all components of the model are implemented, and
- conducting research in dynamic settings in which multiple activities occur daily that affect the project and its successful completion.

Creating working definitions and identifying specific methods for measuring each component of the model have been difficult. Components represent broad concepts, and existing measurement tools and descriptions of professional practice factors tend to be specific and useful — evaluating limited aspects within the concept. Moreover, common definitions for outcome measures such as quality of care and professional identity do not exist.

Quality of care measurement tools are time-consuming to implement. For a comprehensive study in which quality of care is but one element of a multioutcome approach, such tools are not feasible because of the time required for completion. Therefore, we have elected to use hospital nursing standards of practice as our criteria for assessment of quality of care. Although we recognized certain limitations inherent in this approach, we chose this method for several reasons:

- The standards have been approved by the Joint Commission on Accreditation of Health Care Organizations (JCAHO), suggesting that they are adequate to meet the specifications of an agency that is responsible for monitoring quality of care.
- Although the sophistication of the forms varies across institutions, the content is based on the same standards for care delivery.

- This approach was used in the hospital settings prior to the study's introduction and will be used once the study is complete.

In addition to monitoring morbidity, mortality, and changes in length of stay over time, we also are collecting patient satisfaction data as an indication of perception of quality of care. Efforts to identify a useful tool for measuring patient satisfaction have forced us to develop our own. Despite the project team's reluctance to develop instruments during the course of the study and our desire to use existing instruments with proven reliability and validity, our dissatisfaction with available patient satisfaction measures led to this decision. We also considered using tools in existence at each of the institutions, but these were determined to be insufficient to meet our needs. The tool we are developing is based on Swanson-Kauffman's (1986) caring model, and has recently undergone a second round of analysis based on sample patients from experimental and comparison units. Preliminary analysis findings are favorable, and our intent is to reduce the tool to 25 items following additional internal consistency and factor analysis.

Scales measuring existing professionalism (we are using the Snizek adaptation of the Hall Professionalism Scale) focus on attitudes about occupation (Snizek, 1972). Missing are indications of professional practice behavior that clarify how a nurse with strong professional attitudes approaches care delivery and interacts with others. Our definition of professional identity is broader, and includes how fully professional nurses make decisions about care delivery. This concept, similar to Benner's (1984) description of a nurse with expert clinical knowledge, is broader still — implying commitment to patients and colleagues, and a willingness to be creative in developing new approaches to patient care delivery and problem solving.

Keeping the research and demonstration aspects of the project separate has required ongoing discussion. We have debated whether to allow information obtained from the study to be included in decisions about implementation or to use work already underway during implementation activities to guide the research plan. If information obtained from research activities is used to modify implementation approach, the evaluation component becomes part of the intervention. If information about how the implementation is either working or not working is kept separate from implementation activities, the program implementers miss the opportunity to take early corrective action.

Our decision has been to use a middle-of-the-road approach and to consider carefully the implications of our actions each time an issue arises. In general, we are not using quantitative data to measure staff satisfaction, quality of care, or cost in considerations about model implementation. We are using some data identified through focus groups, nonparticipant observation, review of participant logs, and interviews to take corrective implementation action. Most recently, the project director who has primary responsibility for model implementation observed tensions arising during a meeting of experimental unit nurse managers. They were discussing their perceived responsibility for overseeing the work and their adjustments to role changes. Prior to this time, the research plan had included only focus groups to measure staff nurse perceptions about the effect of model implementation. Focus groups had not been planned for the management group. Instead, seminars to discuss strategies for adapting to role change had been designed for these individuals.

The project director's observations led us to believe that the nurse managers needed an opportunity to express their feelings about what was happening around them. As a result, a focus group was implemented for the nurse managers. Although they were not as disclosing during the session as had been hoped, they conveyed perceptions that they had not had an opportunity to meet regularly to offer each other support and to discuss difficult issues. Despite several sessions designed by the project team explicitly for this purpose, they were not perceived by the nurse managers as meeting their needs for support. The project team then implemented measures to assure that nurse manager work sessions were clearly differentiated from nurse manager support sessions. In this example, the demonstration aspect influenced the research aspect, ultimately feeding back to the demonstration. Modifications were made in both components based on information obtained in each.

Establishing consistent data retrieval mechanisms at sites has been difficult. Our original plans to collect data for three years prior to the initiation of the study had to be dropped. The data for most of the variables simply were not available. Particularly difficult to gather was information pertaining to preintervention quality, continuity, and cost of care delivery.

Initial plans to monitor care according to common diagnosis related groups (DRGs) were also a problem. Instead, we have elected to monitor care delivery by a random sampling of all unit admissions. We arrived at this decision because of the difficulty in identifying common DRGs and because of the direction being taken on the units in case managed care for certain patient populations. The patient groups being selected to receive case managed care are not necessarily those with the most frequent DRGs. Consequently, we are concerned that by focusing on one group or another we would overlook important changes in the quality of care delivered to all patients on the unit. Since we are interested in the outcome of the model on patient care delivery on the unit, we are still ultimately concerned with the need to measure its full effect.

Monitoring the model's true effect in dynamic institutions in which retention activities are underway (independent of those associated with the project) has proved to be a major methodologic issue. Although this problem was identified early in the project's development, its potential extent was not. Moreover, nursing leaders at some of the sites have stated that although they are initiating innovations separate from the project, the impetus for the changes comes from the project team in their institutions. The activity of the research team and the team's methods for facilitating change have been the determining factor in actualizing the ancillary activities. This unanticipated effect, which we have identified as "creating an environment for change," is an important consideration for researchers and administrators alike who are contemplating joining research teams with nursing practice.

This positive association between research team and hospital nursing personnel is producing several additional unanticipated effects. Members of the research team have been approached at local and national meetings by colleagues of the study units' staff and leadership. These nurses have heard about the project through their friends and are seeking information about how to implement similar innovations in their own institutions. Experimental hospitals are identifying the project in recruitment advertisements and are marketing themselves to area schools of nursing as being the sites of a major, federally-funded nursing research project. Further, the director of nursing and the nurse manager of the experimental unit at the community hospital have requested information about doctoral study. Although both these nurse leaders are highly motivated and are likely to continue their education at some point in the future, the project and the climate for change it has created have provided the impetus for their immediate actions.

Summary and Recommendations

The Enhanced Professional Practice Model has been designed to remove recognized barriers to control over practice and to encourage staff nurse autonomy, accountability, and professional role identity. Although the issues associated with implementing and evaluating a major innovation in hospitals are considerable, the potential for positive outcomes — both anticipated and unanticipated — is very real.

❏　　❏　　❏

Table 1

ANOVA for Experimental and Comparison Hospitals by Group (Experimental and Comparison) and by Place (Medical Center, Community Hospital, and Rural Hospital)

Variable	(N = 284)	F Value	PR > F
• Age			
Place		3.79	0.02 *
Group		0.47	0.49
• Marital Status			
Place		5.79	0.003 *
Group		2.13	0.15
• Nursing Position			
Place		0.34	0.71
Group		0.19	0.66
• Basic RN Education			
Place		8.86	0.0002 *
Group		0.28	0.59
• Years in Nursing			
Place		2.76	0.06
Group		0.21	0.65
• Usual Shift Assignment			
Place		25.57	0.0001 *
Group		11.66	0.0007 *

*p < .05

Creating and Extending Successful Innovations: Practice and Policy Implications

Susan B. Meister, Ph.D., R.N., F.A.A.N.
Suzanne L. Feetham, Ph.D., R.N., F.A.A.N.
Shirley Girouard, Ph.D., R.N., F.A.A.N.
Barbara A. Durand, Ed.D., R.N.,C., F.A.A.N.

T he ability of the nursing profession to exert direct influence on health policy depends in large measure on convincing policy makers that nursing practice models can ameliorate health problems. Innovative nursing interventions with significant policy implications have emerged in select instances (Brooten, Kumar, and Brown, 1986; Milio, 1970). Frequently, however, knowledge of practice models and their effectiveness remains at the point of service resulting in limited dissemination and influence.

The purpose of this paper is threefold:

1) to present two health policy frameworks in which to analyze innovative nursing practice models;
2) to describe within these frameworks a successful nursing practice innovation focusing on the planning, implementation, and, most importantly, extension of the nursing model; and

The views expressed in this article are those of the author; no official endorsement by The Robert Wood Johnson Foundation is implied or should be inferred.

3) to place this process in a larger context by considering the implications of innovative nursing practice models in terms of practice, research, and national health policy.

This paper provides examples of the types of contributions nurses can make when their innovative ideas and practices are incorporated into institutional and governmental policy. Nurses often are instrumental in the introduction and testing of innovative approaches to patient care problems. However, in this process, new methods of delivering patient care and responding to health care issues rarely become "institutionalized" through policy channels.

Challenge, Context, and Resolution

A primary goal of nursing is to promote the health of all people. To achieve this goal, nurses must act at a number of different levels, including individual, organizational, and societal levels. They must continue to expand their sphere of influence beyond the level of patient/client service (Butterfield, 1990; Milio, 1983; Milio, 1989).

Nurses are becoming increasingly aware of how health policies influence the structure and financing of health care services and their ability to deliver nursing care. This awareness has led to changes in the amount of activity by nurses in the policy-making process, both within their institutions and at all levels of federal and state governments. Although the number of nurses involved in the development and implementation of policy is growing, the full potential of nurse participation in this area has yet to be realized (Milio, 1984; Milio, 1989).

If the contributions or innovations of nurses are to influence patient care, the health care system, and policy, several steps must be taken. The innovations must first be disseminated, replicated, and generalized, then adopted and institutionalized. Dissemination must extend beyond occasional publications in nursing journals or presentations at nursing conferences. Innovations should be shared with other health care professionals, policy makers, and the general public if they are to be available for use by others. Once others know of the innovations, nurses should assist in their adoption by providing technical assistance for replication. Nurses also must take steps to see that nursing innovations become incorporated into the policies of established health care institutions, insurance companies, and federal and state governments. Nursing innovations that are made part of the process or structure of care are more likely to be sustained beyond the period of the project or current administration. Therefore, dissemination and adoption strategies must be considered during the planning and implementation of innovative programs to ensure their institutionalization.

Policy Process and Context

The six-step process used to influence policy outcomes in institutional settings and at any level of government is similar to the six step nursing process for providing patient care. Therefore, developing policy based on innovative approaches to health care issues can be based on the process used during the development of a patient care plan. The context in which the innovation is being proposed must be considered in all phases of the policy process (see Table 1).

The six-step policy process should guide the transformation of nursing innovations from idea to policy. The first step — the identification or formation of the problem — is based on the perception of a need that could be addressed through an intervention applicable to a variety of situations. For example, a nurse working in the inner city recognizes the need for primary care among the children receiving day care and develops an innovative program of total services in collaboration with the Visiting Nurses Association (Milio, 1970). The nurse recognizes that support for the program will have to be provided by the city and state governments. The next step, then, is to enlist the support of governmental agencies and to contact policy makers willing to place this problem on their agendas.

When the problem has been recognized and put on the policy agenda, the policy must then be formulated. Possible solutions are identified and presented as alternatives. In the day care example, the nurse might suggest that present policies do not incorporate health prevention, thus resulting in preventible problems that burden the child, family, and society.

In the next phase of the process, policy makers must be convinced to adopt the proposed innovation by incorporating it into legislation or regulation. After the policy is accepted (for example, a law has been passed), bureaucratic or institutional mechanisms implement the policy.

The final step in the policy and nursing processes is the evaluation phase. In this phase, the effects of the innovation or policy are assessed and then refined and made more appropriate to the needs of the constituents.

Nurses can incorporate policy-related concerns into the conceptualization, implementation, and evaluation of their innovations. To better direct this effort, a few questions must be asked about the difference the innovation may make:

- Will the innovation improve health outcomes?
- What outcome or effect will the innovation have on health care services and their costs?
- Which institutions, agencies of government, and levels of government might be interested in the innovation?
- How will the innovation be shared and disseminated?
- How can the innovation be made a permanent component of practice and/or education?

Meeting the Challenge: Frameworks and Applications

This next section describes an innovative nursing model that was developed, implemented, and evaluated with attention to the institutional and governmental policies that would make it a permanent service for children with chronic illness in two communities.

The essence of an innovation is defined by the service it delivers and the context in which it operates. Often, success in the implementation depends heavily on how well the service model and context were addressed during the planning process. Perhaps less evident, although equally true, is the fact that the planning process can also be designed to support the extension of a successful innovation to larger or more complex applications.

Extension occurs after the innovation has been implemented and is judged to be effective. Extension can take many forms. For example, the service might be extended to another population; the service delivery system might be extended to include other providers or to restructure other services.

Each of these situations would require retesting the innovation unless the first implementation had been designed to define changes in policies affecting beneficiaries, providers, and agencies. Using policy changes to extend successful innovations is more efficient than conducting more demonstration projects; however, this capability must clearly be built into the planning process at the beginning.

Given an appropriate framework, it is not difficult to include both implementation and extension in planning. There is a logical basis for the dual focus. An innovation is created to address the unmet needs of a specific group of individuals. These unmet needs constitute a set of problems related to policy. Disseminating, generalizing, replicating, and institutionalizing — all aspects of obtaining the most from an innovation — require a precise understanding of both the service needs and policy problems.

Components of Planning

There are four principle components of service delivery planning:

1) to recognize the need or opportunity for innovation,
2) to recognize two sets of goals (implementation and extension),
3) to determine what is necessary to achieve each set of goals, and
4) to design the innovation.

Generally the list of components is in chronological order. However, most planning work cycles back over components, adjusting previous choices in light of new information and decisions. The four components are probably best thought of as being interactive rather than linear. The project described in the following section illustrates some aspects of a planning process designed to address both implementation and extension.

Planning the Children's Hospitals' REACH Project

The original program, Rural Efforts to Assist Children at Home (REACH), was developed in the early 1980s in Gainesville, Florida. It was funded by The Robert Wood Johnson Foundation and involved a waiver from the Health Care Financing Administration (HCFA). The leaders of the program included Patricia Pierce, PhD, RN, and Steve Freedman, PhD, of the University of Florida at Gainesville (Pierce and Freedman, 1983; Pierce et al., 1985; Schwab and Pierce, 1986; Pierce and Weiss, 1986).

The aim of this first program was to provide a cost-effective case management service for about 1,000 medically dependent Medicaid children in 16 rural counties in north central Florida. These children suffered from a variety of serious chronic illnesses. Nurses received special training to teach, consult on, coordinate, and supervise services for these children in collaboration with the tertiary care physicians at the university. The nurses served as local resources and community liaisons through home visits.

In the late 1980s, administrative and clinical leaders at two children's hospitals (Children's Memorial Hospital in Chicago and Children's Hospital and Health Center in San Diego) were working on improving services for a group of children with serious, ongoing health problems. Philip Porter, MD, the director of Healthy Children (another project funded by The Robert Wood Johnson Foundation), met with the hospitals' administrators and presented a number of models for consideration that had been distilled from innovations carried out in a wide variety of communities. The innovations were quite different from one other but shared the attributes of being well matched to their communities, designed around a specific group of children, and cost effective. The Gainesville REACH project was one of these models.

The leaders at the children's hospitals in Chicago and San Diego decided that the Gainesville model of the nurse as case manager and direct care provider held great promise for their urban populations. The model was altered so as to focus on children's hospitals rather than on the community because the target population of children was connected to and in need of the hospitals' tertiary services. It was hoped that basing the nurses in the hospitals would increase the resources available to the children and their families (Martinez et al., in press).

Several strategies enhanced the planning phase and contributed to building from the strengths of the original REACH project and meeting the goals of implementation and extension to policy. For example, a nurse from the new REACH project went to Florida to work with the project director of the Gainesville REACH project, and then trained nurses at both sites. Also, consultants in measurement and evaluation and health care financing were included in the planning work.

Each hospital in the new REACH project conducted a two-year pilot program directed by a pediatrician and carried out by two or three nurses. The service component of the pilot ended in mid-1990, followed by data analysis and evaluation.

The new REACH project began with the children's hospitals' efforts to define an effective policy for their existing populations of children on Medicaid. These children had serious ongoing health problems, complex medical needs, and complex social situations. Planning focused on identifying gaps in service — that is, what the children and their families needed. Experienced clinicians and consultants were essential in this identification process. Planning was augmented by information from the literature on chronic illness, case management, and family health.

In retrospect, it is apparent that the REACH planning would have been greatly enhanced if the literature had included a framework within which to unite the clinical and policy dimensions of caring for children with chronic illness. Durand's (1989) analysis of the theory and practice surrounding children with chronic illness and their families provides a framework that can be integrated with Richmond and Kotelchuck's (1983) model of social policy development, which includes three interactive elements: knowledge base, political will, and social strategy. Durand's findings can be analyzed and grouped into Richmond and Kotelchuck's three elements to derive premises and recommendations for projects such as REACH.

The incorporation of elements from Richmond and Kotelchuck's model into Durand's framework for the care of children with chronic illness and their families produces a blueprint which can then be used to guide specific decisions about the program's design. In this fashion, theory and practice merge with the nature of policy development to support the decisions inherent in planning the service and its context.

Knowledge base, the first element of the social policy development model, includes three premises that were basic to the new REACH project:

1) the needs of children with chronic illness and their families are often more social, material, and supportive than medical;
2) the existing policies are fragmented, limited, and uncoordinated; and
3) the care for these children and their families is service-intensive and expensive.

Although REACH was designed before Durand's framework was available, it contains some important implications. Consistent with Durand's recommendations, the REACH project staff determined that it would be important to adopt a model of care that is comprehensive and clearly defined. It also was determined that the outcomes for both the child and his/her family have multiple determinants; therefore, measures of the outcomes should be chosen cautiously. Finally, while the program may not reduce total care costs, REACH would certainly influence the effectiveness side of cost-effectiveness analysis, if not the cost side itself.

Since Durand's framework and the elements of political will and social strategy in Richmond and Kotelchuck's model are consistent with strategies in the REACH project, the latter project could serve as a source of information to policy makers for policy change. For example, the care provided by the REACH nurses was child-centered and family-focused to support the development of the child and family. Second, the services incorporated the family environment, included access to all levels of needed care and education, promoted self-management, and provided financial, respite, and psychological support to the family.

Planning for extension raises a basic question: what kind of service program can produce information to support policy analysis? As with implementation, this aspect of planning is greatly enhanced when it begins with a framework as a guide.

Rossi and Freeman's (1989) Impact Model is an excellent example of such a framework. Causal, intervention, and action hypotheses are determined as part of the Impact Model. The application of the model requires clear statements to define the key variables and their relationships to both the outcomes and the broader social context. It produces a definition of the innovation that is specific to extension, including the procedures by which to monitor the program.

Application of this framework to REACH produced a second set of questions and, in fact, necessitated that the project staff revise their thinking. For example, REACH has two primary outcomes — to prevent avoidable health problems and to make utilization more appropriate.

Tracking the first outcome through the Impact Model produces the following hypotheses. The causal hypothesis states that coordinated multiple services are necessary for these children, but there is no coordinator and there may be no services. The result is health problems that could have been avoided. The intervention hypothesis states that designating a coordinator who is able to provide linkages, access, and direct care will correct some existing health problems and will prevent some avoidable ones. The action hypothesis states that the amount of intervention affects the pattern

322

of health problems, as well as the child's pattern of activity (Meister, 1991). The Impact Model pares down variables and relationships so that the essential mechanisms take center stage. These are the same mechanisms that will form the springboard for policy activities (see Table 2).

After the plan has been put into action, it is important to continue assessing the context and its implications for implementation and extension. Making progress toward both goals requires a dynamic, circular process. However, when that process is based on a set of plans derived explicitly from frameworks tied directly to the goals, decisions can be both consistent and coherent.

The Challenge in the Larger Context

In the previous sections, the application of two frameworks has been described in developing an innovation for children with complex health problems and their families. General implications for nursing innovations will be discussed in the following sections.

To increase nursing's contributions to policy analysis and to policy change, several events must occur:

- Nurses must take a broader view of health care and health delivery issues.
- Nurses must be more deliberate in linking their research to policy.
- Nurses must see how the policy relates to the strengths and knowledge of their practice.

A Broader Perspective

It has been recognized that better health for the American population requires action from many policy sectors beyond health services. Effective employment, education, and agriculture policies also promote health equity. For nursing to influence broader policies, it must command an ecologic viewpoint (Milio, 1989) in which health has the capacity to maintain renewable, balanced relations between the natural and socially-created worlds. This perspective is demonstrated in the REACH project described herein as it addressed the social, financial, and educational needs of children and their families.

The need for a broader perspective in nursing's perceptions and its influence on policy is reinforced by McKinlay (1979) and

Butterfield (1990). They evoke the image of a swiftly flowing river to represent illness where the health professional is so caught up in rescuing the victim from the river that there is no time to find out who or what is pushing the patients into the water. This analogy emphasizes the futility of downstream endeavors that are seen as short-term, individual-based interventions. It is these types of interventions that are most frequently employed in nursing. Nurses need to look upstream to modify broader aspects of the social system — such as economic, political, and environmental factors — that are known to be associated with poor health.

Linkages Between Research and Policy

To increase nurses' influence on policy development, the linkages between research and policy must be recognized. Milio (1984) reports that although research plays a small role in the real work of policy making, it does have some influence, especially in new or controversial areas of public policy. She describes three types of research across the spectrum of policy-relevant research. At one end of the spectrum is broad government-commissioned policy analysis; at the other end is theoretical disciplinary research. As the pace of social and technological change quickens and new institutions are amenable to more than just the wisdom of experience, the necessity for policy-relevant research will continue to increase (see Table 3).

Of the three types of policy relevant research, most nursing research falls in the category of disciplinary research (Milio, 1984). Although the purpose of disciplinary research is not for policy development, this research may have policy implications and may be used by policy analysts. Unfortunately, most investigators conducting disciplinary research do not utilize the policy implications of their findings.

Each type of research in this spectrum of policy-relevant research can contribute to policy development in several ways. First, the research can monitor the course of events that might be relevant to policy. The children's hospitals' REACH projects, for example, kept close tabs on changes in Medicaid policy throughout the projects. Second, the research can forecast emerging problems prior to their occurrence. The sample size in REACH will limit some forecasting analyses, but it is large enough to address issues concerning the increasing numbers of medically fragile children and the increasing demands on the health and social systems to care for them.

A third contribution of policy-relevant research is the identification and analysis of problem-raising situations. REACH did this by focusing on the infrastructure needed to link tertiary and community health resources for the children.

Fourth, research serves as a critique of current policies. For REACH, this was done in retrospect. For example, the project was not planned in anticipation of public laws, such as PL 99-457 (the public law that authorized services for persons with disabilities and health problems), but the outcomes can be related to that law and other emerging policies.

Fifth, research may result in a redefinition of the problem. REACH, as a research/demonstration project, actually transplanted and redefined the intervention from the rural focus of the Gainesville project to an urban and tertiary care context.

The sixth contribution of policy-relevant research to policy development is an analysis in the policy-making process of initiation, development, implementation, outcome, and evaluation. This result was a major objective of the REACH project and the analysis conducted therein serves as an example of policy-relevant research. While this analysis of the new REACH project is in process, preliminary results indicate that the clinicians found the REACH model to be workable and effective (Martinez et al., in press). Additionally, outcomes for the children and families were improved and system health care dollars were saved (Meister, 1991). Thus, the model seems to be a promising one for extension and has been assessed from the four key perspectives of the child and family, the clinician, the institution, and the payer (see Table 4).

There is growing awareness among nurses that the issues of importance to nursing should be framed in policy-relevant terms. However, authors in the nursing literature have focused on how to influence policy (Aiken, 1982; Fagin, 1982; Pillar, Jacox, and Redman, 1989), rather than emphasize the substance of alternative policies and analyze their actual or potential effects (Milio, 1984).

Other countries have a better track record for developing and implementing major innovations for change in health policy and health practices. In this country, there often are small projects that test these changes, but the link between demonstration and policy formation that was forged with REACH appears either not to have been attempted or to have been frustrated (Milio, 1990). When the research demonstration project is transferred to public programs, changes are made that make them less effective (Schorr and Schorr,

1988). This is contrary to the expected outcome of research in which movement from small demonstration projects to larger statewide and/or national programs would occur.

Policy Relevance and Practice

Nursing practice and nursing knowledge contain elements that provide a strong basis by which nurses and nursing can influence policy. Nurses work in multiple contexts and dimensions. From this diversity, nurses should be able to define the interrelated effects of apparently separate policies (Meister, 1989). For example, what are the effects of access, income maintenance, food, and the provision of primary and secondary health care on families of children with chronic illness? Or, in another example derived from the REACH project, what are the effects of costs, access, and professional relationships on various payment systems, such as fee-for-service and capitation?

Because of the multiple perspectives and contexts of nursing practice, nurses also are able to formulate new or neglected questions. As nurses develop experience in policy analysis, they should be defining the policy implications of their practice research and nursing service evaluation and research, while defining the health consequences of those policies, particularly the social and economic ones. Finally, building from their science and the research questions, nurses should be able to address some of the broad methodological issues.

This paper reinforces the principle that policy analysis provides a framework for broader interpretation and influence of nursing practice and research. As nursing research and evaluation begin to take place more often within the context of policy analysis, nurses must move from individual-focused interventions and begin to examine broader based interventions. As nurses assume a broader perspective, the results of their research will provide information for policy formation.

❏ ❏ ❏

Table 1
Steps in Policy and Nursing Processes

Policy Process	Nursing Process
• Identify/formulate the problem.	• Make the assessment/ nursing diagnosis.
• Set the policy agenda.	• Determine goals.
• Formulate the policy.	• Develop the care plan.
• Adopt the policy.	• Adopt the plan with input from the patient and others.
• Implement the policy	• Implement the care plan.
• Evaluate the policy.	• Evaluate the outcomes.

Table 2
Rossi and Freeman's Impact Model

Develop an impact model by defining the following:

- Causal hypothesis —
  Hypothesis concerning how the problem is brought about.
- Intervention hypothesis —
  Hypothesis that specifies the relationship between intervention and the elements in the causal hypothesis.
- Action hypothesis —
  Statement about how to assess whether the intervention is necessarily linked to the outcome.

Prepare to use the impact model by doing the following:

- Define the target population in relation to the impact model.
- Create a blueprint of the delivery system.
- Initiate a formative study or simulation early in the development.
- Specify procedures to monitor program.
- Establish plans for assessing impact and efficiency.

From *Evaluation: A Systematic Approach,* 4th edition, P. H. Rossi and H. E. Freeman, 1989, Sage Publications.

Table 3
Spectrum of Policy-Relevant Research

- Explicit policy analysis research
- Focused policy research
- Disciplinary research

From "Nursing Research and the Study of Health Policy," N. Milio, in *Annual Review of Nursing Research*, vol. 2, H. H. Werley and J. J. Fitzpatrick, eds., 1984.

Table 4
Contributions of Policy-Relevant Research to Policy Development

- Monitor course of events relevant to policy
- Forecast emerging problems
- Identify and analyze problem-raising situations
- Critique current policies
- Redefine the policy-relevant problem
- Analyze the policy-making process

Measurement of Practice Outcomes: The Impact of Certification in Neonatal Nursing on the Outcomes of Neonatal Intensive Care

Rosanne Woods Ed.D., C.P.N.P., F.A.A.N.
Eileen McQuaid Dvorak, Ph.D., R.N.

The Problem

T he major reason for certification is the public belief that outcomes of care delivered by certified practitioners exceed the quality of care delivered by noncertified practitioners. Professional nursing proponents of certification assume that a person who chooses to demonstrate the special knowledge inherent in the role of neonatal intensive care nurse through National Certifying Corporation (NCC) certification can achieve improved practice outcomes. Despite the logic of these assumptions, there is little empirical evidence to support these beliefs (Warren, 1987).

Critics of licensing examinations have questioned the validity of examinations as measures of competence, despite the fact that the instruments demonstrate high content validity (Hogan, 1979). An investigation of the ability of examination scores to measure performance criteria is definitely needed. Without these data, successful test takers could prove to be either competent or incompetent on the job (Chrystal and Crudi, 1985; del Bueno, 1988). In addition, the current emphasis on cost containment and cost benefit analysis demands an answer to the question of the predictive validity of certification. Care delivered by specialists has been associated with increased cost (National Guidelines, 1989). Unless those increased costs associated with certified nurses result in improved care, the public must question the need for certified nurses.

Proposal Development

Although the need for outcome-focused evaluation is clear, literature specifically related to certification is scant. Thus, little direction is available to guide the development of measures that will predict the validity of certification examinations. Conceptual and methodological issues associated with the measurement of practice outcomes also abound. In 1989, the NCC demonstrated its leadership and concern for problems associated with the predictive validity of its certification examinations by funding the formation of a panel of experts. They were responsible for analyzing and synthesizing the "state of knowledge" needed to devise a proposal to determine the predictive validity of the NCC examination in neonatal intensive care nursing. The decision to focus on neonatal intensive care nursing was based on:

- the need for a defined domain of nursing practice,
- the potential availability of a sample of nurses to participate in the investigation, and
- available expertise to identify outcomes of autonomous nursing practices.

Six areas of knowledge were identified as essential to the problem analysis, and included information about:

- generalizing criterion-related validity evidence on certification requirements across situations,
- selecting models to direct the measurement of nursing practice,
- identifying relationships between certification and practice outcomes,
- evaluating existing criterion measures of practice outcomes in general,
- identifying patient outcomes specifically associated with nursing practices, and
- measuring the process and outcomes of nursing actions.

A geographically diverse group of experts in measurement, research methods, neonatal nursing practice, and test development participated in the panel. Each member prepared a concept paper specifically addressing one of the six topics identified in the model. All members received the papers prior to the meeting. Consensus development strategies were implemented to develop a methodology for investigation. The process took approximately one year to complete. The consensus judgment of the panel is reflected in the following discussion.

Summary of the Literature on Certification and Practice Outcomes

Literature on predicting patient outcomes as validation of certification processes, including examinations, is limited. Information on the process and/or characteristics of practitioners is of paramount importance to most of the literature on certification (Dvorak and Woods, 1989). Literature from other professions has not shown evidence that certification is directly and consistently related to the continuing demonstration of professional competence as measured by patient outcomes (del Bueno, 1988; Wilbur, 1979; Wallis, 1987). In his treatise on assessment of competence in optometry, Wallis (1987) states that there are no standards against which an applicant's competence can be assessed, and that a great need exists for objective performance criteria derived from psychometric standards. In addition, Wallis states that there is a need to document competence in specialty areas of practice by objective criteria. The National Board for Professional Teaching Standards has established guidelines that mandate that a teacher's primary responsibility is to assure learning by students (National Guidelines, 1989). According to the guidelines, certification should focus on effectiveness, and not on whether the teacher took the right courses or followed approved procedures. Only one study on relationships between learning outcomes and certification was identified. The results demonstrated that learning disabled and educable mentally retarded elementary students, when taught by teachers whose certification matched child label, made no significantly greater gains than when instructed by teachers with licenses not matching pupil labels (Marston, 1987). Although no relationship between certification and learning outcome was identified, the effort to conduct a predictive validity study is noteworthy.

An investigation conducted by the medical profession attempted to define the relationships between certification and practice patterns, patient satisfaction, and patient outcomes (Ramsey et al., 1989). No significant differences were found. A major limitation of this retrospective study was reliance on chart audits to measure the process and outcome of medical care. Adequate controls were not introduced for case mix, missing data, or other limitations of the medical record. Knaus and Nash (1988) cited a need to identify outcome measures that can be used in clinical studies. They confirmed the need to develop measures of outcomes in patients as a first step in enabling future studies to determine if differences in practice exist dependent on certification. In pharmacy, one study was reported on the predictive validity of certification tests on the pharmacist's ability to appropriately prescribe. The results supported a positive relationship between certification and prescribing appropriateness (McGhan et al., 1982). Specific information on the outcome measure used was not provided. However, the investigation suggests that the more specific an area of study, the greater the likelihood of being able to identify specific outcomes.

Practitioners in infection control have studied certification and recertification. A report from the members of the Association for Practitioners of Infection Control states that one of the three major methods of recertification is evaluation of clinical practice (Pugliese et al., 1986). The report does not identify the components of clinical practice, nor does it indicate that patient outcomes were assessed. The only suggestion that patient outcomes were included appears under "goals and objectives," where the authors state that consumers can choose certified practitioners to ensure that their care comes from qualified practitioners (Pugliese et al., 1986).

Mitchell et al. (1989) have reported on a methodologically and conceptually sound demonstration project to document fiscal costs and patient care effectiveness in a critical care nursing unit characterized by valued organizational attributes. Their results strongly suggest that positive organizational and clinical outcomes coexist with valued aspects of the organizational environments.

Measurement of Patient Outcomes

Measurement of patient outcomes is problematic for several reasons. Currently, outcomes associated with quality neonatal nursing care have not been well defined or reliable, and valid measurement methods remain untested. In addition, neonatal care is not easily divided into categories of nursing care versus medical care. This inability to divide care into discrete categories makes it difficult to measure patient outcomes attributable solely to nursing. However, although measurement of the quality of neonatal nursing care outcomes is difficult due to the lack of specific guidelines and norms of reference for all types of neonatal problems, reliable and valid measurement strategies have begun to emerge.

Problems in evaluating the effects of nursing actions on the neonate include:

- The patient is nonverbal.
- Some changes in nursing actions are based solely on observational methods — such as changes in the patient's color — and are related to a nurse's expert judgement (what has worked in the past with other neonates).
- The nursing process, including neonatal assessment data, is not attributable simply to the discipline of nursing.
- Measurement of physiological parameters, such as vital signs, invite comparisons with standards or norms (but for some parameters, the neonatal intensive unit norms have yet to be developed or verified through research).
- Measurement of physiologic parameters is dependent on accurate instrumentation; however, with very small infants, detection of subtle changes in vital sign measurement are dependent on highly sophisticated technology.
- There is little "science" available to apply to practice (Kenner, 1989; Schraeder, 1989).

Although these problems provide significant challenges for the profession, progress toward definition of quality outcomes is underway. In addition, funding agencies, third-party payers, accrediting bodies, and the public have identified outcome evaluation as a priority concern.

Identification of Measurable Quality Outcomes

It is not apparent from review of the literature that any nursing group can yet identify patient outcomes associated with quality nursing care. However, the American Association of Critical Care Nurses (AACN) has convened a task force to develop patient outcome standards (Haller, 1989). The AACN project is progressing in four stages:

1) development of patient outcome standards,
2) assessment of the utility of the standards in a quality assurance model,
3) implementation of clinical trails to test the effect of nursing intervention on patient outcomes, and
4) development of standards to measure the quality of care in collaboration with other disciplines.

Within this model, the unit of analysis for quality assessment is the nursing unit rather than the individual practitioner. Nurses are assumed to be collectively accountable for patient outcomes.

Work measures also have been designed to systematically assess responsibilities of practitioners. Scoring rules and observation checklists must be developed for each measure (Cline, 1985). Measures consist of identified patient outcomes that achieve ratings of agreement by expert judges. Linacre (1989) has designed a precise Rasch measurement model for rank-ordered data and a many-faceted approximation for small data sets. This model would enable judgments about patient care outcomes to be ranked within one standard error by relatively untrained personnel.

In analyzing evaluation studies done on neonatal intensive care unit care, nurses, patients, and families revealed few pertinent studies (Jalowiec, 1989). Because of this, salient information from evaluation studies on pediatric, obstetrical, and general populations was also considered. It was assumed that measurement approaches in other settings might be adapted to the neonatal intensive care unit (Jalowiec, 1989). Measurement variables identified included the following:

- Structure — Staffing patterns, adequacy of orientation programs and in-service education, salary and benefits, presence of a clinical ladder for advancement, amount of decision making and autonomy allowed the nurses, facilitation of collaboration between medicine and nursing, adequacy of support services, safety of the work environment, type of performance appraisal process, and adequacy of technological support.
- Process — Record review or audit of charts, flow sheets, and nursing care plans.

- Outcome — Patient, family, nurse, other provider, and institution.

Models Used to Measure Nursing Practice

There are several types of models used in measuring nursing practice — decision-making models, evaluation models, nursing-process models, and nurse socialization models (Strickland, 1989). Each model has certain advantages and disadvantages, given its specified purpose. Since this study is concerned with the ability of certification in neonatal intensive care nursing to predict the quality of practice outcomes, the more direct approach suggested by the Donabedian (1966) evaluation model has been used.

The Donabedian model defines specific criteria, goals, and/or objectives against which the quality of nursing care or the nurse's performance is measured. The model focuses on whether nursing care goals and objectives were met, and whether the practicing nurse is capable of providing high quality care. The model is concerned with nursing care goal attainment and the knowledge and performance level of the nurse. It is primarily outcome oriented, with the focus on process rather than on quantification of process. Outcomes are stated in measurable terms based on common nursing care problems found in neonatal intensive care nursing. Scales are constructed to represent the criteria on a continuum, with the nursing care problem appearing on one end and the most favorable possible outcome at the other (Inzer and Aspinall, 1981; Wilson-Barnett, 1981).

Outcomes selected for this study are contingent on nursing care behaviors, therefore assuming that the more skillful and competent the nurse, the higher the quality of nursing care provided.

Situational Factors and Predictive Validity

Several situational factors must be considered in investigating predictive validity (American Psychological Association, 1985). These factors are:

- the way in which the predictor construct is measured,
- the job involved,
- the type of test taker, and
- the time period in which the study was conducted.

The Predictor Construct. The predictor construct is a passing score on the Neonatal Intensive Care Nursing Examination. The competency statements and content outline for this examination were developed and validated by a geographically representative group of expert neonatal intensive care nurses. A study of this examination's content outline revealed substantial content validity (Perez-Woods, 1990).

Framework for Identifying Patient Outcomes (the Job Involved). All measures are related to the care provided in neonatal intensive care units. The framework for identifying patient outcomes will be composed of selected indicators of quality care outcomes. Outcomes in this study are defined as resulting from the application of science by neonatal nurses using knowledge and psychomotor skills (Schraeder, 1989). Specific outcomes include infant physiological stability and growth, reduced complications, and improved behavioral and interactional competence; and improved family satisfaction and confidence at discharge.

The outcomes to be measured were selected by members of the expert panel commissioned by NCC. Practitioners, measurement experts, academics, and neonatal nurse researchers constituted the group. The outcomes selected constituted a set of hypotheses which assume that the nursing structure (including certification) has an effect on patient status (Haller, 1989). Donabedian's model posits that outcomes result from both structure and process of care. The interaction of these two components results in both process (i.e., light, sound, patterns of care) [Blackburn, 1989] and structure (i.e., work environment, satisfaction with work environment, staffing patterns, turnover, patent nurse ratio, ongoing clinical updates of knowledge, presence of clinical ladder, etc.) [Jalowiec, 1989]. Hegyvary and Haussman (1988) have reinforced the need to measure both process and outcome variables to determine if a relationship exists between the nursing practice and patient outcome. The collective responses of the individual neonates in the neonatal intensive care unit assigned to each of the study groups comprise the unit of analysis in terms of physiological response to care (Kenner, 1989).

Target Population (Test Takers). Members of the study and comparison group met the eligibility criteria for the NCC neonatal intensive care certification examination. The unit of analysis was the study group of nurses, rather than the individual practitioner. Nurses are seen as collectively responsible for patient outcomes; therefore, out of two groups of nurses, one group will be comprised of certified nurses and the other of noncertified nurses. Infants are randomly assigned to a group following informed parental consent. Both groups of nurses practice on the same unit on different teams.

Time Frame. All data for the pilot study will be collected within a six-month time frame. Cluster studies are recommended following the pilot. If the results of the cluster studies yield similar results, then confidence in the validity of the context of neonatal intensive care will be forthcoming.

Methods

The question raised by the literature review asks if there is a difference in patient and family outcomes (primarily resulting from nursing practice) dependent on the certification of nurses by NCC in the specialty practice area of neonatal intensive care nursing. The independent variable is NCC certification in neonatal intensive care nursing. The dependent variable is practice outcomes in the neonatal intensive care unit. Certification is the demonstration of a designated level of knowledge in neonatal intensive care nursing, exemplified as a passing score on the NCC certification examination in neonatal intensive care by a majority of the nurses on a designated nursing unit.

The hypothesis that follows states that there is a significant difference in practice outcomes on a unit where the majority of nurses ($>50\%$) are certified in neonatal intensive care nursing compared to a unit staffed by noncertified but certification-eligible nurses.

Research questions include:

- Are the process and structure variables similar in both groups?
- What are the practice outcomes for each group?
- Is there a significant difference in practice outcomes dependent on process and structure variables?
- If differences exist in practice outcomes dependent on structure and process variables, are these differences associated with type of group?
- Can relationships between certification and practice outcomes be generalized from one weight group of infants to another?

Design and Procedure

A prospective correlational two-group comparative design will be used. Following informed parental consent, newly admitted subjects that meet the eligibility criteria will be enrolled in the study. Infants then will be randomly assigned to a study group (a team of certified or noncertified nurses) by opening a sealed envelope which contains the assignment. The sample size for the pilot study will be 30 infants per group. Power sampling techniques based on the results from the pilot study will be used to estimate numbers needed for generalizing the results in a multisite study following completion of the pilot phase. Following Institutional Review Board approval, collection of data for the pilot study is anticipated to take six months. An additional six-month period is devoted to analysis and dissemination of the findings. All data will be collected by trained research assistants at the site of implementation.

Subjects

The dependent variable — quality of outcomes for neonates and their families — will be measured in two groups of inborn neonates ($\geq$ 800 - 1,200 grams; $\geq$ 1,201 - 2,500 grams). These neonates will demonstrate no significant congenital anomalies or evidence of perinatal infection. They will be from English-speaking families admitted to the two designated neonatal intensive care units. Infants transported to the neonatal intensive care unit from another agency or whose mothers have a history of substance abuse will be excluded due to the potential for variability in nursing management prior to transport affecting outcomes. The unit of analysis will be the collective responses of individual neonates and families.

The independent variable will be the nursing care team. One team will consist of nurses who are certified by NCC in neonatal intensive care nursing. The other team will consist of unit staff nurses who are noncertified. The unit of analysis will be the group of nurses to which the infants are randomly assigned.

Measures

Quality of practice outcome measures will include the following:

Neonate.

1) Physiological Stability — Thermal stability (number of times outside normal range; documented on admission and daily or when charted), pulse oximetry (number of times + or − normal range; measure at admission, and daily or when charted), glucose level (number of times + or − normal range; measure at admission, and daily or when charted), growth (number of times greater than 10% deviation in normal curve for preterm infant; measure weekly), weight gain (ounces), occipital frontal circumference (centimeters), length (centimeters).

2) Cost of Care — Total cost, mean cost per patient day, number of neonatal intensive care unit days (based on all bills rendered for the infant's hospitalization; measure at discharge).

3) Number of Deaths During Hospitalization — Standardized mortality ratio; 100% times observed/expected used with the chi-square distribution to test the significance of the difference from a ratio of 100%.

4) Number of Neonatal Intensive Care Unit Days.

5) Number of Rehospitalizations — Within one month of discharge.

6) Number of Nonroutine Health Visits — Within one month of discharge.

7) Complications — Number of self-extubations; acquired limb/digit deformities, timed glucose level + or − normal range, nosocomial infections (diagnosed by positive culture); burns, skin sloughs and abrasions; central line occlusions/ displacements; infants with necrotizing enterocolitis requiring surgical intervention — all to be measured weekly.

8) Behavior at Discharge — Cluster score on Brazelton Neonatal Behavior Assessment Scale; measured at discharge.

Nutrition.
1) Maternal Desire to Breast-Feed — Yes/no; measured at admission.
2) Number of Weeks Infant Breast-Fed — Measured weekly.

Family.
1) Maternal-Infant Interaction at Discharge — Score on Nursing Child Assessment Feeding Scale (Barnard, 1978).
2) Satisfaction — Score on satisfaction scale at time of discharge (score on Woods' Neonatal Intensive Care Unit Parent Satisfaction Questionnaire).
3) Confidence at Discharge — Score on Woods' Neonatal Intensive Care Unit Satisfaction Questionnaire at time of discharge.

Process Variables and Measures.
1) Patterns of Care — Record review or audit of charts and flow-sheets (type of plans present, observations charted, interventions charted — i.e., content and methods of teaching), and evaluations charted; proposed score on the Woods' Chart Review Form for the neonatal intensive care unit (Woods, 1990).

Structure Variables and Measures.
1) Nursery Environment — Blackburn Nursery Climate Survey (Blackburn, 1990).
2) Work Environment — Organizational structures: clarity and autonomy subscales of the Moos Work Environment Scale [WES] (Moos, 1986), influence subscale of the Charnes Organizational Diagnosis Survey [CODS] (Charnes, 1983).
3) Unit Organizational Processes — Unit process, coordination, conflict management, and physician opinion questionnaire of the CODS.
4) Unit Organizational Outcomes — Nursing Organizational Climate Description Questionnaire [NOCDQ] (Duxbury, 1982), relationship and maintenance dimensions of the WES. Satisfaction: Minnesota Satisfaction Questionnaire [MSQ] (Weiss et al., 1979). Morale: esprit dimension of the NOCDQ and burnout inventory of the CODS.

Measures of process and structure variables are included because these variables have been associated with practice outcomes in the literature. Estimates of homogeneity between groups in relationship to these variables will be described. The primary purpose of the pilot is to test the feasibility of the methods, develop reliable and valid measures, and provide a foundation for the planning and development of a grant for a group of cluster studies.

Analysis

Analysis will involve estimates of instrument reliability and validity, descriptive and correlational statistics, and tests of significant difference. Procedures will be selected dependent on the level of data under analysis. The use of sophisticated multivariate procedures is not anticipated in the pilot phase.

❏   ❏   ❏

Part VII

Education and Differentiated Nursing Practice

Education for Differentiated Practice: A Rural University's Experience

Kay Carr, Ed.D., R.N., C.S.
Beverly Siegrist, M.S., R.N.,C.

Abstract

This paper presents one educational program's curriculum design for differentiated practice and the implementation of this model. Western Kentucky University is a moderate-sized university in south-central Kentucky serving a rural population. The school of nursing is in its 26th year and has an associate degree program and a baccalaureate in nursing program, which was established in 1976. Four years ago, the baccalaureate program was revised from an upper-division program for registered nurses to a generic program with a track for the RN. The resulting curriculum models demonstrate this university's attempt to promote education for differentiated practice. This paper has two focuses: to briefly describe the associate and baccalaureate curriculum models, and to discuss challenges and barriers in implementation.

A Rural University's Experience

For 14 years, Western Kentucky University has had two nursing programs — an associate degree and a baccalaureate program for registered nurses. In 1976, when the RN-BSN completion program was initiated, studies indicated that there were sufficient numbers of associate degree nurses in the area, but a need remained for baccalaureate degree nurses. Program evaluation indicated that this need was still prevalent in 1985. The number of associate degree graduates entering the baccalaureate program had been low, and many of the baccalaureate graduates had migrated to the surrounding urban areas. In 1988, to increase the number of baccalaureate graduates, the faculty redesigned the nursing program toward a more generic baccalaureate program with a track for the registered nurse.

Revision of the baccalaureate curriculum reawakened associate and baccalaureate faculties' philosophical differences about nursing education and practice. A grant from a service agency permitted faculty to bring a consultant on campus to present seminars on differentiated practice. As a result of these seminars, faculty became more aware of the need for differentiation of competencies of the graduates from each program. They were able to reach a consensus that both a technical and a professional role could be delineated. Both programs began curriculum revisions to clarify the roles, responsibilities, and skills of the technical versus the professional nurse. Although the process of curriculum differentiation of the associate and baccalaureate degree nursing programs is not complete, progress has been made in developing program philosophies, conceptual frameworks, terminal objectives, and practice roles. Accomplishing this curriculum revision continues to cause conflict, challenges, and satisfaction for the faculty.

An Educational Model

The first step in the curriculum revision was to review the philosophies. The faculty revised the overall departmental philosophy to reflect their beliefs about nursing education. Faculty were able to agree that both associate degree nursing and baccalaureate degree nursing education should occur in institutions of higher learning, and that education is an ongoing process. Both faculties believed that they had a responsibility to provide the educational patterns to accommodate career goals within nursing. The faculties also agreed that the associate degree prepares the graduate to enter technical nursing practice, while the baccalaureate degree is the first professional degree in nursing and provides the knowledge base for graduate study in nursing. In addition, the faculties believed that the associate degree is not a terminal degree; therefore, the associate degree nurse can pursue the baccalaureate degree in nursing. These beliefs also are reflected in the philosophies of the individual programs.

Differentiation in nursing role and practice settings is more specifically identified within individual program philosophies. The associate degree philosophy states that the graduate is prepared to work primarily with individuals in a secondary care setting under the supervision of a professional nurse. The baccalaureate degree philosophy describes the role of the professional nurse as a generalist who cares for clients from diverse cultures, throughout the life cycle, in a variety of health care settings.

The two programs function on different conceptual models. The conceptual framework of the associate degree program is based on basic human needs, while the conceptual framework of the baccalaureate degree program is based on stress, adaptation, and systems theory. Associate degree nurse graduates matriculating into the baccalaureate program have had no difficulty in making the transition from a framework based on needs to a stress, adaptation, and systems model.

From these conceptual frameworks, the associate and baccalaureate nursing faculty independently designed terminal objectives which differentiated the graduate's role in relation to nursing processes, roles, practice settings, and clients.

Faculty from both programs elected to use a five-step nursing process model:

1) assessment,
2) nursing diagnosis,
3) planning,
4) implementation, and
5) evaluation.

Differentiation occurs within each step of the model. To perform assessment, the associate degree nursing student collects data using a structured assessment format, while the baccalaureate nursing student expands the data base to identify complex health care problems of individuals, families, and groups.

For the second step, the associate degree faculty established a list of selected nursing diagnoses from the North American Nursing Diagnosis Association's (NANDA) classifications that they viewed as appropriate for technical nursing. Faculty then assigned these diagnoses to specific courses. In each course, the student was expected to use the new nursing diagnoses in addition to the ones learned in previous courses. The baccalaureate nursing students could select from the NANDA list those diagnoses they deemed appropriate for their clients, but they were not limited to this list.

To fulfill the final steps of the nursing process, the associate degree student was expected to identify goals and interventions that are short-term and consistent with the overall comprehensive nursing plan of care. The baccalaureate degree student was expected to develop a comprehensive plan of care with the client to achieve the most optimal state of health. Both associate degree and baccalaureate students were expected to implement, evaluate, and revise the plan of care. Evaluation was further expanded for the baccalaureate student and included structure, process, and outcome evaluation. The students were also introduced to quality assurance models, including utilization review and risk management.

The roles of the nurse, as defined in the terminal objectives, differ in number but not context. The role statement for each terminal objective identifies the difference in practice of associate and baccalaureate degree graduates. The associate degree program defines the roles of the nurse as:

- member of the profession
- teacher
- coordinator/manager
- communicator
- provider of care

The baccalaureate program identifies the roles of the professional nurse as:

- provider
- collaborator
- manager
- teacher

Although "communicator" and "member of the profession" were not identified as specific roles for the baccalaureate graduate, the baccalaureate faculty found that communication and professional accountability were inherent in all professional nurse roles.

This role differentiation can be easily exemplified by comparing the teacher role for each program. The associate degree terminal objective states that the graduate will utilize basic teaching — learning principles by modifying and implementing a standardized teaching plan. The baccalaureate degree terminal objective states that the baccalaureate degree nurse will design and implement teaching plans for clients. The differentiation between the technical and professional nurse teacher role is readily evident and further clarified in the level objectives.

In each program philosophy, the appropriate setting for nursing practice is clearly identified. The associate degree graduate is prepared to practice in structured clinical settings, while the baccalaureate degree graduate is prepared to practice in a variety of health care settings. Though some agencies are used by both programs, the clinical focus remains within the parameter of technical or professional practice. For example, both programs utilize the public health department's prenatal clinic. The focus of the clinical experience for the associate degree nurse is on uncomplicated prenatal care for pregnant women. The baccalaureate degree student focuses on the individual, but includes family and multiple complex situations. The baccalaureate student may participate in educational classes for pregnant women in the preterm labor program and provide home visits for prenatal and postpartum nursing care of high-risk pregnant women.

Further program delineation can be seen in the type of client the student is prepared to care for and the related goals of nursing care. Both programs prepare the graduate to provide nursing care for ill clients throughout the life cycle. The associate degree program focuses on the ill individual within the context of the family. The goal of the associate degree program is to provide nursing care to restore the client's health. The focus of the baccalaureate program is on both ill and well clients of diverse cultures. In addition, the baccalaureate degree program's client might be an individual, a family, or a community. The baccalaureate nursing student is expected to provide nursing interventions to achieve promotion of health, prevention of illness, restoration of health, and rehabilitation of the client.

After development of terminal objectives, the faculty defined level objectives. The terminal objectives of the associate degree program are comparable to the first-level baccalaureate objectives, and describe the competencies of the technical nurse graduate. The second-level baccalaureate degree program objectives describe the competencies expected of the professional nurse. Both programs are in the process of implementing these revisions to the curriculum.

Barriers to Change

In our community, we have two primary employing agencies — one rural medical center with 294 beds, and a private corporation hospital with 211 beds. Other employing agencies in the surrounding area are mainly small rural hospitals with 10 – 30 beds, and long-term care facilities. With the exception of the rural medical center, the nursing managers are primarily associate degree nurses. Most, if not all, of the nursing supervisors and staff nurses in the agencies are also associate degree nurses. Therefore, involving community service agencies in educating nurses for differentiated practice is a challenge. Community service agency representatives were invited to the seminar on differentiated practice, but attendance was poor. Our faculty must continue to educate nursing administrators and staff about the need for and importance of differentiated practice.

Only recently have graduates from the baccalaureate nursing program remained in the area to practice nursing. One reason for this traditional exodus may be that 50 miles from the school is a large metropolitan area that offers higher salaries; more flexible scheduling, reimbursement, and graduate education opportunities; and the opportunity to practice in the role of the professional nurse. Another problem could be that only two of the local employing agencies offer salary differentiation for the baccalaureate nurse. One of these agencies is the public health department, which offers the lowest starting salary in the area. The other is a specialty agency that employs a small number of nurses. This has resulted in a lack of baccalaureate-prepared nurse role models for the baccalaureate degree graduates.

Moving Toward Differentiated Practice

Despite the barriers, faculty believe that there is a potential for differentiated practice in this rural area. Several changes have occurred that we believe will help us move toward differentiated practice. In one major employing agency, a master's-prepared nursing administrator motivates the hospital staff to pursue a baccalaureate degree in nursing. Secondly, the number of applicants for the generic baccalaureate degree nursing program is excellent. The number of registered nurse applicants each year was approximately 30, with two-thirds of the students enrolling. Currently, the number of applicants for the generic baccalaureate nursing program is 150, and the number of registered nurse applicants is 15. The class size is limited to 70 students. Hopefully, these graduates can be encouraged by nursing faculty and service agencies to remain in the area. Without the appropriate number of baccalaureate-prepared nurses, differentiated practice cannot occur.

Kentucky nursing leaders are assisting in educating community agencies about differentiated practice. The Kentucky Board of Nursing sponsored a nursing conference on differentiated practice, and in October 1989, submitted a proposal for a statewide demonstration project using a differentiated nursing practice model (Kentucky Board of Nursing, 1990).

From our perspective, education alone will not accomplish differentiated practice. Several things must occur before it becomes a reality. First, there needs to be a separate licensing examination for associate and baccalaureate degree nursing graduates. Second, there must be professional consensus about the different competencies expected for each type of nursing graduate. Third, there must be more research and published articles describing differentiated practice models. In the mean time, we will continue our efforts to promote education for differentiated practice.

❏   ❏   ❏

Differentiated Practice: Integrating Education and Service

Patricia H. Foster, Ed.D., R.N.

The development of a collaborative partnership between the University of North Florida's Department of Nursing and St. Vincent's Medical Center has linked nursing education and practice for the benefit of students, nursing staff, and the community. Integrating education and practice was essential in developing the Patient-Oriented Delivery Model to enhance nursing practice and prevent inappropriate utilization of nurses in an acute care facility.

The University of North Florida in Jacksonville, Florida has a baccalaureate in nursing program, offering both an RN–BSN and a basic nursing track. In 1987, the department of nursing approached its advisory council for assistance with faculty funding to increase the enrollments of baccalaureate nursing students. Collaborative partnerships were explored, and St. Vincent's Medical Center in Jacksonville answered the request by agreeing to fund a 12-month faculty line (later named the St. Vincent's Professorship).

A "memorandum of understanding" was drafted and signed by the appropriate parties. The focus of the agreement was clearly the instruction and supervision of nursing students. The agreement outlined the expectation that students would be brought to the medical center for appropriate clinical rotations. Certain courses would be offered on-site, and faculty members were to participate in developing and conducting nursing research, and to participate in appropriate medical center committees. The St. Vincent's professorship was accorded all rights, privileges, and support by university faculty. This line was designated nontenure-earning. Recruitment for the professorship was a joint endeavor. Faculty from the university and nursing administrators from St. Vincent's Medical Center served on the search committee. The individual who was selected had a master's degree in nursing with a specialization in adult health and gerontology. She had teaching experience at the baccalaureate level and a strong clinical background.

Tenure-earning faculty at the university are assigned a certain percentage of time for teaching, research, and service. Although this line was not tenure-earning, the behavioral expectations were similar in that teaching, scholarly activity, and service are hallmarks of professional practice. A major service commitment for the St. Vincent's professor was to work on medical center committees, on the department of nursing's curriculum committee, and on the admissions committee.

During the first two years, the St. Vincent's professor held staff development workshops at the medical center, offered electives, was visible in the medical center, and maintained high visibility with baccalaureate nursing students. However, it was not until the medical center steering committee began to explore a new model of differentiated practice that the St. Vincent's professor's role in integrating education with service began to take on new significance. As a member of the medical center's steering committee, which was charged with the task of differentiating practice according to education, experience, and competence, the St. Vincent's professor began to stand out as one who articulated the roles and behaviors that professional nurses would be expected to demonstrate in a differentiated model of patient-oriented care. Under this model, the baccalaureate-prepared nurse was expected to assume the professional role of case manager who would make the pre- and post-admission contact, coordinate daily team rounds, investigate variances in outcomes, initiate and ensure patient and family education, attend to quality assurance and utilization review, and maintain a close liaison with the attending physician. The St. Vincent's professor also helped define the differences in expectation, knowledge, skill, and educational preparation for different roles of technical nurses and other members of the team. The American Association of Colleges of Nursing has taken the stance that education for professional nursing practice is a function of the first professional degree. This role must be clearly delineated and set apart from the role of nurses without such credentials (Felton, 1990).

The St. Vincent's professor was in an unusual position of "insider-outsider," as she was not employed by the institution in the same way as other staff. She had no secondary gains or hidden agendas, although she had a vested interest in the success of the project. She was a powerful advocate for professional nursing practice and patient-oriented care. As an insider-outsider, she could challenge members of the group without fear of retribution. She was objective, well informed, up-to-date about nursing practice nationwide, and could assist in negotiations for win win solutions.

Given her background as a nursing educator with a master's degree in adult health and doctoral coursework in curriculum and instruction, the St. Vincent's professor was accustomed to teaching nursing process, nursing diagnosis, goal setting, and charting using the SOAP format. Her role was exceedingly valuable in developing a documentation form used by the multidisciplinary team, and in persuading reluctant factions of the committee to consider using a common format.

Her work continues as care plans are being developed according to patient outcomes, with patient and family education forming a significant aspect of patient management in view of the emphasis on length of stay and minimizing patient care costs. The St. Vincent's professor will continue to work closely with the nurse managers to review teaching/learning theory and application; encourage the case managers to routinely assess teaching/learning needs; and write outcome objectives and measure goal attainment in terms of the cognitive, behavioral, and affective domains.

The patient-oriented delivery concept facilitates the integration of home care pre- and post-admission into a continuum of care, and fosters patient and family education, reinforcement, and evaluation. The goals of the patient-oriented delivery system are to:

- Decrease the number of caregivers who come in contact with the patient.
- Maximize the highest skill level of the caregiver roles.
- Bring services closer to the patient.
- Coordinate care to increase efficiency.

The Professional Practice Committee

At the same time that the St. Vincent's professor was gaining recognition on the steering committee, she was also integrating education and practice through her participation on the medical center's professional practice committee. This committee serves to:

- Identify major practice issues.
- Promote excellence in practice.
- Present recommendations to nursing management.

Members of this committee included three baccalaureate nursing graduates from the University of North Florida. These nurses were enthusiastic participants who became the core group of advocates for new models of practice. They were informed about issues and knew the change process from a theoretical and experiential point of view. Serving on this committee gave them a vehicle to put their ideas into practice. In fact, the committee has gained such status that staff compete for membership on it. The committee structure was composed of nursing administrators and nursing staff. Again, in the role of insider-outsider, the St. Vincent's professor acted as a consultant when practice issues became emotionally charged and the administrators and staff argued from different viewpoints.

The benefits of integrating education and practice are numerous, both in terms of education and clinical practice. Nursing faculty sometimes become isolated from practice issues, even though they take students into the clinical setting and might also practice in the institution. Serving on a committee that addresses patient care issues, while at the same time serving on a steering committee of administrators and top-level management responsible for patient outcomes and organizational leadership, provides the professor with a reality base to bring into the classroom. The St. Vincent's professor also brought the institutional perspective to departmental curriculum meetings and heightened the clinical awareness of faculty who wrestle with theoretical bases, clinical applications, and legal practice issues. She brought an academic perspective to the clinical practice setting, and at the same time presented the reality of the acute care setting to nursing education. This bridging helped the medical center develop an environment in which the multidisciplinary staff could delineate roles and develop skills to their full potential.

It takes time to build relationships between the "ivory tower" of the university and the clinical setting. Through active participation on committees, the St. Vincent's professor began to gain trust and acceptance by the medical center staff, and to earn recognition and power in decision making. Over time, she gained legitimate status as a part of the group. She was able to help create an environment for differentiated practice that is good for patients, family, and staff, as well as for student nurses.

The implications for nursing curricula are vital to the future of nursing education. If professional nurses are to be accountable for supervising support staff, they need to be taught supervision skills The implications for impact on leadership theory and style, management skills, team building, group process, accountability, delegation, organizational communication, etc. are glaringly obvious.

As pointed out in *Current Issues and Perspectives on Differentiated Practice*, the success of differentiating nursing practice is "directly related to the involvement and responsiveness of nurse educators" (Murphy and DeBack, 1990).

Throughout the country, there are examples of health care facilities that are involved with educational institutions to develop new practice models and select research criteria for their evaluation. At the same time, nursing faculty are beginning to redesign curricula in an effort to prepare students for the new roles that will be assigned to them (Murphy and DeBack, 1990).

As was the case in the St. Vincent's model, nursing educators have become active members of steering committees of medical centers, meeting on a regular basis to design and implement differentiated practice and to prepare new graduates for the roles they will be expected to assume. This process also calls for establishing clinical experiences that will foster the development of practitioners for differentiated roles (Murphy and DeBack, 1990).

Issues for Research

The development of a differentiated practice model in which roles are redesigned and delineated provides numerous opportunities for research and evaluation. The differentiated practice model raises the following questions about goal attainment:

Is there a relationship between the Patient-Oriented Delivery Model and:
- Continuity of care?
- A reduction in patient transfers?
- Patient satisfaction?
- Staff satisfaction/retention?
- Reduction in length of patient stay?
- Reduction in readmission of patients?
- Increased patient education?

Other questions may be asked about the multidisciplinary team approach to patient care in a test unit of the medical center:
- Is communication enhanced?
- Are professional relationships strengthened?
- Is respect for other professions increased?
- If so, what are the criteria for success?
- Does role blurring begin to occur as team members speak the same language and work closely over time?
- If role blurring does occur, is the phenomenon one to be valued or is the effect perceived as negative?
- What are the unanticipated side effects of the patient-oriented delivery model?
- What are the stories to be told that will guide us as we look to the future?

Integrating education and practice is one answer to the challenge.

❑   ❑   ❑

Part VIII

Looking at the Past and Defining Practice Models for the Future

Parallels and Paradoxes: Differentiated Nursing Practice

Rosemary T. McCarthy, D.N.Sc., R.N., F.A.A.N.

One of George Washington's first acts after taking command of the army at Cambridge in July 1775 was to write to the President of the Continental Congress, then assembled in Philadelphia, requesting that they take action to ensure a well-regulated medical system. In response to Washington's request, Congress established a Medical Department by Act on July 27, 1775. The law provided for one director general and chief physician, four surgeons, an apothecary, 20 surgeon's mates, a clerk, two storekeepers, a nurse to every 10 sick, and occasional laborers as needed (Fitzpatrick, n.d.).

The nurses, both men and women, were to attend the sick and obey the matron's orders (Ford et al., n.d.). The tasks of the nurse centered on housekeeping, laundering, distributing the linens and clothes, keeping the environment clean by washing and sweeping the floors, emptying the refuse jars, washing dishes, and providing extra nourishment or more delicate fare than the rations allowed. In some instances, the nurse even dressed wounds. Who were these nurses, "one to every 10 sick"?

Even though there were no schools of nursing in colonial America, there were men and women who were regarded by themselves and others as skilled in the attendance of the sick and injured. Apprenticed or self-taught, they served their neighbors — their service being both voluntary and commercial. They learned their craft through observation and practice. Ideas, remedies, and techniques spread informally, and in some instances, were circulated by the press. The press also served as the recruiter for those hired by the director general.

On March 4, 1776, subscribers to the *Boston Gazette and Country Journal* read:

> Wanted for the General Hospital, a number of nurses for the houses at Cambridge and Roxbury, the preference will be given to Boston and Charlestown women, and some men laborers, as assistants to the nurses (those belonging to the distres'd seaport towns would be the persons that the Director General would chuse [sic],) and as soon as may be. A quantity of herbs of all kinds for baths, sage and baum, rags, fine tow, honey and beeswax, thread & c. rosin, malt, hops and wheat bran, is also wanted . . . . Thomas Carnes, Q.M. & Steward, Convalescent Hospital, Cambridge, Feb. 22 (Boston Gazette, 1776).

No doubt these advertisements met with some success. However, the recruitment of female nurses was not sufficient to meet all the requirements for nursing personnel, and soldiers were supplied to make up the difference. The shortage and uncertain supply of nursing personnel was a continuing problem for the hospitals, both general and regimental. The major effort made by the Continental Congress to combat the shortage of nurses was through periodic increases in salary. However, no amount of pay was able to counteract the lack of a skilled nursing personnel pool.

Between the War for Independence and the Civil War, the status of the Medical Service was improved. The mere fact of the medical officer's rank made it easier for him to advise commanders on matters concerning the health of the command. The stability of the steward's position helped improve the management of hospitals. The supervisory control by the stewards over wardmasters, who in turn controlled soldier nurses, was clearly established within the military structure. The employed matrons and female nurses continued outside that structure (Rules and Directions, n.d.).

In 1861, very few Americans were educated — i.e., trained as nurses. Indeed, outside Protestant and Catholic nursing orders, little training was available. A few had "walked the wards" in the large hospitals, and some English women who had served with Florence Nightingale in the Crimea had immigrated to this country. However, when the Civil War broke out, many women wished to help the soldiers both in the North and South. Even though the official nursing force continued to be made up of detailed men and convalescents supervised by the stewards, women with limited experience found work through a variety of avenues — contract, certification, and volunteering. As Nutting and Dock (1907) so eloquently stated:

> The War washed away the petty anchors which had kept
> the majority of women carefully moored in the quiet remote
> little bays of domestic seclusion, and they floated out upon
> a stream of public duties.

The exact number of women who served as nurses for the Union Army is not known, but has been estimated to be about 3,200 (Ramsey, 1927). The tasks of the nurses are best exemplified by Emily Parsons in a letter to her mother:

> I have direct and complete control over the female nurses,
> I also direct all the male nurses; I do the latter work mostly
> through the ward masters who are here simply head nurses.
> They have the care of directing all the cleaning of wards and
> changing the patients' linen. I tell these men what I wish to
> have done, how I wish to have it done and when they are
> to see that it is done; I tell the nurse myself if necessary.
> I have now to train the female nurses. . . . They are to give
> all medicines, see that the special diet patients get all they
> are ordered and that it is properly served out to them,
> and to watch the patients and do for them whatever they
> require. . . (Parsons, 1880).

Emily Parsons had two years of study under Dr. John Warren, the superintendent of the Massachusetts General Hospital, and truly saw her role as that of nurse administrator.

Others, including Sophronia Bucklin, were more direct in the type of service they provided. Bucklin (1869) described her care for a patient with erysipelas:

> His eyes were shut with swollen lids, and every feature
> swollen to immense proportions. . . . I bathed his scaled face
> in a cooling preparation, combed out his hair and cleaned
> his fingernails, removed dead scales from his cheek and
> forehead, and laid over the whole a damp cloth.

All nursing was influenced by the realities of the situation. Whether in the field or general hospital, on a train or transport ship, clinical practice was dictated by the state of medical knowledge and the intuitive ability of the nurse. Memoirs of soldiers and nurses alike frequently refer to the reading of Scripture by the nurse as part of care. Nurses wrote letters for the patients or directly to their families urging their presence at the bedside of a dying soldier. Several stories of amateur theatrics and patriotic song-fests attest to the social aspects of caring (Lee, 1942).

Although some improvement occurred during the Civil War in the ongoing action and function of the Medical Department, it was never able to establish a corps of hospital men under the direct control of the medical officers, so that an official system of nursing within the Medical Department never developed.

The female nurse, along with the unofficial nurses sponsored by the various associations and commissions of relief, quickly disappeared. Custom, like the waves at the shore, washed away their tracks. Nonetheless, their Civil War work had changed the image of the female nurse from pest-house attendant to lady of healing, and opened the field of nursing as a socially acceptable occupation for middle-class women. Many who served during the war were to take an active part in the establishment of the early schools of nursing in America.

However, it was the performance of the contract nurses during the Spanish-American War that convinced the army and the nation that a corps of women trained as nurses was required for the welfare of American servicemen. It was also the first conflict in which the soldier nurses were under the direct command of the Medical Department.

In actual fact, the Spanish-American War was a military and political victory, but a medical disaster. In response to public pressure, President William McKinley requested the Secretary of War to appoint a commission to investigate the conduct of the war. Headed by retired General Granville Dodge, the commission held 109 meetings and heard testimony on all aspects of the conduct of the war. A major portion of the testimony had to do with the work of the female nurses, which stood the test of scrutiny and led to the recommendation to secure a corps of trained nurses ready to serve in an emergency. The Army Reorganization Act of February 2, 1901, written by Dr. Anita Newcomb McGee, established the Army Nurse Corps (Female) as part of the Army Medical Department (Army Reorganization Act, 1901).

Even without an emergency to respond to, there was still a need for trained nurses to be actively involved in the care of military patients. The first appointed (not commissioned) members of the Army Nurse Corps were drawn from the 220 contract nurses on duty at the General Hospital in San Francisco, the Tuberculosis Hospital at Fort Bayard, New Mexico, and several small installations in the Philippines. They were graduates of hospital schools of nursing with varied educational backgrounds. Only the superintendent was required to have graduated from a two-year program. Some of the nurses were better able to adjust to the requirements of the position than others. Mrs. Dita Kinney, the first superintendent, suggested that each nurse be assigned to the hospital at the Washington Barracks (Fort McNair), where their suitability could be observed. However, it was not until 1911, during the tour of Jane Delano, that such a program was initiated (Office of the Surgeon General, 1911). The program was informal, as nurses were recruited in small numbers and arrived sporadically. It was, in fact, more of a trial than an educational experience.

Because they were appointed and not commissioned, the nurses held no rank or authority over the enlisted hospital corps, and the system of management of patient care continued with the steward as the director of military (soldier) nursing personnel, and the female nurse as the director of the appointed nurses. The overall control was provided by the medical officer. Even at the ward level, the organization continued to be dual in nature.

Many conflicts developed between the Army Nurse Corps nurses and the enlisted nurses. From the start, however, there was an implicit differentiation of practice in that army nurses were assigned to duty at all army hospitals where the cases were of such a nature as to require the care of trained nurses. No more than two were assigned to a hospital of less than 20 beds (Manual of the Medical Department, 1900). As time went on, the Army Nurse Corps' tenuous foothold was strengthened by its members' superior knowledge. When disputes over patient care arose, they were resolved by the ability of the female nurses to influence the ward officers. By 1916, local ward rules gradually identified the Army Nurse Corps as the preferred leader of the nursing service. In 1917, Dora E. Thompson, superintendent of the Army Nurse Corps, inserted a statement into the Medical Department regulation that gave female nurses authority in patient care matters after the medical officer.

When the United States entered World War I in April 1917, 403 army nurses were on active duty. By June, there were 1,176; one year later, there were 12,186 (2,000 regular and 10,186 reserve) at 198 stations worldwide. The majority of these nurses came with the affiliated hospital units. Although these affiliated units represented the best of medical and nursing practice, they were totally ignorant of the military aspects of war service. For example, Base Hospital No. 18, the Johns Hopkins Unit, left for Europe on the 19th of June, 1918 with only a briefing from Clara Noyes, Chairman of the Bureau of Nursing Service American Red Cross. In an effort to overcome this lack of knowledge, the army set up mobilization stations. Chief nurse Edith A. Mury was assigned to the station at Ellis Island in New York Harbor. Along with Assistant Chief Nurse Mina Keenan and two other regular army nurses, she attempted to orient the chief nurses awaiting assignment, especially those of the affiliated units. Their time was limited, the program informal and demanding. As Mury said, "I often expected the chief nurse to acquire in a single day . . . methods it had taken me one year to learn" (Mury, n.d.)

The introduction of these affiliated units infused the U.S. Army Medical Department with the latest in medical-surgical knowledge and techniques. The nurses who were part of these teams were experienced and respected coworkers, skilled in operating room procedures and ward management. Anne Penland of U.S. Base Hospital No. 2 (Presbyterian Hospital, New York) was the first trained nurse anesthetist to arrive in the British sector. Her work so impressed the British Surgeon that she was soon employed in training the British Sisters. The course length consisted of two months didactic and supervised practice at the base hospital and one month supervised practice at the casualty clearing stations (Maxwell, 1918).

In the United States, the first clinical courses open to army nurses were in the administration of anesthesia, and were conducted at the Mayo Clinic in Rochester, Minnesota. Army nurse graduates were expected to teach other nurses and corpsmen the techniques they had learned, for the Surgeon General urged the broadest possible dissemination of these skills (Stimson, 1927).

As the war progressed, the country was faced with increased demands for nursing services, both military and civilian. Early in 1918, at the request of the Committee on Nursing, United States Council of National Defense, Annie Goodrich was appointed Chief Inspecting Nurse of Army Hospitals. She toured military hospitals and compared the quality of bedside care with that currently available in civilian hospitals staffed by active schools of nursing. Her report was negative. The military hospital had too few trained nurses to provide the needed care, the corpsmen were indifferent and poorly trained, and the supervision was minimal. She accompanied her report with a formal proposal for the establishment of an Army School of Nursing. Goodrich believed that a well supervised group of student nurses would provide the military patient with better care than was currently available or could be received from another group of partially trained personnel, no matter how well motivated.

She proposed that the school be headquartered in the Office of the Surgeon General, that the faculty be presided over by a dean, and that the plan of instruction be based on the National League of Nursing Education's new *Standard Curriculum for Schools of Nursing* (National League of Nursing Education, 1917). The program was to be three years in length; upon completion, the graduates would be eligible for state registration and become members of the regular Army Nurse Corps as positions opened up. After a lengthy debate, the plan was endorsed by the three national nursing organizations: the American Nurses Association, the National League for Nursing Education, and the National Organization of Public Health Nursing. With the support of these groups, the proposal weathered the legislative mill and was approved by the Secretary of War on May 25, 1918. Annie Goodrich was named director of the Army School of Nursing.

The school was unique — a consortium of independent units with their own faculty. Created out of need, it centered its work on control of curriculum, and standards of practice and procedures.

The students of the Army School of Nursing contributed much to the improvement of care in the army hospitals where they were located, and relieved some regular army nurses for service elsewhere. The obvious advantage of the school, the persuasive arguments of Annie Goodrich, and the influenza pandemic of 1918 probably saved "The School" from termination following the November Armistice. In December 1918, out of 10,597 applications received, 5,858 had been accepted and 1,462 students were on duty at 32 units. A survey showed that 80% wanted to complete the course. The school was continued, and in June 1919, Julia C. Stimson was appointed dean. In December, she was appointed to succeed Dora Thompson as superintendent of the Army Nurse

Corps. She held both positions until the school was suspended in 1933 (Office of the Surgeon General, 1920a).

The National Defense Act of June 4, 1920 authorized relative rank in the grades of second lieutenant through major, and Julia Stimson was the first nurse to wear the insignia of major on her uniform. Like all new members of an exclusive club, the nurses were scrutinized for their military bearing and demeanor. In fairness to the nurses, and obviously in response to their critics, the Surgeon General called for classes to be taught in the methods and requirements of saluting (Office of the Surgeon General, 1920b).

One outcome of the award of relative rank was the eligibility of Army Nurse Corps officers for schooling in civilian schools. From 1921 to 1939, more than 60 nurses attended courses at Teachers College, Leland Stanford University, and George Peabody College in Nashville, Tennessee. Enrollees included Ruth I. Taylor in administration at Stanford, 1922; and Julia O. Flikke, Maude C. Davidson, and Mary W. Tobin in administration at Teachers College, 1925. The majority of these early educational opportunities went to actual or potential instructors at the Army School of Nursing. Army nurses attended courses in dietary administration, basal metabolism testing, laboratory techniques (i.e., x-ray technology), psychiatric nursing, and some business courses (Office of the Surgeon General, 1923).

The importance an organization places on an activity such as education can be evaluated by the "institutionalization" of that activity. The first step in that process, as it applies to nursing, was the separate identification of the teaching activities of the principle chief nurse in Army Regulation 40-20, Army Nurse Corps, General Provisions dated October 6, 1930. These duties included the following instruction to army nurses:

> . . . in their duties peculiar to Army work with emphasis on Army Regulations that relate to the Army Nurse Corps; any necessary matters pertaining to the work of nursing, and when required by the Commander of the hospital the instruction in practical nursing of enlisted men on ward duty (Department of the Army, 1930).

This regulation indicated the gradual shift in the role of the Army Nurse Corps officer in relation to the enlisted technicians assigned to the wards of the army hospitals where more complex care was required. It identified the need for corpsmen with patient care skills, in addition to those needed in the field during in time of war. The experience with the affiliated units may have convinced the regular Medical Department leaders that more training was needed by the enlisted technicians to make them as useful as the civilian assistants had proven to be during the war. Therefore, the army nurse continued to move into a position of leadership in patient care through education, both administrative and clinical.

Six months after Japanese planes bombed Pearl Harbor, there were 12,000 nurses on active duty. Not many had any military experience. As Theresa Archard observed, "Nurses . . . were more apt to raise their right hands, take the oath, put on their white uniforms, and find themselves, in no time flat, on the ward up to their ears in work" (Archard, 1945).

The first mandatory military training for Army Nurse Corps members was developed by the Nursing Division of the Office of the Surgeon General and published in October 1942. The course was designed for the Army Nurse Corps in the theater of operation, and was to be carried out at the various staging areas. Four weeks of 44 hours each were divided into 16 hours of ward duty; the other 160 hours were devoted to classes — in army medical organization, military courtesy, and custom; uniform regulations; dismounted drill; physical fitness; defense against air, chemical, and mechanized attack; military administration; and first aid and field sanitation. The program was not very well carried out because of the diversity of support and lack of facilities at the staging areas. The need for nurses to care for the ever-increasing number of patients took precedence over training.

In contrast to basic military training which could not be conducted efficiently in hospitals, clinical training courses could be, provided that proper emphasis and priority was given to the program. In the spring of 1942, anesthesia courses were given at Walter Reed, Army-Navy, Fitzsimmons, and several station hospitals.

By mid-1944, nearly 100 nurses had completed the program; in 1945, over 2,000 Army Nurse Corps members were qualified as nurse anesthetists (Mullins and Parks, 1974).

Before World War II, psychiatric patients at army hospitals were kept only long enough for arrangements to be made for transfer to St. Elizabeth's, or other long-term care facilities near their homes. In World War II, there were many such patients. One out of every 12 admitted to army hospitals was admitted for psychiatric reasons, and approximately 400,000 soldiers were discharged with psychiatric diagnoses.

Lieutenant Kathleen Otto, who had been superintendent of nursing at McLean Hospital, Waverly, Massachusetts, prepared a program guide for use at the School of Military Psychiatry, Lawson General Hospital, Atlanta, Georgia. By the end of 1945, 589 Army Nurse Corps nurses and 296 cadet nurses had completed the program (Glass and Bernucci, 1966).

Most nurses who joined the army in World War II had training in basic operating room procedures and techniques. Their unused skills were sharpened with on-the-job experience. However, it was necessary to develop programs to broaden the management and supervisory roles, as well as provide classes in methods of instruction for the teaching of enlisted technicians.

Flight nurse training was initiated at Bowman Field, Kentucky, in November 1942 under the control of 349th Air Evacuation Group, and remained under its control until the group was deactivated and redesignated as the Army Air Force School of Air Evacuation in June 1943. Flight nurse training was the only school required for assignment to a specific specialty during the war (Air Evacuation Program, 1944).

Colonel Florence A. Blanchfield summed up the problems of training in World War II in a memo she wrote to the chief of professional administration service:

> The one problem . . . (is) that the training has not been approved on an Army Service Forces level, and the nurses taking this training have not been relieved from assigned duties to a degree that enable them to secure the maximum benefit from such courses. Furthermore, . . . it has not been possible to standardize the programs (Blanchfield, 1945).

In 1944, Public Law 350 enacted by the 78th Congress granted army nurses temporary commissions in the U.S. Army, with full pay and privileges of the grades second lieutenant through colonel, for the duration of the emergency plus six months. Colonel Blanchfield continued to campaign for permanent rank for army nurses and enlisted the help of Representative Frances Payne Bolton and Senator Margaret Chase Smith. Together they sponsored the Army-Navy Nurse Act (Public Law 36, 80th Congress), which passed on April 16, 1947, just two months short of the limitation of the previous law. This act established the Army Nurse Corps (Female) in the Medical Department of the Regular Army, with permanent commissioned officer status in the grades of second lieutenant through lieutenant colonel, and established the Army Nurse Corps section of the Officer's Reserve Corps. Provision was made for the chief of the Army Nurse Corps to serve in the temporary grade of colonel during her statutory tour. Florence Blanchfield was given the service number N-1.

During this postwar period, the Army Nurse Corps was able to formalize and standardize courses. In 1947, anesthesia nursing was offered at Brooke, Letterman, Fitzsimmons, and Walter Reed hospitals, which led to preparation for examination and certification by the American Association of Nurse Anesthetists. In the same year, operating room technique and management was offered at Letterman and Walter Reed (the Walter Reed program affiliated with Catholic University); in 1946, psychiatric nursing was offered at Brooke General Hospital.

For the first time, the Medical Field Service School, which moved from Carlisle Barracks to Fort Sam Houston, Texas in February 1946, included nurses in its program. The faculty prepared an eight-week basic course for women officers with no army service. The first class entered in the spring of 1947. Plans for inclusion of women in the advanced courses started immediately. Thus, when the first technical manual on career planning was published in June 1948, the relationship of training to position was clearly outlined (Department of the Army, 1948).

The administrative realization of the need for standardization, which grew out of the wartime effort to mold over 57,000 individual nurses into a unified force that could function flexibly in a variety of settings under constant change, led Colonel Blanchfield to assign five Army Nurse Corps officers to develop a procedural guide. The resulting *Department of Army Technical Manual: Professional Nursing Techniques* proved very helpful in the orientation of newly-assigned Army Nurse Corps officers and became the textbook for the training of enlisted medical technicians (Army Nurse Corps, 1949).

Army nurses were assigned to the Medical Field Service School to direct and teach two enlisted technicians' courses: basic and specialty. The size of the teaching staff increased as the number of medical officers declined, and the medical officer training became more academic — competing with civilian schools for interns and residents. Programs also attracted a wide variety of medical specialists to provide the clinical leadership required to meet residency training program accreditation and requirements for certification.

By 1954, the army nurse had officially replaced the ward officer as first-line unit administrator. The board-certified physician-medical officer had moved to chief of service, paralleling the civilian teaching hospital arrangement. The head nurse was responsible for the nursing service on one or more units, reporting to the medical officers for the execution of medical orders, and to the chief of nursing service for guidance on the standards of nursing care rendered (Department of the Army, 1959). Her regular rank as an aide to management gave her authority over the enlisted medical technicians, who themselves were receiving more formal and complex instruction.

In 1949, a pilot course for enlisted personnel on the practical nurse level was begun at the Army Medical Center, Washington (Walter Reed). The director and the faculty were Army Nurse Corps officers. Additional courses were started at other Army medical centers to meet the patient care needs throughout the hospital system and to provide technical leadership to the medical soldiers. The addition of the military practical nurse (9IC-clinical specialist) augmented the nursing team, and they proved their worth as soldier nurses in the field, MASH, and station hospitals of Korea. Promotion opportunities helped to ensure that the men and women selected to attend the military practical nursing programs were the best available (Shields, 1981).

The department of nursing in the army medical treatment facility had evolved into a team of nursing personnel prepared by education and training to meet the nursing care needs of the military patients. The department was headed by the chief nurse and enlisted noncommissioned officers who supervised and provided patient care and maintained the physical environment where care was provided (Adams-Ender and Hudock, 1989). This organization has remained stable, although the increased demands for care created by the Korean and Vietnam Wars without full-scale military and industrial mobilization necessitated increased use of civilian personnel. Civilian counterparts can now be found for most job titles or positions on the nursing units.

The 1950s were years of professional growth for the Army Nurse Corps. Not only did research and practice receive recognition, but the educational aspects of service were also emphasized. The position of "nursing instructor" as a separate role was identified in 1954 (Army Regulation 40-20), and that of "educational coordinator" was identified in 1959 (AR 40-6). By 1969, the title of "instructor" was used to designate Army Nurse Corps officers assigned as instructors for authorized U.S. Army Medical Department courses. The position of "educational coordinator" was expanded to "chief, nursing education and training services," and was charged with the management of all nursing education programs conducted at medical treatment facilities. To be assigned as chief, nursing education and training, an Army Nurse Corps officer was required to have at least a master's of science in nursing. Doctorally-prepared nurses were given preference for this key assignment.

After the suspension of the Army School of Nursing in 1933, attempts were made to reestablish the program in 1940, 1945, 1948, and 1958; all were unsuccessful. However, on March 20, 1963, General Leonard D. Heaton (the Surgeon General concerned with the continuing decline in strength of the Army Nurse Corps), noting the shortage of nurses nationwide, directed that a study be initiated to determine the feasibility of reopening the Army School of Nursing. General Heaton received formal approval for the proposed School of Nursing from the Department of Defense in August 1963. The approval came in the form of a memo from the Secretary of Defense and said, "O.K. Bud, you can have your School."

The University of Maryland Board of Regents approved and forwarded the plan to the Surgeon General, whereby the university would accept responsibility for the development and supervision of an upper division nursing curriculum for the Army Institute of Nursing at Walter Reed Army Medical Center (WRAIN) on March 13, 1964. The school operated until June 1978. The last class of 91 nurses graduated and was commissioned at a Walter Reed rose garden ceremony during which the WRAIN unit flag and crest were retired and donated to the Army Nurse Corps for display in the Army Medical Museum. Closed because of the high attrition rates, high cost, and budget constraints, the school never met the expected recruitment and retention objectives (Heaton, n.d.).

In addition to the WRAIN program, several other initiatives were developed to reduce the shortage of military nurses generated by the buildup in southeast Asia. On December 30, 1965, the Secretary of Defense authorized each military department to offer warrant officer appointment to civilian registered nurses having two years of training — that is, associate degree graduates of National League for Nursing (NLN) approved schools. At the same time, Draft Call #38 was issued to provide 700 male nurses between fourth-quarter fiscal year 1966 and fourth-quarter fiscal year 1967.

Provisions were made to increase the number of civilian nurses at stateside facilities and to enlist licensed practical nurses as sergeants. Professional nurse recruitment efforts were intensified.

Recruitment of technical nurses began on January 11, 1966, and the warrant officer nurse program was officially approved and became effective on April 12, 1966. The Office of the Surgeon General requested that 100 technical nurses be obtained for fiscal year 1966 and a total of 400 be obtained for fiscal year 1967. Accessions of these nurses fell far short of these objectives. In November 1967, only 83 (66 males and 17 females) were on active duty. All told, only 90 nurses were commissioned under this program (Department of the Army, 1967).

Duties of the technical nurse fell under three categories:

1) surgical technical nurse,
2) technical nurse anesthetist, and
3) general technical nurse.

These duties involved practicing technical nursing under the direct supervision of a professional nurse in hospitals of 200 or more beds. In the case of the technical nurse anesthetist, supervision was to be by a professionally-certified registered nurse anesthetist or physician. Most were classified as general technical nurses. Less than 21% of the Army Nurse Corps commissioned officers on active duty during the duration of the warrant officer program were baccalaureate graduates. Although the duties of the warrant officers were clearly defined, in actuality they frequently found themselves expected to practice without direct supervision and to assume some administrative tasks during the evening or night tours of duty.

In 1968, A. M. Hays studied the perceptions of selected warrant officer nurses and their immediate nursing supervisors regarding effective and ineffective nursing behaviors of warrant officer nurses and aspects of practice which these nurses were best and least prepared for in their nursing education program. The sample consisted of 19 (24%) warrant officer nurses assigned as technical nurses in clinical units in the U.S. Army Medical Service and their immediate supervisors (in this case, head nurses). There was a great deal of difference between the nurses and the supervisors. Most of the warrant officers were men; most of the supervisors were women. The median age of the warrant officers was 26; that of the supervisors was 39. All but one of the supervisors were graduates of diploma programs. Warrant officers were perceived as those best prepared to give direct nursing care and as liking this aspect of nursing most. They also were perceived to be least prepared in ward management duties and to like this aspect of nursing the least. One of the major findings of the study was that the warrant officer nurses were not utilizing those functions for which they were prepared educationally and for which they were directed by the regulations governing them. Another conclusion was that the system was not ready for their inclusion. The Army Medical Department (the Army Nurse Corps) was not ready or able to provide a structure in which the technical nurse could ideally function. Therefore, the concept of technical and professional roles could not be implemented in a system where the majority of the corps were, in fact, only technically prepared (Hays, 1968).

Because the program failed to meet the manpower objectives, and due to the fact that only three of 83 surveyed responded positively to the question concerning their desire to remain on active duty, the warrant officer program was suspended with the expiration of the authorizing circular on April 3, 1968. The last warrant officer nurse was discharged from active duty in April 1971 (Army Nurse Corps Career Activity Office, n.d.).

The failure of the warrant officer nurse program also served to strengthen the Army Nurse Corps' resolve that the appropriate basic education for a professional nurse and officer of the corps was at the baccalaureate level. Every effort was made to encourage those army nurses on active duty to achieve the BS through part-time or full-time study. Steady progress toward that goal was made a matter of record for evaluation and advancement. By 1971, 42% of all Army Nurse Corps members were prepared at the baccalaureate level, at least. The Army Nurse Corps was ready to comply with the army's guidance, and in 1972, the bachelor's degree was made a requirement for appointment on active duty (Rexrode, 1978).

Early in 1971, under the leadership of Brigadier General Anna Mae Hays, chief of the Army Nurse Corps, a task force developed a coordinated plan for advanced training in clinical specialties to prepare nurse clinicians for specific and definitive roles. The task force outlined their belief that increasing the availability of health care services was essential to the promotion of health and reduction of morbidity in the military community, and in keeping with the mission of the Medical Department "to conserve the fighting strength." They described the expanded scope of nursing as being three-dimensional.

First are the nursing skills, techniques, judgments, and interventions that have been taught as nursing. Second are those medically-delegated functions and responsibilities, many of which were already being practiced. Third are those functions that increase participation in interdisciplinary planning for formulating comprehensive health plans for patients and their families and providing for their continuity. This approach to health care is necessary to provide benefits to all the health clients and to ensure that health care goals, as defined by each member of the team, are complementary.

In 1972, courses in the Army Nurse Corps clinician program included ambulatory care/adult health, obstetrics and gynecology, pediatrics, and nurse midwifery. The advanced operating room, anesthesia nursing, and army health nursing courses were modified to include the nurse clinician role in 1973. By 1974, 245 army nurses had completed the program — 169 in army schools and 75 at civilian programs (Travers, 1972).

During September, October, and November of 1973, a study of the practice effectiveness of army nurse clinicians was conducted to determine quantity and quality of services provided patients, and to assess acceptance of nurse clinicians as primary health care providers. A sample of 96 nurse clinicians functioning in ambulatory care settings who provided a variety of services to the patient with both acute and chronic conditions, as well as well-person check-ups, indicated that they were well accepted by their patients. Both the psychiatric-mental health and intensive care nurse clinicians had difficulty with the role of clinician as primary caregiver. The intensive care nurses considered themselves specialists in intensive care and felt that the clinician role was too limited. The psychiatric-mental health nurses frequently felt that, because of the organization of the setting where they worked, it was not possible to use a clinician's skills unless assigned to a special program — such as a day care center.

The study concluded that those clinicians practicing primarily in an ambulatory care setting were practicing as prepared and providing direct care to a large number of patients. Of the 96 surveyed, 50 were monitored for number of patient contacts during the study month. These clinicians saw 10,926 patients — approximately one per working hour. Another encouraging finding was the large number of patients who reported an increased understanding of their illness or condition, medications, and medical treatment (Russell and Williams, 1976).

Similar patient acceptance was found by Rexrode (1978) in a survey of 28 nurse practitioners (clinicians), 28 professional (nonclinician) nurses, and 84 patients assigned to each nurse group. The degree of acceptance was proportional to the amount of contact the patient had with the practitioners. During the third quarter of fiscal year 1980, 162 army nurse practitioners saw 35,457 adult medical-surgical patients; 50,829 pediatric patients; 33,250 obstetric and gynecologic patients; 5,544 psychiatric patients in the ambulatory care setting; and 280 normal deliveries were performed by nurse midwives — a sizable contribution to the health care of the military community.

However, not all aspects of the army nurse clinician program were positive. One of the first complications arose when the program change request of 1971 granted funds without an increase in authorized spaces. This meant that existing resources would be expected to provide personnel for the expanded services. Thus, shortages in the acute care setting were increased, and the nurses working on the hospital units perceived the program as competitive, not complementary. At the same time, those nurses who were functioning as clinicians found the experience very rewarding. They enjoyed the one-to-one experience and the challenge of increased autonomy. Chief nurses were under constant pressure to increase the number of nurses assigned to the hospital units and to ambulatory care settings. The clinicians were perceived as inflexible.

A second problem was created by the diverging perceptions held by nursing and medicine of the nurses' roles. One of the reasons the army nurse clinician program was so well received by the medical leadership of the U.S. Army Medical Department was the fact that it was introduced at a time of need for physician augmentation due to the end of the physician draft. In spite of carefully worded statements about the expansion of nursing, the main feature of the program which received acceptance and reward was the physician extender aspect.

In September 1976, a "working conference" was held to make recommendations to the chief of the Army Nurse Corps as to the future direction of the army nurse clinician program.

Recommended changes included:

- That prerequisites for admission to the course be a baccalaureate degree in nursing and the achievement of career status in order to ensure a better base of experience and commitment.
- That the title of those graduating from these courses be changed to "nurse practitioner," in keeping with the practice in the civilian nursing community; and the title of "clinical nurse specialist," be reserved for army nurses who have a master's of science in clinical nursing.
- That the courses be examined and revised as necessary to prepare for beginning specialty practice in both the acute and ambulatory care settings to increase flexibility of assignment.
- That in the event of mobilization, nurse practitioners revert to their basic medical-surgical specialty unless large numbers of women and children are involved in the mobilization/disaster setting; that first priority for course conduct during mobilization be assigned to courses in operating room, anesthesia, intensive care, and psychiatric-mental health nursing; that second priority be assigned to obstetrical and gynecological nursing; and all others as resources allow.

In this way, the working conference affirmed that the goal of the Army Nurse Corps is to maximize professionalism in the practice of its members, lending support to the mission of the Army Nurse Corps as a contributing member of the U.S. Army Medical Department (Army Nurse Corps Career Activity Office, 1976).

The goal of a Army Nurse Corps qualified at the baccalaureate level has been achieved. Currently, 30 Army Nurse Corps members (0.7%) have doctoral degrees; 1,350 Army Nurse Corps members (30%) are prepared at the master's level; and an active worldwide program of continuing education is in force to ensure the clinical and military nursing leadership of the professional nurse (Bartz, 1990).

Since its inception, the Army Nurse Corps has used education to meet the requirements of its mission. Clinical education has advanced the practice, whereas military education has emphasized the readiness of army nurses to assume the heroic posture for which the corps is maintained. Vagts (1959) once said, "Every war is fought, every army maintained in a military way and in a militaristic way." He further contrasted the two:

> ... the military way as limited in scope, confined to one function (the winning of specific objectives efficiently and with the lowest possible expenditure of men and material), and scientific in its essential qualities. In contrast, the militaristic way is frivolous, full of customs, interests, actions and thoughts which glorify the trappings of war and sacrifice the means of war for the glory of individuals and nations (Vagts, 1959).

For an army to perform in a military way, each member of the force must have a special place in the structure of that force, specific functions in the process of the operation, and sufficient knowledge and power to perform efficiently. Symbols of status (rank) are used to place individuals in the structure. Directives, orders, manuals, job descriptions, and standards are used to guide functions, and education is used to provide the individual with the skills and abilities needed for efficient functioning and advancement. Today, the U.S. Army Nurse Corps has its place in the structure, its specific functions, and a body of knowledge which gives it power to contribute to the winning of victory.

This paper describes the emergence of the Army Nurse Corps as a component of the U.S. Army Medical Department, and highlights the role of education in the differentiation of the practice of nursing in the army health care system. Throughout the paper, several themes have emerged as instrumental in this process: public demand and political action, the demands of war and system constraints, and scientific knowledge and power.

Public demand and political action are exemplified by the call from George Washington and the response made by the Continental Congress to the needs of the sick and injured at Cambridge in 1775 which established the Army Medical Department. It is further illustrated by the actions the nation took in response to the findings of the Dodge committee investigation of the medical activities during the Spanish-American War which led to instituting the Army Nurse Corps (Female) in 1901. The struggle by nursing leaders within the Army Nurse Corps for rank is another example of political action that had a remarkable effect on establishing nursing as a bona fide expression of army health care.

The unprecedented war demands for nurses in the military (particularly during World War II) and, as a consequence, in the civilian community, called for the differentiation of practice not only within nursing, but also in the use of post-graduate training in the clinical specialties of anesthesia, operating room, trauma, and psychiatric-mental health nursing, as well as by teaching and delegating selected nursing tasks to the enlisted technicians.

System constraints on nursing in the army health care system are the same as those experienced by nursing everywhere — primarily in the control of health care by the medical profession, but also in the perception of the status of nursing as an agent of medicine. This control is culturally and socially determined by the status and expectations attached to medicine by the public which, to a large degree, have been determined by the possession of scientific knowledge. In our society, medical knowledge is perceived to be of a higher order, and those possessing it have been awarded the power to control the systems through which it is delivered.

In the U.S. Army Medical Department, the power which resides in the organization is possessed by the medical officers who fill the leadership positions and hold the military rank commensurate with their responsibility and authority. Over the years and in response to the demands of the public, they have delegated many responsibilities and shared some of their authority with the leadership of nursing. Although most of this response has been perceived as meeting the needs of the clients, the methods have always included individual professional protectionism. The advance of nursing in the army is the result of seized opportunity and demonstrated worth. Army nursing has also exerted its power, whether conferred by rank or knowledge, over the practice of nursing in the army health care system — an action that can be considered both a parallel and a paradox.

However, within the limits of its bureaucratic boundaries, the U.S. Army Medical Department illustrates differentiated health care practice, career advancement, job security, and personal growth — an evolution that has occurred over a 200-year period. There is a need to accelerate, continue, and share this process. As Virginia Henderson has said:

We should get health workers attuned to the idea that they've got to sit down and say: "What are our health problems? Who do we have to deal with them? How can we divide this job up so that the patient will be well served?" . . . Until we can get rid of our vanity about who we are and what we do, that's not going to happen (Henderson, 1978).

The story of the development of nursing practice in the U.S. Army Medical Department shows that Henderson's call can be implemented. It is time to make it happen and continue into the twenty-first century.

❏   ❏   ❏

Differentiated Nursing Practice: Historical Parallels and Paradoxes in Public Health Nursing

M. Louise Fitzpatrick, Ed.D., R.N., F.A.A.N.

C ommunity health nursing in the United States has been stimulated by environmental and social forces. It also has been conditioned by the economy and changes in the major health problems of populations to which it has responded. Yet community health nursing has been limited in the full expression of its mission and the accomplishment of its goals by the lack of an organized system of health care delivery and health care financing nationwide. It has been constrained by the focus on hospital care that has dominated the latter half of this century, and it has been both assisted and impeded by developments in nursing education.

It is serendipitous that this topic should be discussed at a meeting in Charleston, South Carolina, because visiting nursing in this country dates back to 1813 when the Ladies Benevolent Society of Charleston organized a volunteer service to provide nursing care and food to the sick poor during acute stages of illness, especially during epidemics of yellow fever. Like other early responses by the Women's Board of the New York City Mission, various Protestant church groups, and the secular humanities of the Ethical Culture Society of New York City, such services typically employed one or two nurses. However, between 1894 and 1905, there were 171 such ventures in 110 cities and 445 nurses were employed. For the most part, these nurses were local women and graduates of a variety of hospital-based schools with sponsorship provided by philanthropic organizations (Waters, 1909).

This volunteerism gave way to a more organized approach to providing care to the sick and sick poor at home, as well as through community-based dispensaries in the larger cities. Such services proliferated during the beginning of the twentieth century. In Boston, Philadelphia, Baltimore, Detroit, Cleveland, Rochester, Buffalo, Chicago, and New York, as well as in the smaller cities of the East and Midwest, visiting nurse services evolved.

Although variations in the emphasis of programs existed, a major thrust was the delivery of care to large numbers of immigrants, many of whom were poor and in need of preventive services as well as sick care. In 1905, the hospitals in New York cared for approximately only one-tenth of the city's sick (Wald, 1906). Lillian Wald and other pioneers of the visiting nurse movement established their services — including care of the sick — on a basic premise that to prevent illness and monitor well-being, it was vital to teach people how to care for themselves. The nurse, as the primary instrument of the public health movement, was to also be a nurse and a health teacher who made scientific discoveries regarding the transmission of disease applicable to the daily lives of the average citizen.

Note, if you will, the inclusion of the word "instructive" in the names of some of the early visiting nurse associations, such as that in Boston (1886). From the earliest point in their history, the role of the community health nurse included an educative function. C.E.A. Winslow, a driving force behind the public health movement in America, believed that, "The visiting nurse was the most important figure in the modern movement for the protection of public health" (Winslow, 1923). Adelaide Nutting not only disagreed, but commented that:

> The public health movement did not create the public health nurse; it found her at work in her district, nursing the sick, watching over families and the neighborhood, and teaching in the homes those sanitary practices, those measures of personal and home hygiene, which do much to prevent disease and promote health (Nutting, 1923).

Not unlike our present situation, the early development of public health nursing practice existed within an environment characterized by a high incidence of communicable disease, cultural diversity, poverty, and limited resources. These small, spontaneous responses to the society's health needs gave rise to the development of bureau-cratic structures, which were organized and designed to provide better care in a more efficient manner. All over the country, sponsor-ship eventually shifted from philanthropic organizations to reim-bursement from insurance companies, and then to local tax support which emerged with the rise of local health depositories in the 1930s. Later, this gave way to reimbursement through federal pro-grams such as Medicare in the 1960s, and to a combination of pri-vate insurance and tax dollars upon which we rely at the present.

The need to finance care and support these services, and the limitations to service and practice resulting from the consequences of change, has spawned the return of grass roots efforts. In this sense, community nursing services were part of a spontaneous response to the needs of people unserved (see the many examples of projects addressing the needs of the homeless, AIDS patients, and various "new" immigrant groups).

Although a greater dichotomy now exists between organized community nursing services and their financial sponsorship and the volunteerism of these newer projects, our era is replete with par-allels and paradoxes when contrasted with the beginning of the cen-tury. Even the present shortage of adequately prepared personnel to meet the nursing and health needs of society, and the controver-sies that arise when standards and qualifications must be balanced with numbers of people available to engage in such work, are not new phenomena. Inherent in the historical development of the pub-lic health nursing role has been the tension between the need to provide care to the sick at home and the larger role of preventive and health education at both the individual level and the policy level, with a focus on planning for the needs of aggregates within the population. Another parallel is the educational preparation of the nurse who functions outside the hospital and the requisite knowledge and skill required for independent action and autonomy in such practice roles. Still another related issue which finds its roots in the early part of this century is the question of whether commu-nity nursing is best delivered as a generalized or specialized service, or whether in today's environment the nurse should be a generalist rather than a specialist. Assuming a variety of nurses now practicing outside the hospital, upon what basis should practice be differentiated?

The precedent for differentiated practice in community health nursing is a very strong one, based on sound theoretical rationales as well as experiential and empirical evidence. Yet the experience of community health nursing with differentiated practice is not extensive.

When the visiting nurse or public health nursing movement was in its early development, all preparation for nursing took place in hospital-based schools which were proliferating at a phenomenal rate. Three prevalent issues emerged. The first involved the legal protection of the public and the nurse. The licensure movement was in its infancy and the differentiation between skilled and unskilled caretakers of the sick was of major consequence for organized nursing. A second issue centered around the major focus of the practice role of the visiting nurse. Its emphasis was that nurses who were enthusiastic about their roles in health teaching and preventive care might abdicate their responsibilities to those who were sick and in need of bedside care. A third issue concerned education for practice, with a strong belief on the part of nursing leadership and public health activists that nurses in community work needed a foundation in hospital care, plus a broader education in subjects such as culture, economics, and politics that affected the lives, health, and welfare of their patients.

This focus on educational preparation as the premise for differentiated practice or appropriate background for work in community health nursing became such a strong belief that, as recently as the 1960s, many diploma school graduates gave their reason for returning to school to complete a BSN as the desire to practice as a public health nurse. They responded, therefore, to the necessity to meet the basic educational requirement for that practice. So strong was the belief that additional education was a necessity for nurses practicing in the community that as early as 1910 a university course preparing graduate nurses for community work was established at Teachers College, Columbia University in affiliation with the New York School of Philanthropy and the Henry Street settlement. Courses included psychology, hygiene and sanitation, bacteriology, food economics, cultural health practices, social agencies and resources, principles and practices of organization and administration, and social aspects of charities (Christy, 1970). It was taught by an interdisciplinary faculty and established the preferred pattern of preparation which endured for nearly 30 years. The program required that hospital school graduates entered one of a variety of postgraduate courses in public health nursing, some of which awarded a certificate to practice in community nursing. The

National Organization for Public Health Nursing (which existed from 1912 until the reorganization of nursing associates in 1952) assumed guidance in a very deliberate manner over the development of education and the practice and development of administrative structures to provide for delivery of care (Fitzpatrick, 1975). Since then, the incorporation of community health nursing into basic baccalaureate nursing programs has become an expectation.

Since 1910, there has always been a discrepancy between the supply of "prepared" public health nurses and the demand from individuals, regardless of nursing preparation, to engage in this sphere of practice. As early as 1917, the National League of Nursing Education recognized that not all nurses who would work outside the hospital would be as adequately prepared as was recommended. The National Organization for Public Health Nursing was enlisted to develop an outline for basic preparation in public health nursing which was included in the 1917 curriculum guide. This guide and the others that succeeded it in 1927 and 1937 were, of course, designed to encourage conformity among hospital-based programs in the hope that standardization would occur, thus distinguishing better schools from the many others that had developed without benefit of qualified faculty or students. The fact that hospital preparation included the best clinical education that could be provided was not considered to be sufficient preparation for work in visiting nursing. This agreement was widely accepted by nursing leadership and used as a stimulus for staff development and employment throughout larger, more sophisticated hospital agencies.

World War I had a profound effect on this educational development by creating a demand for more nurses on all fronts. Of major consequence was rural health care, communicable disease control (especially in areas near military installations), child health, the influenza epidemic of 1918, polio prevention, and maternal-infant nutrition. The Vassar Training Camp, which offered a three-month preliminary nursing program for college graduates prior to entering an accelerated two-year nursing program, produced some of public health nursing's strongest leaders in the 1930s and 1940s (Clappson, 1964).

The demand for nurses to meet mounting community needs gave way to the development of shortened postgraduate courses in public health nursing and the use of nonprofessional workers and volunteers to assist nurses. Strain and some conflict resulted when organized nursing approved the use of unskilled nonprofessionals in public health who were being hired as attendants (Thwing, 1919). These attendants were encouraged to take on additional responsibility by physicians, but technically were not under nursing's supervision. Conflicts arose based on perceived threats to public safety and perhaps some self-protectionism, which meant that professional nursing saw the possibility of losing control over its practice.

Physicians were particularly interested in the preparation of a new kind of health worker to assume the preventive aspects of service, which posed a threat to public health nursing. There was widespread dissatisfaction with hospital training schools and, despite the curriculum guides, there was resistance to incorporating public health nursing concepts into the three-year training programs. In the community nursing agency, the balance between bedside care and preventive care was difficult to strike. Unhappily, our current situation reflects that dilemma, since reimbursement for services frequently dictates the priorities of nursing practice.

The foremost proponent of the new worker was Dr. Haven Emerson, commissioner of health in New York, New York. During World War I, Emerson had worked with health visitors in England and had trained similar indigenous workers in France. His experiences convinced him that what was needed was neither a nurse nor a health teacher nor a social worker, but a new combination of health worker who would deal directly with families, agencies, charities, and courts to coordinate and plan care and provide education in public health (Nursing Archives, n.d.). Emerson saw the ideal health worker as a female high school graduate with an 11-month program in hospital and medical services who had performed field work in the Bureau of Child Hygiene and Preventive Disease, attended lectures at the School of Philanthropy, and conducted practice case work in charitable organizations. After two years of work on the job, a degree in public health service would be awarded, with those who were already college graduates receiving a modified program and special grooming to assume leadership positions.

Leaders in organized nursing, such as Adelaide Nutting and the National Organization for Public Health Nursing, voiced their concerns about the eventual licensure of such individuals, admitting that the available nursing education was inadequate for the role that had developed. They contended, however, that a nursing background was necessary and appropriate for teaching prevention, but that more education, not less, was required for adequate public health teaching. They argued that such teaching was part of nursing's role at the bedside as well as in other settings, such as school health, well-child clinics, and industry. Postgraduate education was viewed as an achievable short-term goal, but long-term public health preparation needed to be included in basic nursing programs.

It was this threat of a new health worker that stimulated the Rockefeller Study of Preparation for Public Health Nursing which soon evolved into the classic study, *Nursing and Nursing Education in the United States* (Goldmark, 1923). It seemed that the prophetic comment by Ella Crandall, executive director of the National Organization for Public Health Nursing, had been fulfilled: "It may be reasonably expected that findings of the committee will one day be recognized as the first forward-looking step toward the reorganization of nursing education" (National League for Nursing, 1918).

From an administrative standpoint, development of public health nursing services was enormous during the 1920s and early 1930s. Whenever possible, standards for employment of public health nurses and additional education became a common expectation. This added to the prestige of the practice field and reinforced a generalized approach to the organization of services, although specialized public health practice in tuberculosis and child care continued to exist under the umbrella of "community health nursing." Qualifications for public health nurses were published and experiments in the training and use of subsidiary workers in public health roles were conducted by companies such as Metropolitan Life Insurance Company and others in collaboration with the National Organization for Public Health Nursing and its leadership. The content of nursing visits as assessed by audit were analyzed, the need and type of nursing supervision required was assessed, and cost studies were conducted to determine practice variations in various parts of the country — leading to more effective ways to operate agencies. A ratio of one supervisor to 10 nurses was recommended, and experiments were instituted with non-nurse managers to free nurses for supervision of clinical practice in the field. Rather than emphasizing specialized services, specialist nurse consultants to nurses in generalized practice became a popular model, with specialists in maternal-child health, mental health, rehabilitation, and nutrition being typical (Fitzpatrick, 1975).

In agencies utilizing auxiliary workers who were not nurses, role differentiation was clear. The norm was a full staff complement of registered nurses, with an ideal pattern being a staff of nurses with postgraduate preparation in public health nursing. Even when this was not possible, such preparation for supervising nurses was expected. *A Curriculum for Schools of Nursing* further introduced public health principles and urged their integration into basic nursing programs (National League of Nursing Education, 1927). Fledgling baccalaureate programs which included public health nursing as part of the basic education were encouraged.

Innovation in practice characterized the era. Experimental models of comprehensive service, that combined under one roof the services of a variety of social and health agencies and were neighborhood-based in areas of high need, were useful demonstrations of role development and, occasionally, role ambiguity for public health nurses. Interdisciplinary in their thrust, centers for such demonstration projects included one in Cattaraugus County, New York; the Frontier Nursing Service in Kentucky; and two in New York, New York — the Bellevue-York Project and the East Harlem Nursing and Health Project. These were useful not only in the development of collaborative models of care delivery, but also in underscoring the role of the public health nurse in the coordination and planning of care and the utilization of a myriad of resources to assist those in need in the community. Considered to be the forerunners of the neighborhood community health centers of the 1960s and early 1970s, these projects involved consumers in planning but did not use indigenous workers to deliver care, as did the more recent models. The restriction of this kind of sophisticated practice to those considered appropriately prepared for the work was reinforced, and so prevailed.

Despite the gains that public health agencies made in their employment practices and the utilization of nurses, the Depression severely affected the traditional agency, its work force, and the financing of care. Yet, out of the crisis, there emerged a new set of needs for service and approaches on how to meet them.

Agencies which had continued to receive their primary financial support from philanthropy lost sponsorship and, in some cases, their endorsements. Insurance reimbursement for services was curtailed or severely limited.

The Federal Emergency Relief Act of May 1933 and, later, the establishment of the Civil Workers Administration — both responses to the Depression — encouraged relief projects for unemployed nurses, the use of subsidiary workers, and free care for the poor in their homes. Federal funds were allocated for nursing, augmenting state and local funds. The resulting projects stimulated eventual tax support of public health nursing services through the development of such services in the growing numbers of official agencies (as seen in public health departments of municipalities). The Social Security Act of 1935 stimulated these developments, and government involvement in health care at local, state ,and national levels emerged as a strong focus of relief projects.

The threat to voluntary agencies and to preferred hiring practices was real. Projects were developed to better deliver care, and in so doing, employed nurses in community-based services without concern for their educational preparation for this kind of practice. Sorting out the dichotomy which was rapidly developing between the voluntary agency — which continued to practice bedside care — and the tax-supported agency — which focused more on ambulatory care, preventive, and health teaching measures — presented a formidable challenge. It is still not totally resolved today (Fitzpatrick, 1975).

Whenever it was possible, contracting for services from established nursing agencies became the norm and provided a reasonable model which was commonly adopted. In this way, a subsidiary for voluntary agencies as payment for services from tax-supported health departments was provided.

There was a risk, however, that the progress made to ensure a better prepared nurse in public health work would be eroded by an influx of diploma school graduates who lacked the additional preparation. The considerable astuteness of Pearl McIver, the Public Health Service's chief nurse consultant, greatly helped to prevent that erosion from occurring, and assisted in enacting an education standard for professional practice in public health nursing. At the time, approximately two-thirds of those involved in public health work were unprepared for it. McIver's interpretation of the Social Security Act and its provisions for scholarship assistance to prepare health workers created a climate and a mechanism for subsidizing large numbers of nurses to attend postgraduate educational programs as preparation for the public health work in which they were already engaged.

Through this federal legislation and the influence of McIver, Surgeon General Parren, and Naomi Deutsch (a Henry Street nurse who later became chief nurse at the Children's Bureau), a plan was put into motion. It met with great success, thereby averting a diminution of qualifications and standards in public health nursing practice which inevitably would have occurred as a result of the federal projects. By 1938, there were 22 National Organization for Public Health Nursing-approved postgraduate courses in public health nursing. These continued into the 1940s. In addition, there was more preferred hiring of "prepared" nurses by public health agencies under both voluntary and public auspices, and greater emphasis on ongoing staff development (Tobey, 1939).

When World War II again depleted the civilian nursing staffs, the response was reflected in student recruitment projects such as the federally-funded Cadet Nurse Corps. There was a movement for consolidation of services and agencies, and pressure was exerted for care of the sick to again become part of a generalized service or to be purchased from existing agencies.

Nursing standards of the American Public Health Association, the National Organization for Public Health Nursing, and the National Nursing War Council for Nurse Services explored new models for financing and delivering care. The development of generic baccalaureate programs in nursing, such as that at Skidmore College, which in 1944 was the first to receive National League of Nursing Education and National Organization for Public Health Nursing accreditation for beginning practice in public health nursing, accelerated. Interest in specialization developed as a result of the war, and with it, school nurses and mental health nurses became more identified with their own groups than with the generalist public health nurse.

Another significant development was the National Nursing Council's belief that practical nursing provided a solution for improving the quality of care. The Russell Sage Foundation study chaired by Esther Lucille Brown and called *Nursing for the Future* posited differentiation in nursing education and public roles and encouraged further differentiation among nurses as a consequence of educational preparation and intended function (Brown, 1948).

Throughout the 1940s and 1950s and well into the 1960s, the preferred employment of qualified public health nurses was generally maintained. The proliferation and development of basic college programs in nursing which included theory and practice in public health and which awarded the BSN degree, supported the implementation of these standards, making it possible to supply agencies with adequately prepared professional staff, although this was not universal. Simultaneously, the further development of graduate education in nursing assured more highly qualified supervisory and administrative staff.

The socially oriented government programs of the 1960s, such as President John F. Kennedy's "New Frontier," which came to full development in President Lyndon B. Johnson's "War on Poverty," created challenges as well as confusion for public health nurses. Use of demonstration projects to deliver care in innovative ways, consumer involvement in both the neighborhood control of services and as indigenous workers to deliver the care, and increased use of trained home health aides added to the complexities of practice in community health nursing. Most significantly, the passage of the Social Security amendments of 1965 — specifically Medicare legislation — created a financing mechanism to underwrite home care for the elderly. Although supply and demand frequently dictated the employment of nurses for public health work, the preferred use of the prepared professional nurse who had additional and special preparation for this kind of practice was an enduring characteristic of the larger and better developed agencies.

When funding for experimental projects ceased, many of those nonprofessionals who had participated in home and community care under such experiments found their way into community-based agencies for employment. The growing numbers of elderly in the population, the reimbursement mechanism in Medicare legislation, and changes in the economic climate and social agenda of the country gave rise to the proliferation of entrepreneurial enterprises of home health care. Today, the shifting control of home care has created a situation which is no longer chiefly influenced by nursing leadership. Nursing practice, roles, and functions are largely influenced by proprietary agents of the employing firms and reimbursement policies.

There are large numbers of diploma and associate degree prepared nurses in such practice today, as well as large numbers of nonprofessional workers in auxiliary positions. Traditional agencies that have survived find that these nurses have been forced into services that are reimbursable, thus diminishing their role in health education and preventive work. The needs, demands, and realities of the system may be far from what is deemed desirable, but we are faced with a system that may not conceivably change — yet one that can probably be better managed. The numbers of BSN-prepared nurses have increased in recent years. Despite the nursing shortage, a larger number of professional nurses are actively employed.

Technology has also changed home health care. The need for technically proficient nurses and specialty nurses may outweigh the need for those with a broader educational orientation. It would seem that a reasonable approach to the model which has emerged is to fully prepare and develop the management role for community nursing services.

Clearly, we are not in a position to meet all the pressing health needs in the community. Limiting our services is difficult, both practically and philosophically. From nursing services to a wide range of home health services, from small agencies to large companies resulting from mergers — the field has expanded and developed. As with all growth, there are new issues and concerns to be addressed. What remains clear is that there is an even greater need and role for the prepared public health nurse in the future. The public health nurse is the pivotal person in the determination, evaluation, planning, implementation, and coordination of resources for support of the patient and family, and in the management of resources and reimbursements in a safe but cost-effective manner.

The professional who can provide continuity in care today is still, as was the case 100 years ago, the public health nurse. With the exception of the clinical nurse specialists who are needed for increasingly complex home care, professional nurses of the future — though fewer in number — will assume case management/integrative roles, with larger numbers of associate degree and nonprofessional health care workers assuming the responsibility for direct care. That is why it is important to differentiate nursing roles with deliberateness, rather than simply permitting things to happen.

❏   ❏   ❏

Parallels and Paradoxes: Differentiated Nursing Practice in Psychiatric Care

Olga Maranjian Church, Ph.D., F.A.A.N.

Defining nursing and, in this case, differentiated nursing practice is a lifelong pursuit which can provide those who persist with a vast assortment of perspectives and insights into the human condition.

Examples from the past may seem quaint, but the descriptive labels that were once used in all seriousness now challenge the imagination. In psychiatric care, for example, prior to the development of an organized specialty education, those who were caretakers of the afflicted were called, "mental nurses" who practiced "nervous nursing."

During the first decade of this century, the newly developing specialty was known, at least for a period of time, as "psychopathic nursing." Simply from the labels, one can, with some degree of clarity, perceive the parameters or the limits of the knowledge that prevailed in addressing a particular aspect of health or illness.

For example, the term "alienists" was used to label the role of the physician whom we now would call a psychiatrist. This term might seem appropriate, given that the condition to be treated was considered at the time to be a form of mental alienation. There is an elegant simplicity in that description. As for psychotherapy, it has been described as an "undefined technique applied to unspecified cases with unpredictable results. For this technique, rigorous training is required" (London, 1964).

Some may take issue with this last definition, but the idea of the nurse as psychotherapist has had an intriguing history which is directly related to the topic of differentiated practice. This idea conjures up the notion of rigorous training and education that serve to define and determine the qualifications for certain aspects of psychiatric-mental health nursing practice.

Multiple forces have shaped the evolution of psychiatric practice, and within the confines of this brief paper, it may be useful to examine some of the critical forces that gave rise to its transition from custodial caretaking to professional practice. I also will review the variety of roles, responsibilities, and settings in which current practitioners function in the name of nursing.

The concerns we have today for control over practice and education were apparent prior to the turn of the century. There is ample documentation of the struggle for educational autonomy by nursing leaders. Their visionary efforts to align themselves with those they cared for through education and preventive measures contributed to the ultimate development of the informed consumer.

In early psychiatric nurse training programs, which were isolated from the rest of nursing, limitations were imposed by physicians who sought to medicalize the asylums. Dr. Edward Cowles determined in 1894 that it would be "the nurses of a new order in our hospitals that make possible the new and better modes of treatment" (Cowles, 1895).

Twelve years earlier, in 1882, Cowles had established the "first formally organized training school within a hospital for the insane in the world" (Massachusetts General Hospital, in 1921). In so doing, he managed to both praise Nightingale ("that noble reform") and insult her efforts. Cowles ignored Nightingale's basic principle of autonomy in establishing training programs. Instead, he insisted that the McLean Hospital Training School be one which was part of the hospital organization itself, independent of "outside" influences.

Cowles' approach was indicative of the historical imperatives that relate to traditional concerns of the workplace, such as professional boundaries, economics, and education, which in turn reflect the Victorian notion of working women intruding on a man's world.

By 1913, the first nurse-organized training program for psychiatric care was established by Effie J. Taylor, at the Johns Hopkins Phipps Clinic. Taylor's crusade for developing psychiatric nursing concepts as part of the general educational program for nurses demonstrates her commitment to establish a foundation of comprehensive knowledge on which all nursing care could be based.

A comparison in the orientation and scope of practice expected by graduates from Phipps with the graduates from McLean provides early examples of the differences in the prevailing treatment-oriented medical ideology with the health promotion and disease prevention nursing ideology of that period.

At McLean, the training and employment of nurses served many critical purposes. Not only was the nurse important as a symbolic manifestation of converting the asylum into a hospital, but as Cowles emphasized in his reports, nurses as women provided a great asset, value, and moral and curative influence by their presence on the wards. The nurses' natural "motherliness," together with their "acute womanly intuition," were essential to the work of the physicians.

During this period, Taylor and other nurse educators spoke up for the nurse's role as one that included more than cooperating with the physician. For them, it was essential to acknowledge that the nurse was instrumental in decision making. The rhetoric of Taylor's training program included such phrases as "the nurse is instructed to think for herself and use her own judgment, keeping in mind how she would wish a thing done were she the patient herself" (Taylor, 1926). By 1914, the rhetoric of respected and influential nursing leaders advanced the scope of practice as one which permitted considerations of prevention and the promotion of mental and physical hygiene.

Yet the medical/curative ideology prevailed and continued to limit the development of a broader scientific and academic perspective for schools of nursing. It would take major social and political forces to bring about significant changes in the development of nursing education, research, and practice in psychiatric care. Sociopolitical events, such as wars, together with natural disasters, traditionally play a part in organizing societal responses to a given need. For psychiatric nursing, an Act of Congress (the 1946 Mental Health Act) marked the beginning of significant federal support for nursing education. It ultimately led to opportunities for graduate education and the development of a leadership core of psychiatric nurses.

The changes that were hoped for as a result of federal intervention moved with guided deliberation. For example, the Committee on Psychiatric Nursing of the American Psychiatric Association, which was established in 1906, included in their 1947 report definitions of the term "psychiatric nurse." Although a rather inclusive description was provided, in the final analysis the psychiatric nurse, according to the committee's wisdom, was "the one that carries out the orders of the physician" and served as a "hostess on the ward" (American Psychiatric Association, 1947). Nowhere is there a discernible view of the nurse as a professional peer. Instead, the image of the nurse as "mother" to her charges and "obedient wife" to her master, the physician, prevails.

By mid-century, nursing education leaders convened to formally define psychiatric nursing and to describe the characteristics of its practitioners. Participants at the Conference on Advanced Psychiatric Nursing and Mental Hygiene Programs, which was jointly sponsored by the National League of Nursing Education and the University of Minnesota, articulated the scope of psychiatric nursing. They determined that psychiatric nursing was concerned with the total nursing care of psychiatric patients through the development of interpersonal relationships, the application of nursing skills, and the development of therapeutic situations (Peplau, 1956).

Postwar technological and methodological advances in psychiatric care created expectations for well-educated personnel to carry out improved therapeutic programs. This period has been identified as the beginning of the third revolution in the development of modern psychiatry. Traditionally, the three major "revolutions" are considered to have occurred:

1) at the end of the eighteenth century and during the Enlightenment, which inspired humanism and the moral methods of treatment;
2) at the close of the nineteenth century, when Freud hypothesized his theories of mental development; and
3) during the mid-twentieth century with the emergence of the community mental health movement, which developed as a direct result of chemotherapeutic interventions made possible by the discovery and development of psychoactive drugs.

The underlying assumption for the community mental health movement had been that, with the help of more modern treatments such as drug therapy and group therapy, psychiatric patients could be treated on an outpatient basis. For some, hospitalization could be prevented altogether. Thus, prevention and treatment modalities never before possible could be attempted with the appropriate use of drugs and support systems in the community (Deloughery, Gebbie, and Neuman, 1971).

It was at this point that nurses became more directly involved in organized therapeutic interventions in psychiatric care. Psychiatric nursing, as a special entity to be understood and integrated within the nursing profession, became increasingly complex.

According to a report published in 1950 by the National Committee for the Improvement of Nursing Services, "An adequate psychiatric nursing experience was defined as 12 to 16 weeks on a service with 25 patients or more. A total of 70 percent of the nursing schools met this standard. . . ." The report also indicated that, "11% of all the schools offered psychiatric nursing experiences which did not meet the standard(s)" (National Committee for the Improvement of Nursing Services, 1950).

Not unrelated to the above was the professional consensus enacted by the National League for Nursing* that all students have an experience in psychiatric nursing. Thus, organized nursing, via the National League for Nursing, launched an extensive educational experiment by including the behavioral sciences in basic undergraduate nursing programs.

According to L.S. Bermosk (1963) another interesting development occurred when, in 1954, funds were made available by the National Institute of Mental Health to "finance a special project, 'Integration of Mental Health — Psychiatric Concepts into the Basic Curriculum,' within baccalaureate programs in nursing in an effort to erase (recognized) limitations."

Subsidized by financial support from the government, the psychiatric nurses of the early 1950s had ample opportunity to demonstrate their unique professional capabilities. Paradoxically, the efforts to integrate psychiatric nursing content threatened to diminish the unique and specialty qualities of this segment of the profession.

Federal funding for psychiatric integration projects, which were designed to introduce psychiatric concepts into all the basic nursing education curriculums, indicated an acknowledgment of the necessity for an informed psychological orientation in dealing with the patient population for all nurses.

---

*By 1952, the National League for Nursing Education had become the National League for Nursing as part of the postwar reconstruction of nursing organizations.

The ultimate value in the development of the integration projects to psychiatric nursing was questioned later. Although the study of human behavior was basic to all nursing, the need for deeper and more inclusive preparation in specifically caring for the emotionally disturbed patient would eventually become apparent:

> According to Esther A. Garrison, between 1954, when the first project of this kind was inaugurated, and 1965, the federal government made grants to 119 colleges and universities for such projects, and foundations provided support for an unknown number of others. During this period, the federal grants alone amounted to approximately $11 million. If in addition to this sum the foundation donations and the college and university contributions in the form of faculty time are taken into consideration, it is probable that the investment . . . in psychiatric integration totals in the neighborhood of $20 million (Schmal, 1966).

The integration projects were to address the long-standing problems in the preparation of nurses — in particular, the preparation of psychiatrically-oriented nurses. This type of orientation would prepare those who had the potential for professional skill in interpersonal techniques and would enhance psychological aptitude, or awareness of the self, in the interpersonal process.

There were many who questioned the value of the integration projects and whether, given the vast amounts of time, energy, and financial backing required, the results were worth such expenditures. In the final analysis, the value of the projects was in their revelation to nonpsychiatric faculty members of the rationale and special skills inherent in psychiatric nursing practice.

However, the questions remained: was the integration movement an effective means to an end of more and better-prepared general nurses? If so, was it successful? And to what extent would such preparation alleviate the need for more and better-prepared specialists in the care of psychiatric patients? Given the conservative tenor of the 1950s and the traditional guarded response to all things psychological, the very fact that a sustained effort was made with varying degrees of success was in itself an accomplishment. It is well to remember that, "The success of a movement depends much less upon the force of its arguments or upon the ability of its advocates, than upon the predisposition of society to receive it" (Rossi, 1973).

The need for specialist preparation persisted, as did undergraduate experience in psychiatric nursing.

Our history is replete with inspired nursing reforms and leaders who sought educational advancement while facing the diverse challenges of economic fluctuations, legal constraints, and political realities. Reports that documented the awareness of "the powers that be" did not necessarily lead to enlightened action; yet, these reports continued to serve as evidence in the case for competency-based curricula and competency-based job descriptions in describing and defining the roles and responsibilities of nursing practitioners.

Such findings as the *Goldmark Report* (Goldmark, 1923), the report of the Committee on the Grading of Nursing Schools (Committee on the Grading of Nursing Schools, 1934), the Ginsberg Report (Ginsberg, 1949), and the Brown Report (Brown, 1948), gave thoughtful testimony to the status quo and offered suggestions for change. In addition, psychiatric nursing leaders also documented their special concerns in reports such as the Bailey Report (Bailey, 1936) and *Facing up to Changing Responsibilities* (American Nurses Association, 1964).

By 1948, preparation of large numbers of nursing specialists had not occurred "because specialization requires unhurried time for intellectual and emotional growth, and because most graduate nurses did not have an academic base on which specialization might be built" (Brown, 1948).

With regard to mental hospital education for nursing, Brown's critique was direct and to the point. Saying that "no school in a public hospital for the mentally ill . . . was nearly satisfactory" and that "specialized psychiatric nurses, desperately needed not only for the successful direction of nursing service and nursing education but for the care of patients, are negligible in number" (Brown, 1948), she recommended changes that would do away with such schools. She maintained that the existing system did not produce an adequately prepared practitioner:

> At best, these schools produce nurses who are skilled in the care of psychotic patients according to the standards of practice in their parent hospitals . . . (instead) . . . of giving the student a deep understanding of the emotional component of all physical disease.

Brown encouraged the use of these facilities as places for affiliating students from other programs, saying that, "One of the most encouraging developments in nursing education in recent years is the increased emphasis upon requiring of *all* students some three months of clinical experience in psychiatric nursing" (Brown, 1948).

The topic of differentiated practice has evolved naturally from the changing realities in nursing's domain. For Peplau (1967) among others, the psychiatric nurse was "a registered nurse who has completed a program of study in psychiatric nursing in a university setting and who, therefore, holds a master's or doctoral degree." Thus, the definition of the psychiatric nurse would be determined by virtue of her educational credentials and competency. In other words, the nurse who happened to be working in a psychiatric setting did not automatically qualify for the role of psychiatric nurse.

Recent developments in addictions nursing provide more food for thought along these lines. Psychiatric mental health nursing would seem to be a natural specialty to accommodate addictions nursing as a subspecialty. Yet, there are many excellent, competent practitioners who are addictions specialists without having prepared first as a psychiatric nurse who would argue the point.

Certainly, addictions as health problems are pervasive throughout nursing practice. Yet there are different levels of preparation and skills inherent in the role(s) of the nurse generalist and the nurse specialist in the care of clients with addictions (American Nurses Association, 1988).

Within the past year, certification examinations have been developed and administered which will serve to identify a particular level of addictions nursing practice. How well this development will meet the needs of the marketplace is yet to be determined. Given the fact that the nurses functioning in the field prior to the recent development were expected to qualify as certified alcohol and/or drug counselors through study and/or examination from other non-nursing disciplines, it is a proactive stance that hopefully will serve nursing's interest.

On another note, it is interesting that psychiatric-mental health nursing has only recently developed supportive organizational structures in the guise of professional organizational associations such as the Society for Education and Research in Psychiatric-Mental Health Nursing and the American Psychiatric Nurses Association, to name a few. Since psychiatric nursing began as a specialty, it is paradoxical that there was no movement toward organizing as a specialty.

Having developed in isolation and been separated from the overall development of general nursing, psychiatric nurses sought to become integrated into the mainstream of nursing rather than to separate themselves organizationally. Yet, the threat of dissolution through integration (i.e., losing the specialty by sharing its unique attributes with the rest of nursing) has been a constant concern. Given the complexities of contemporary living and the great expectations that will come with the turn of the century, delineating the universal responsibilities from the specialty-specific facets of nursing practice is a major imperative.

We need to remember that shaping the future requires an awareness of our shared past. Together, we can begin to develop a communal consensus for a future vision where competence determines the provider with an informed compassion as the nurse who will meet society's health care needs.

❏　　❏　　❏

Part IX

The Challenges and Opportunities of Different Paths to Differentiated Practice

Differentiated Practice: Response from a Researcher

Joanne Comi McCloskey, Ph.D., R.N., F.A.A.N.

T his paper will focus on three areas: the research that reveals whether nurses with different types of education perform differently; the reformulation of the differentiated practice role through the use of case managers and nurse extenders; and, lastly, the need for research on the new delivery of care models.

Research Reveals Whether Nurses with Different Types of Education Perform Differently

The concept of differentiated practice has, until recently, been related to the entry into practice issue and has focused on different roles for the BSN and the ADN nurse. The underlying research question has been, "Do baccalaureate nurses perform better, or at least differently, than associate degree nurses, and in some cases, diploma nurses?"

While there has been much interest in nursing performance for several decades, few studies have, in fact, documented how nurses actually perform. Most of the research on nurse performance focuses on perceptions of a group's performance rather than on measuring individual performance. Despite this and other methodological problems, there are some conclusions to be drawn from the existing research. The following five conclusions have been drawn from my own and others' research.

First, education does affect performance but not to the same degree as the number of years of education, including years in non-nursing degree programs and the amount of continuing education (McCloskey, 1983; McCloskey and McCain, 1988b).

Second, the type of performance needs definition. Baccalaureate nurses do somewhat better with communication, problem-solving, and teaching skills (Johnson, 1988). Leadership skills are unclear (Yes: Bottoms, 1988; McCloskey and McCain, 1988b; No: Johnson, 1988). Autonomous skills are not high (Johnson, 1988) and critical care (technical) skills are low (McCloskey and McCain, 1988a; 1988b).

Third, *all* nurses are better at professional development and interpersonal relationships/communication than at teaching/collaboration, planning/evaluation, and leadership skills (McCloskey and McCain, 1988a).

Fourth, job performance is a complex phenomenon with multiple determinants (McCloskey and McCain, 1988b). The type of education a nurse has is not a very good predictor of his/her practice performance. Education apparently accounts for less than 5% of the variance in job performance (McCloskey, 1983; McCloskey and McCain, 1988b).

Fifth, while research evidence is sparse due to limitations in sample size, it appears that master's-prepared nurses do perform differently (at a higher level) than nurses with less education (McCloskey, in press).

Having reviewed the question of baccalaureate nurse performance, I have come to a conclusion regarding the entry into practice issue. An article I read several years ago by Roemer (1981) helped. Roemer outlined three social theories that explained the relationship of higher education to work:

1) Functionalism — Education provides knowledge and skills directly related to work.
2) Status-competition — Education provides the cultural attributes associated with high status, and thus improves the competitive position of an individual.
3) Legitimacy — Education legitimizes certain knowledge and encourages the creation of new knowledge which expands practice.

The research on nurses' job performance relates to the functionalist theory. Using only the functionalist or competency theory, there are too few differences among associate, diploma, and baccalaureate nurses to argue that a role differentiation should be made based on education alone. However, there are reasons to differentiate based on the status competition and legitimacy theories. That is, the promotion of advanced education for nurses requires the profession to build a knowledge base which will legitimize the profession, will help secure our place in the health care system, and will allow nurses to have more influence on redirecting the focus of health care in this country toward illness prevention, health maintenance, and consumer responsibility and choice.

With the foregoing as a brief background of the more traditional view of the differentiated practice issue, we may review some recent developments.

Expanded Roles and Nurse Extenders

In the aftermath of DRGs and in the presence of a national nursing shortage, two phenomena are helping us to reformulate the issue of differentiated practice — case management and nurse extenders.

While case management has been practiced by community health nurses for decades (American Nurses Association, 1988), case management in hospitals is a recent innovation. Many models of case management are being proposed and implemented; however, after a review of several such models, members of my doctoral class and I decided that each model incorporates four key concepts: standardization, efficiency, continuity of care, and interdisciplinary collaboration.

The driving force is to maintain quality during a shortened length of hospital stay. The case manager should be someone with good communication and management skills, and who works well with other disciplines. In this expanded role, which often covers the patient from preadmission to postdischarge, a baccalaureate- or master's-prepared nurse works with several other unit-based nurses who perform the day-to-day treatments and who may be assisted by various types of nurse extenders. Critical paths, which highlight each day's procedures and treatments, and variance analyses are used as management tools.

In Kramer's (1990) report on revisiting magnet hospitals, she points out how this new role differentiation differs from previous ones. In the past, Kramer says, we defined and attempted to differentiate professional and technical nursing by having the BSN nurse perform the supportive, teaching, and expressive interventions, while the ADN nurse performed the instrumental or technical interventions. That is, we differentiated the roles by "splitting" the interventions. In the new differentiated practice models, the case manager devotes the majority of his/her time and energy to planning and evaluation, while the case associate specializes in intervention. That is, we are differentiating the roles by splitting the steps of the nursing process.

What research we have to date on the effectiveness of case management is mostly anecdotal. It does appear, however, that using case managers helps to decrease length of stay (Ethridge and Rusch, 1989) and to increase nurse autonomy (Ethridge and Rusch, 1989), but that it can be expensive to implement and is probably not justified for all patients (American Nurses Association, 1988; Morlock, 1990).

Another reemerging phenomenon is that of nurse extenders, defined by Aydelotte (1988) as individuals who enable the nurse to provide a larger volume of services. Aydelotte has defined six types of extenders:

1) Traditional — Aides, orderlies, ward clerks.
2) Modified traditional — A "super aide," usually with a new title, such as "patient care assistant."
3) Unit assistant — As in the Rush Presbyterian model, a person who assists with unit activities but has no clinical tasks.
4) Technician — An OR technician, for example.
5) Primary partner — Manthey's definition of an aide or LPN who works as assistant to the primary nurse.
6) RCT — AMA's proposal for three types or levels of assistants.

Nurse extenders are once again in vogue because we cannot find enough nurses to fill needed positions, at least not at the current salaries. The salaries of unfilled budgeted nurse positions are being used to hire more LPNs and non-nurse assistants. Most of the extender models use lesser-prepared personnel to deliver clinical routine care to patients and to assist with routine unit housekeeping chores. In these new emerging delivery models, nurses delegate tasks to different types of assistants, similar to the model of team nursing. Once again, the need to define nursing comes to the forefront. That is, what nursing tasks, treatments, and decisions can be performed by non-licensed personnel with limited education? Interestingly enough, this delegation of parts of the primary nursing role comes at a time when research (Hartz et al., 1989) demonstrates that at least one patient outcome — that of decreased mortality — correlates with the percentage of nurses who are RNs.

The new features of role differentiation are illustrated in the previous papers and in an interesting model called ProACT (Professionally Advanced Care Team), which has been described in at least four publications (Brett and Tonges, 1990; Tonges, 1989a; Tonges, 1989b; Tonges, 1990). ProACT has been implemented and evaluated on one unit at the Robert Wood Johnson Hospital in New Jersey. In this model, a baccalaureate- or master's-prepared nurse with at least two years of experience works as case manager on a schedule correlated with resident coverage. Other nurses work as primary nurses to manage nursing care on a 24-hour basis. LPNs work as associate nurses, and aides help primary and associate nurses with clinical tasks such as bathing and feeding. A new worker, called a "support service host," carries out hotel functions for a specified group of patients and makes unoccupied beds, distributes water and linen, and checks the unit's supplies. A unit-based pharmacy technician supervised by a pharmacist prepares all medications, organizes them by time of administration, changes IV tubing, and hangs the IV piggybacks in the patient's room for the nurse to administer. The nursing department's budget pays for all the services.

Need for Research on New Delivery of Care Models

There is no question that we have and will continue to have new models of care delivery due to the increasing fiscal demands in the health care environment. These models are in an early stage of implementation and evaluation. Research evaluating their effectiveness is still incomplete. There are several aspects of the research needed that I would like to address, but I will only make five points briefly.

First, we need to carefully define the model or innovation that is being implemented. The concepts may be similar but the characteristics of implementation differ greatly. We need to know exactly what was done so we can determine whether differing results are due to differing independent variables. For example, are the outcomes due to the use of a case manager, the use of critical pathways,

411

the alignment of nurses with physicians, or the staff's level of education and experience?

Second, control (either through measurement or design) of possible intervening variables is essential. There is a great need for this research and, indeed, for all nursing administrative research to use standardized measures of organizational variables. Standardized measures would help us to determine whether the results were, in fact, due to innovation, or due to certain environmental features. Also, we need standardized measures so that we can accumulate and tabulate the results of separate studies done in different organizations. This research by necessity will be mostly case study research. A standardized approach to the definition and measurement of possible intervening variables is highly desirable. To facilitate this effort, some colleagues in Iowa are in the beginning stages of defining a Nursing Management Minimum Data Set (NMMDS). Modeled after Werley's idea of the nursing minimum data set (Werley and Lang, 1988), they are attempting to define a minimum number of variables used by nurse administrators on a regular basis to make decisions in such areas as cost of services, allocation of personnel, and comparison of care delivery models. The concept is that these variables would be uniformly defined and measured in all institutions so that data can be aggregated and compared. Variables come from several levels — the individual patient, the nursing unit, and the institution.

Third, these changes in delivery models are being implemented swiftly due to economic considerations. Busy administrators who are focusing on the change process and conflict resolution may lack time to carefully consider design and measurement issues. Sometimes changes are implemented without any baseline measures of important outcome variables being done. Institutions with a director of research are at an advantage, and those with directors who know something about administrative research have a particular advantage. As hospitals experience economic cutbacks, temptations arise to eliminate nonessential positions. I urge our directors of nursing not to consider their directors of research as nonessential; they are anything but that.

Fourth, hospitals need to define the outcome measures they are seeking. What nurse-sensitive patient outcomes can be easily measured, or for what outcomes do we have data already collected? How will cost be measured? Are there good measures of nurse satisfaction, extender satisfaction, physician satisfaction, and patient satisfaction already being used? What instruments can be used? A variety of outcome measures should include quality, cost, and staff satisfaction and retention. Using nurse extenders *will* keep beds open and revenues up, but what else does it do?

Finally, I would like to advise nurse executives in hospitals to implement some method of regular data collection on selected variables. With so many changes happening so quickly, it is impossible to design a separate study to examine every change. For example, if we already had standardized data collected at regular intervals on organizational demographics, units, staff satisfaction, commitment, professionalism, and intent to stay, we would be able use these data to determine the effectiveness of new innovations. We do have some standardized data mandated by JCAHO on patient outcomes, but are these variables helpful to nursing, or should other measures be collected?

In summary, the new models of differentiated practice provide many research opportunities and challenges. The research has moved from questioning the educational level as it affects job performance to questioning the impact of different models of care delivery on staff and patient outcomes. It is important and interesting research, but it is fraught with many difficulties. Conferences like this help to illuminate some of the issues through discussion.

❏   ❏   ❏

An Educator's Response to Models of Differentiated Practice

Rosalee C. Yeaworth, Ph.D., R.N., F.A.A.N.

Based on review of all of the other papers in this book, and after doing some reading on my own, my overall impression is that the more we change in nursing, the more we revisit previous ideas, concepts, and practices with a slightly different focus or new twist.

My initial preparation was in one of the first baccalaureate programs in this country, and most of my career has been in education. I value education, so the idealist side of me says that nursing should not offer educational preparation at any level lower than the baccalaureate. However, I am also a realist and a pragmatist. When I was invited to accept the deanship at the University of Nebraska, I did a lot of soul searching because it had a very successful, accredited, articulated ASN/BSN program. I knew that during periods of shortages, the response has been to try to prepare people in less time. My undergraduate class was the second to enter the baccalaureate program after it had been temporarily discontinued to prepare cadets for World War II. I knew that there were some people who, for financial and personal reasons, believed they could not commit to more than two years of educational preparation at a time, even though they might continue later. I strongly believe in educational mobility, and while I do not discount the importance of professional socialization, I believe that we should acknowledge the education people have received in other than formal courses.

I am also struck by how nursing education is determined not so much by the philosophy and values of nursing leaders and educators, but by legal, economic, and social situations. The Nebraska legislature and board of regents mandated the University of Nebraska to start an associate degree program in an effort to respond to a nursing shortage in the state. It was designed on the terminal degree model, which was separate from the baccalaureate degree. When it was recognized that the associate program applicants looked much like the baccalaureate program applicants, and that many of the associate degree graduates wanted to pursue a baccalaureate degree, the faculty developed the articulated model which encompassed the ASN within the BSN. They also added more science and humanities courses to the associate degree program than are found in many other programs.

Just as the state legislature and the nursing shortage forced the college into designing an associate degree program, the absence of a shortage and economics forced the program out of the college. In 1983, with the advent of DRGs, the Midwest experienced a tight job market. Our associate degree graduates were working in restaurants and department stores while pursuing a baccalaureate. When faced with cutting the college's budget, we fought closing our Lincoln, Nebraska division and agreed to cut the associate degree program. We believed this would allow us to concentrate our resources on the baccalaureate and master's degree programs and on developing a Ph.D. in nursing.

Machiavelli (1513) is credited with saying:

> There is nothing more difficult to plan, more doubtful of success, nor more dangerous to manage than the creation of a new system. For the initiator has the enmity of all who would profit by the preservation of the old system and merely lukewarm defenders in those who would gain by the new one.

We have gained the enmity of those who would profit by the preservation of the old system, but few nurses' reactions to implementing two levels of entry into practice can be classified as "lukewarm"!

While differentiated practice may differ from two levels of entry into practice, it did not suddenly materialize from the efforts of the National Commission on Nursing Implementation Project. It represents a change of focus, a new direction in the ongoing goal of increasing professionalism in nursing and controlling our education and practice.

JoEllen Koerner (1990) also stated that, "The process of change cannot be forced." Nevertheless, I recall the painful transition of going from a master's program in psychiatric nursing to a doctoral program in sociology. One faculty member used a systems approach and stressed the idea of central control and power to create change in behavior. Accordingly, cognitive dissonance would operate to restructure attitudes and beliefs to fit the behavior. I proposed that education, persuasion, and rational means were viable methods to change attitudes and beliefs to create a change in behavior. The faculty member eventually said, "Suppose the United States was attacked by an unfriendly nation — would you try to raise an army by going out and educating and persuading people to join, or would you institute a draft?"

Nursing leaders have had to progress on the belief that if we could just give rational reasons to change and show substantiating data for our beliefs, we could convince people and implement the needed changes. It was acknowledged that nursing education had to occur in a college or university and that the minimum level of preparation for any occupation with professional aspirations had to begin with a baccalaureate degree. However, we lacked the central control or power to require such a minimum level, so we continued to have diploma schools. With educational, political, social, and economic values favoring accessibility to education and the community college concept, we soon discovered that the primary educational preparation occurred at the associate degree level.

At the University of Nebraska, with our articulated ASN/BSN program, we carefully formulated differentiation statements about what we were preparing our graduates to do, and constructed curriculums accordingly. In letters of reference, we specified what our graduates were prepared to do, but explained that we could not control the practice setting. Like other nursing educators, we found that our graduates were used interchangeably in acute care settings and paid the same because their job descriptions were the same.

The 1965 American Nurses Association position paper on nursing education specified two levels of entry (American Nurses Association, 1965). Nebraska, like most states, tried to secure legislation or board of nursing regulation to force two levels of entry. As the immediate past chair of the Nebraska Nurses Association's Cabinet on Nursing Education, I expended a great deal of effort trying to

417

implement the resolution on entry, which the association set as its highest priority — it looked so easy. There was only one diploma program in the state and all the practical nursing education was in community colleges. Despite task forces, assemblies, and developing separate sets of rules and regulations to govern the two levels, we did not have the political power to accomplish the goal. The current shortage and the RCT proposal convinced us that we could not continue to expend our energies and resources on this effort. Besides, we were convinced that we needed two different exams for licensing two different levels, and the exams had to be based on actual practice.

As Lucille Joel (1990) said, "Differentiated practice will be an impetus to redesign nursing care delivery systems, nursing education systems, and nursing data systems." If differentiated practice is implemented in enough settings, then perhaps we can develop two different exams using acute care and other settings. With differentiated job descriptions, we can develop differentiation in pay. It sounds rational and persuasive, but I wish I had the power and control to mandate these changes and see the corresponding changes in attitudes, beliefs, and expectations that would follow.

Margaret McClure stated in her paper that she was beginning to believe education should arise from practice. Certainly, we need close collaboration between nursing service and education; nursing education must be relevant to practice. However, education should lead practice because of the time needed to plan and implement a curriculum that produces graduates. The leaders in nursing practice today must help us prepare for the nursing practice of the future. It should be noted that education can arise from practice near the end of the educational program. More and more programs are using senior practicums, preceptorships, and externships between the junior and senior years as ways to immerse students in practice.

During the summer of 1990, faculty at the University of Nebraska College of Nursing implemented a trial summer externship on an elective basis. A community hospital in Lincoln has been hiring our junior and senior students as aides. They not only put them on salary, but pay part of their tuition as well. This has been a successful recruitment effort for the hospital; however, both the nursing service personnel and the students have been frustrated by the fact that the nursing practice act prevents students so hired from doing anything more than aides would do.

At the hospital's request, therefore, we designed an elective summer externship which we implemented in two different hospital settings. The hospitals were involved in selecting the students who could participate. They paid the students at the aide rate, paid tuition for the course, and paid half the salary of the faculty involved. Under faculty supervision, students could assume much more responsibility and gain an experience comparable to that of a staff nurse. Not only did the students learn a great deal, they were of much more assistance to nursing service. Everyone involved was very positive about the externship and its future expansion.

From the papers presented herein and from other sources, nursing educators have heard that baccalaureate-prepared nurses must be problem solvers; conceptual thinkers; sensitive, articulate communicators; good managers of time, resources, and people; collaborators; risk-takers; priority setters; computer literate; as well as flexible, ethical, caring, creative, empowered, and committed. These are high expectations for baccalaureate-level education or, for that matter, any level of education. I am reminded of my seven-year-old granddaughter who, when being praised for doing well in school, said, "Grandma, I think I want to be a nurse. I've got the brains for it." Brains it will take!

We must end our struggle over titles. It is confusing to have the same role identified by several titles, and very difficult when planning a curriculum to prepare a nurse for a certain role if several different role descriptions match the same title. Titles like "case manager," "professional nurse," and "primary nurse" are used interchangeably. I was relieved to learn that staff at Sioux Valley Hospital changed titles from case manager to primary nurse and from case associate to registered nurse. Case management has been defined as advanced practice and the preparation has been part of many master's programs. I am bothered by calling nurses case managers when they have not even completed their baccalaureate degrees and we are defining that as master's-level content.

We have had so much difficulty getting the baccalaureate-level nurse accepted as a professional that I wonder if we have been aiming too low? Social work and physical therapy now require master's-level preparation. Differences in practice are easy to distinguish between RNs with the various undergraduate levels of preparation and RNs with master's preparation in nursing. We shall continue to have large numbers of associate degree-prepared nurses who continue to learn and grow in the practice setting, but who also want to pursue advanced preparation. Perhaps our goal should be the generic master's and the RN-to-master's, thus making a clear distinction between two levels of practice — associate degree and master's.

In the meantime, these projects have shown that differentiation of two types of practice has produced positive outcomes for patients and institutions, and increased satisfaction for nurses. It is very encouraging to know that differentiated practice can mean use of baccalaureate competencies in acute care settings, and appropriate preceptors and role models for baccalaureate and AD students.

The associate degree is very attractive to nontraditional students who are now becoming the traditional or at least typical students in nursing. The short time commitment required to qualify for an almost guaranteed job makes it a goal which they can envision. The RN upward mobility program described herein by JoEllen Koerner fits with the concept of allowing RNs to maintain the expertise associated with their practice setting while continuing to learn on the job. It could prove to be another means of strengthening the relationship between education and practice.

I find myself struggling to balance what is necessary to maintain standardization and quality control of nursing education with the creativity that gives people credit for what they know, utilizing activities to fit the style of the learner. If we are to produce flexible graduates, we cannot do it with an inflexible curriculum. Yet, nursing faculty expend tremendous amounts of time and energy tinkering with curriculum. Faculty do need to keep learning on the job to keep clinically current and move from the traditional teaching methods to the adult learning principles and techniques that promote active, self-directed learning.

Koerner quotes Erik Erikson's observation that timing is critical to change. Times of turbulence and crisis are also times of opportunity. The American people desperately want to change the present health care system. As Koerner stated, "This is nursing's moment." If properly directed, it can increase access to health care and reduce costs. The nursing "shortage" has given us wide media attention. The leadership of the Tri-Council has enabled us to present a united front for nursing. Nursing has succeeded in becoming much more of a political force at all levels of government. We now have a supply of well-educated, articulate, energetic, and politically astute leaders. Despite the fact that we have not yet accomplished our goals in controlling our practice and education, we have made progress.

John F. Kennedy once said that in his experience in government, when things were noncontroversial and beautifully coordinated, there was not much going on. In nursing, we can safely say there is a lot going on!

❑   ❑   ❑

An Administrator's Response to Three Models of Differentiated Practice

Karen S. Ehrat, Ph.D.

L et me begin by acknowledging the efforts of the Dartmouth-Hitchcock, Maryvale Samaritan, and Sioux Valley hospitals and the quality, or "value added," of their respective differentiated practice projects. As presented herein, the projects stand on their own merit. My paper will provide an administrative response to the models presented by Dr. Cronenwett, Ms. Malloch, and Ms. Koerner. I will attempt to highlight the components of those three models that I find most interesting or most representative of change. My administrative remarks may include educational and research issues.

Carol Cox, president of the Committee for a Responsible Federal Budget, said, "The federal budget is just a metaphor for the difficulties we are having making the system of government work." In health care, achieving a balanced budget or a positive margin is just a metaphor for the difficulties in making hospital systems work. The health care system is intransigent. Role differentiation trials and successes represent a distinct departure from the past. In many instances, nursing innovations in differentiated practice are the drivers for total organizational change.

I admit a bias in believing that health care today is largely a function of historical artifact and inertia. The historical artifact underlying nursing is evidenced in tasks, mindsets, rote patterns of behavior and practice, and bureaucratic policies and procedures that lack a scientific or logical basis.

I salute the ongoing efforts of the aforementioned institutions to achieve a more rational basis for rendering nursing care and for capitalizing on the intellect and abilities of individual nurses. These projects were driven by staff competency rather than basic education considerations. Lest we become overly confident of our progress, however, I would remind the audience that in this last century, America has moved from an agricultural society, through an industrial era, and into an information age. Acute infectious diseases have given way to chronic maladies. Men have walked on the moon. Fax machines can transport information at a faster rate than locomotives. Nursing, on the other hand, has moved from case management to case management.

I appreciate the diversity represented in these three approaches to differentiated practice. While endpoint objectives are similar, the pathways are distinct and appear to incorporate the uniqueness of each setting. Presently, we lack a singular methodology for achieving value-added and cost sensitive care. Eclectic institutional efforts, assisted by the field experiences of others, will likely yield a multitude of nursing approaches that better capitalize on the education and skills of registered nurses.

I believe it would be most effective for my response to highlight select components from each of the three models.

I was struck by the nonclinical nomenclature "RN length-of-stay accountability" in the Dartmouth-Hitchcock model. As I reviewed their experience, I concluded that length-of-stay accountability was, indeed, an overriding construct that could encompass all elements of care. Further, in this model (as well as in the others), differentiated practice was only one interacting variable producing a positive change. In this instance, case management, salaried patient care managers, selective scheduling, attending physician buy-ins, and the professional practice council added to the differentiated practice efforts. Perhaps most noteworthy in the Dartmouth-Hitchcock model was the consensus-building process around shared values. It would seem that, regardless of the future innovations and inventions in care, these shared values underlie all efforts.

The Maryvale experience, while focusing on similar outcomes, partly measured success on the basis of a decrease in negative patient outcomes. The author acknowledged that indicators of quality patient outcomes were less easily defined and difficult to quantify.

I was reminded of the amoeba analogy in Robert Pirsig's (1974) *Zen and the Art of Motorcycle Maintenance*. Pirsig essentially said that if you put an amoeba on a petri dish and slowly drip sulfuric acid on the dish, the amoeba will back away. If it could talk, the amoeba would say that the environment had poor quality, even though it had no knowledge of sulfuric acid or petri dishes. In a similar vein, consumers recognize poor quality, though they understand little about the complexities of care routines and therapeutics. Using this same logic, if the patient says the care is good or that quality exists, we should accept his/her conclusion.

Though I strongly support the search for measurable correlates of quality, patient outcomes will not be improved through internal efforts to quantify what is nonquantifiable. Maryvale appears to have accepted quality improvements at face value and has moved forward using financial and risk avoidance indicators as measures of success.

Maryvale's planning philosophy incorporated the elements of collaboration, change theory, and commitment. Anwar Sadat once said, "He who cannot change the very fabric of his thought will never be able to change reality." As part of its strategy, Maryvale is changing reality — as evidenced by pairing BSN students with case managers and ADN students with case associates. Further role clarification in nursing will necessitate role clarification in ancillary and support departments of the hospital as well. Patient care is multidimensional. The innovations in nursing must encompass other disciples.

The Sioux Valley project has incorporated differentiated practice, case management, and shared governance to achieve a professional business partner role for nursing. Koerner noted that, "The industry is in such a state of turbulence that individuals and groups with the most innovative ideas have the greatest chance of influencing the changes needed to maintain viability." Simply stated, after the feeding frenzy of diversification, corporate restructuring, "night of the living MBAs," and strategic planning, the move is back to basics — providing quality patient care.

America is interested in quality. The auto industry is slowly learning that neon paint, digital electronics, and monotone voice-alert systems do not sell automotive design and performance; America wants a Miata. The health care industry is slowly learning that mauve wall coverings, designer linens, and slick advertising campaigns do not sell mediocre patient care. The business winners of this decade will be those organizations that focus on doing it right, and after that, doing it better.

Clearly, Sioux Valley and the state of South Dakota are to be recognized for their innovative efforts. The work redesign at Sioux Valley acknowledged the need for reconfiguring support services in a more decentralized mode. Whether support services are centralized or decentralized, it is clear that gross inefficiency and rework presently exist both intra- and interdepartmentally within acute care institutions. Simplification is an inexact method for making complex data more understandable. My simplified method for evaluating rework and organizational inefficiency is to count the number of steps required to make a discharge bed "admit ready."

Implicit or explicit in all three models is the notion that prescriptive thinking inhibits innovation. Clearly, education and service have to foster prescriptive thinking. It is very difficult to think innovatively when behavior is controlled by policies, procedures, prescriptive curricula, and bureaucratic norms. I support the premise that "differentiated practice is a function of communication and critical thinking competencies rather than increasing technical skills."

Beyond critical thinking competencies, I believe there are a series of general or liberal competencies that are required to support professional innovation and movement. The list in Table 1 depicts the concurrence among randomly selected service and education representatives regarding the general skills required for the professional practice of nursing — whether gleaned through education or experience.

The three differentiated practice models have addressed staff skill building in these general skill areas. The successes of these three projects are dependent, in part, on the capabilities and credibilities of the leaders, managers, and project champions who often possess certain common traits (identified in Table 2).

In conclusion, I would like to return to my bias. In *What They Don't Teach You At Harvard Business School*, Mark McCormack (1984) presents a wonderful "historical artifact parable":

> A circus keeps a baby elephant from running away by chaining it to a stake. When the animal pulls at the chain, the cuff chafes its leg, and the baby elephant concludes that to avoid pain it best stay put. But when the elephant grows up, the circus still chains it to the same small stake. The mature elephant could now pull the stake out of the ground like a

toothpick, but the elephant remembers the pain and is too dumb to use the new set of facts — how circumstances have changed. The tiny stake keeps a two-ton elephant at bay just as effectively as it did the baby. Many executives are too dependent on old facts, on outmoded conventions, or are still basing decisions on what worked 20 years ago. This is elephantine decision making.

The innovation efforts at Dartmouth-Hitchcock, Maryvale Samaritan, and Sioux Valley represent the antithesis of elephantine decision making. Their efforts demonstrate both rationality and creativity.

In *Future Perfect*, Stanley Davis (1987) told us that rationality and creativity are not contrasting characteristics:

Rational types focus on facts, and facts are about the past. Theory, in contrast, is about the future. Once theory is accepted as fact, it then relates to the past. The more you revere facts, therefore, the more resistant you are to change. The faster things change, the less you can use facts and the more you need imagination (so . . . creativity is rational . . . it may even be scholarly!)

Similar to the efforts discussed herein, the profession must continue to redefine practice and redesign work. Ideas must be implemented. Even if you have the world's best idea, it is of no use unless you act on it.

❑   ❑   ❑

Table 1
General/Liberal Skills

- Inspire followers
- Theorize
- Master uncertainty
- See the whole in the parts
- Inspire confidence
- Accept criticism
- View change with anticipation
- Capitalize on mistakes
- Appreciate the accomplishments of others
- Make value judgments and integrate values
- Act and respond nonjudgmentally
- Create a sense of unity
- Listen with empathy
- Analyze and synthesize information
- View opportunity as development
- Acquire knowledge independently
- Plan work effectively
- Adapt to changing circumstances
- Facilitate consensus among divergent groups
- Present rational discourse and reasoned arguments
- Judge alternatives in accordance with custom and history
- Think critically and constructively
- Read, write, and speak effectively
- Distinguish and relate subject matter
- Manipulate matter, quantity, and motion
- Be sensitive to changing behavior

From K.S. Ehrat, 1985, *Liberal Education Skills in the Field of Nursing,* unpublished dissertation.

Table 2
Leader Characteristics/Traits

- Humility
- Introspection
- Vision
- Commitment
- Passion
- Political astuteness
- Sensitivity
- Self-motivation
- Wisdom
- Optimism
- Character/personal presence
- Influence
- Concern for the greater good
- Self-discipline
- Persuasion
- Ability to challenge
- Creativity
- Humor
- Nurturing ability

From K.S. Ehrat, 1985, *Liberal Education Skills in the Field of Nursing,* unpublished dissertation.

References

Aaron, H.J. and Schwartz, W.B. 1985. Hospital cost control: A bitter pill to swallow. *Harvard Business Review* 63:160-167.

Abbey, J. and Shepherd, M. 1989. The Abbey-Shepherd device education model. In *Nursing and technology: Moving into the 21st century*. Washington, D.C.: U.S. Government Printing Office.

Ackoff, R. 1974. *Redesigning the future*. New York: John Wiley & Sons.

Adams-Ender, C.L. and Hudock, J.M., Jr. 1989. The army nurse care team. *Nursing Management* 20 (March):63-64.

Agency for Health Care Policy and Research. 1990a. *Medical treatment effectiveness research*. Rockville, Md.: Agency for Health Care Policy and Research.

_____. 1990b. *Nursing advisory panel for guideline development: Summary*. Rockville, Md.: Agency for Health Care Policy and Research.

Aiken, L. and Hadley, J. 1988. *Factors affecting the hospital employment of registered nurses*. Report to the Secretary's Commission on Nursing, Department of Health and Human Services. Washington, D.C.: U.S. Government Printing Office.

Aiken, L. and Mullinex, C. 1987. Special report: The nurse shortage — myth or reality? *New England Journal of Medicine* 316(10):641-646.

Aiken, L.H. 1982. The impact of federal health policy on nurses. In *Nursing in the 1980s*, eds. L. Aiken and S. Gortner, pp. 3-20. Philadelphia: J.B. Lippincott.

Air Evacuation Program. *The Army Nurse*. June 1944.

Alan Guttmacher Institute. 1987. *Blessed events and the bottom line*. New York: Alan Guttmacher Institute.

Alexander, C.S.; Weisman, C.S.; and Chase, G.A. 1982. Determinants of staff nurses' perceptions of autonomy within different clinical contexts. *Nursing Research* 31:48-52.

Allison, S.E. 1985. Structuring nursing practice based on Orem's theory of nursing: A nurse administrator's perspective. In *The science and art of self-care*, ed. J. Riehl-Sisca. Norwalk, Conn.: Appleton-Century-Crofts.

Ambrose, E. 1917. How and where should attendants be trained? *Public Health Nurses Quarterly* 9 (July):260-268.

American Academy of Nursing. 1983. *Magnet hospitals: Attraction and retention of professional nurses*. Kansas City, Mo.: American Academy of Nursing.

American Association of Hospital Nurses. 1988. *Standards of occupational health nursing practice*. Chicago: American Association of Hospital Nurses.

American Hospital Association. 1989. *Hospital nursing personnel surveys: 1988 summary of major findings*. Chicago: American Hospital Association.

American Nurses Association. 1964. *Facing up to changing responsibilities*. New York: American Nurses Association.

_____. 1965. *Educational preparation for nurse practitioners and assistants to nurses: A position paper*. Kansas City, Mo.: American Nurses Association.

_____. 1973. *Standards of nursing practice*. Kansas City, Mo.: American Nurses Association.

_____. 1978. *Entry into nursing practice*. Kansas City, Mo.: American Nurses Association.

_____. 1980. *Nursing: A social policy statement*. Kansas City, Mo.: American Nurses Association.

_____. 1984. *Career ladders: An approach to professional productivity and job satisfaction*. Kansas City, Mo.: American Nurses Association.

_____. 1987a. *The scope of nursing practice*. Kansas City, Mo.: American Nurses Association.

_____. 1987b. *Standards of addictions nursing practice with selected diagnoses and criteria*. Kansas City, Mo.: American Nurses Association.

_____. 1988. *Nursing case management*. Kansas City, Mo.: American Nurses Association.

American Nurses Association, Drug and Alcohol Nursing Association, and National Nurses Society on Addictions. 1987. *The care of clients with addictions: Dimensions of nursing practice*. Kansas City, Mo.: American Nurses Association.

American Organization of Nurse Executives. 1990. *Current issues and perspectives on differentiated practice*. Chicago: American Hospital Association.

American Psychological Association, American Educational Research Association, and National Council on Measurement in Education. 1985. *Standards for educational and psychological testing*. Washington, D.C.: American Psychological Association.

American Psychiatric Association. 1947. Report of business meeting of the committee on psychiatric nursing of the American Psychiatric Association. American Psychiatric Association Archives, Committee on Nursing Files, box no. 2.

Anderson, R.; Chen, M.; Aday, L.A.; and Cornelius, L. 1987. Health status and medical care utilization. *Health Affairs* 6(1):136-156.

Andrews, H. and Roy, C. 1986. *Essentials of the Roy adaptation model.* Norwalk, Conn.: Appleton-Century-Crofts.

Archard, T. 1945. *G. I. Nightingale.* New York: W. W. Norton & Co.

Army Nurse Corps. 1949. *Diary Army Nurse Corps.* National Archives RG112. Washington, D.C.: Army Nurse Corps.

Army Nurse Corps Career Activity Office. 1976. *Report of the working conference on the nurse practitioner in the army medical system.* Anapolis, Md.: Army Nurse Corps.

_____.*Summary of warrant officer nurse program.* Army Nurse Corps Archives, U.S. Army Center of Military History, folder no. 117. Washington, D.C.: Army Nurse Corps.

Army Reorganization Act. Section 19, 31 Stat 753. 2 February 1901.

Atwood, J. and Hinshaw, A. 1981. Job stress: Instrument development program results. *Western Journal of Research in Nursing* 3(3):48.

_____.1984. *Nursing job satisfaction: A program of development and testing.* Research in Nursing and Health.

Atwood, M. 1985. *The Handmaid's Tale.* Fawcett-Crest, Valentine Books.

Aved, B. 1987. The Monterey County health initiative — A postmortem analysis of a California Medicaid demonstration project. *Medical Care* 25:35-45.

Aydelotte, M. 1988. *Nurse extender models: Long-term strategies.* Iowa City: The University of Iowa.

Bailey, H. 1936. The Bailey report: Nursing schools in psychiatric hospitals — Report of a survey. *American Journal of Nursing* 36.

Bailey, J.T.; Steffen, S.M.; and Grout, J.W. 1980. The stress audit: Identifying the stressors of ICU nursing. *Journal of Nursing Education* 19(6):15-25.

Barnard, K. 1978. *Nursing child assessment satellite training project manuals.* Seattle: University of Washington School of Nursing.

Barnum, B. 1989. Anger and creating one's world. *Nursing and Health Care* 10(5):235.

Barry, C.T. and Gibbons, L.K. 1990. DHHS nursing roundtable: Redesigning patient care delivery. *Nursing Management* 21:9-66.

Bartz, C.C. 1990. Army Nurse Corps, Professional Development Officer, Nursing Education, Branch Office of the Surgeon General. Personal communication. Washington, D.C.

Bayer, R.; Caplan, A.L.; and Daniels, N. 1983. *In search of equity: Health needs and the health care system.* New York: Plenum.

Bazzoli, G.J. 1986. Health care for the indigent: Overview of critical issues. *Health Services Research* 21(3):353-393.

Benner, P. 1984. *From novice to expert: Excellence and power in clinical nursing practice.* Menlo Park, Calif.: Addison-Wesley.

Bermosk, L.S. 1963. Preparation for psychiatric nursing in the baccalaureate program. In *Education and supervision in mental health and psychiatric nursing,* p. 20. New York: National League for Nursing.

Berwick, D. 1986. Techniques for assessing the impact of new technologies in the neonatal intensive care unit. *Respiratory Care* 31:524-531.

Betz, M. 1981. Some hidden costs of primary nursing. *Nursing and Health Care* 2:150-154.

Beyers, M.; Mullner, R.; Byre, C.; and Whitehead, S. 1983. Results of the nursing personnel survey: RN salary and fringe benefits, part 3. *Journal of Nursing Administration* 13(6):16-20.

Blackburn, S. 1989. Measuring nursing management of the environment. Chicago: National Certifying Corporation.

———.1990. Personal communication

Blanchfield, F.A. 1945. Col. Florence A. Blanchfield, Superintendent Army Nurse Corps, to the Chief Professional Administration Service. Memorandum. National Archives RG112. Washington, D.C.: Office of the Surgeon General.

Blendon, R.J. and Taylor, H. 1989. Views on health care: Public opinion in three nations. *Health Affairs* 8(1):149-157.

Bodnar, E.M. 1988. Occupational health nurses emerge as future corporate care managers. *Occupational Health and Safety* (April):21-24.

Boston, C.M. 1990. Introduction. In *Current issues and perspectives on differentiated practice,* ed. American Organization of Nurse Education. Chicago: American Hospital Association.

Boston Gazette and Country Journal, 4 March 1776.

Bottoms, M.S. 1988. Competencies of liberal education and registered nurse behavior. *Journal of Nursing Education.* 27(3):124-130.

Brett, J.L.L. and Tonges, M.C. 1990. Restructured patient care delivery: Evaluation of the ProACT model. *Nursing Economic$.* 8(1):36-44.

Brimm, J. 1987. Computers in critical care. *Critical Care Nursing Quarterly* 9:53-63.

Brooten, D.; Kumar, S.; and Brown, L.P. 1986. A randomized clinical trial of early hospital discharge and home follow-up of very low birth-weight infants. *New England Journal of Medicine* 315:934-939.

Brown, E.L. 1948. *The Brown report: Nursing for the future.* New York: Russell Sage Foundation.

Bucklin, S. 1869. *In hospital camp: A woman's record of thrilling incidents among the wounded in the late war.* Philadelphia: J. E. Potter and Co.

Buerhaus, P. 1987. Not just another nursing shortage. *Nursing Economic$* 5:267-278.

Burgess, M.A. 1928. *Nurses, patients, and pockets.* New York: Committee on the Grading of Nursing Schools.

Butterfield, P.G. 1990. Thinking upstream: Nurturing a conceptual understanding of the societal context of health behavior. *Advances in Nursing Science* 12(2):1-8.

432

Caliandro, G.B. 1970. The visiting nurse movement in the Borough of Manhattan, New York City, 1877-1917. Ph.D. dissertation. Teachers College, Columbia University, New York, N.Y.

Callahan, D. 1990. *What kind of life? The limits of medical progress.* New York: Simon & Schuster.

Campbell, J. and Patton, M. 1986. External evaluation report of the St. Anthony Block Nurse Program. Unpublished report.

Can You Afford to Get Sick? *Newsweek*, 30 January 1989.

Capra, F. 1982. *The turning point: Science, society, and the rising culture.* New York: Simon & Schuster.

Center for Devices and Radiological Health. 1989. Panel I: The technological, regulatory, and legal factors that impinge on the nursing environment. In *Nursing and technology: Moving into the 21st century,* ed. Department of Health and Human Services. Washington, D.C.: U.S. Government Printing Office.

Centor, R. and Schwartz, J.S. 1985. An evaluation of methods for estimating the area under the receiver operating characteristic (ROC) curve. *Medical Decision Making* 5:149-158.

Charnes, M.P. and Schaefer, M.J. 1983. *Health care organizations: A model for management.* Englewood Cliffs, N.J.: Prentice-Hall.

Christy, T.E. 1970. *Cornerstone for nursing education.* New York: Teachers College Press.

Chrystal, C. and Crudi, C. 1985. Recertification: Toward the development of standards for assuring continued competence. *Journal of Allied Health* 13:252-262.

Clappson, G.C. 1964. *The training camp for nurses at Vassar College.* Lake Mills, Ia.: The Graphic Publishing Co.

Clark, K. 1990. Supply, demand, and salaries. *Journal of Nursing Administration* 20(3):4-30.

Clark, R.B. 1988. Fast track. *Annals of Emergency Medicine* 17:544-545.

Cleland, V. 1971. *Part-time nurses.* Detroit: Wayne State University

_____.1978. A human resource model for nursing. In *Entry into Nursing Practice,* pp. 39-46. Kansas City, Mo.: American Nurses Association.

_____.1990. Wage and salary principles. In *The economics of nursing,* pp. 87-135. Norwalk, Conn.: Appleton & Lange.

Cleland, V.; Bass, A.; McHugh, N.; and Montano, J. 1976. Social and psychological influences upon employment of married nurses. *Nursing Research* 25:90-97.

Cleland, V.; Bellinger, A.; Shea, F.; and McLain, P. 1970. Decision to reactivate nursing career. *Nursing Research* 19:446-451.

Cleland, V.; Quinn, M.E.; and Eggert, A. 1988. *Report of part-time nursing study.* University of California-San Francisco.

Cline, C.S. 1985. Credentialing and job practice in environmental health: An empirical study. *Public Health Reports* 100:427-432.

Clochesy, J. 1987. Introducing new technology: Biomedical engineers and staff nurse involvement. *Critical Care Nursing Quarterly* 9:53-63.

Coates, S.A.; Cyr, J.; Meislin, H.; and Valenzuela, T. 1988. Fast track: Urgent care within a teaching hospital emergency department — Can it work? *Annals of Emergency Medicine* 17:453-456.

Committee on the Grading of Nursing Schools. 1934. *Nursing schools: Today and tomorrow.* New York: Committee on the Grading of Nursing Schools.

The Commonwealth Fund. 1990. *Report on the nursing shortage.* New York: The Commonwealth Fund.

Coser, L.A. 1977. *Masters of sociological thought,* 2d ed. New York: Harcourt-Brace-Jovanovich.

Costs for Health-Care Plans Shoot Up 18.6 Percent. *Seattle Times,* 31 January 1989.

Cowles, E. 1895. Progress in the care and treatment of the insane during the half century. *American Journal of Insanity* 51:22.

Cronin-Stubbs, D. 1977. Job satisfaction and dissatisfaction among new graduate staff nurses. *Journal of Nursing Administration* 7(12):44-49.

Curtis, R. 1986. The role of state governments in assuring access to care. *Inquiry* 23:410.

Darling, H. 1986. The role of the federal government in assuring access to care. *Inquiry* 23:286-295.

Davis, S.M. 1987. *Future perfect.* New York: Addison-Wesley.

Deckert, B.; Oldenburg, C.J.; Pattison, K.A.; and Swartz, S.L. 1984. Clinical ladders. *Nursing Management* 15(3):54-62.

Deets, C. and Froebe, D.J. 1984. Incentives for nurse employment. *Nursing Research* 33:242-246.

del Bueno, D.J. 1988. The promise and reality of certification. *Image* 20:208-211.

_____.1990. Experience, education, and nurses' ability to make critical judgments. *Nursing and Health Care* 11(6):290-294.

Deloughery, G.W.; Gebbie, K.M.; and Neuman, B.M. 1971. *Consultation and community organization in community mental health nursing.* Baltimore, Md.: Williams & Wilkins.

Department of the Army. 1930. *Medical department: Army Nurse Corps, general provisions.* Army regulation 40-20. Washington, D.C.: Department of the Army.

_____.1948. *Department of the Army technical manual: Career management for army officers.* TM20-605. Washington, D.C.: Department of the Army.

_____.1959. *Medical service: Army Nurse Corps.* Army Regulation 40-20. Washington, D.C.: Department of the Army.

_____.1967. *Warrant officer program for army medical service.* Circulars no. 601-15. and 601-20. Washington, D.C.: Department of the Army.

Department of Health and Human Services. 1989. *Report of the 1989 NIH task force on nursing research*. Washington, D.C.: Department of Health and Human Services.

Departments of Social Services and Labor. 1984. *Collective labor agreement for the health care system*, pp. 101-106. The Netherlands.

Division of National Cost Estimates, Office of the Actuary, Health Care Financing Administration. 1987. National health expenditures, 1986-2000. *Health Care Financing Review* 8(4):1-36.

Division of Nursing, Health Resources and Services Administration, Department of Health and Human Services. 1990. *Registered nurse population, 1988*. Washington, D.C.: U.S. Government Printing Office.

Donabedian, A. 1966. Evaluating the quality of medical care. *Milbank Memorial Fund Quarterly* 44:166-180.

Donaldson, S.K. and Crowley D.M. 1989. The discipline of nursing. *Nursing Outlook* 9:113-120.

Donovan, L. 1980. What nurses want (and what they're getting). *RN* 43(4):22-30.

Dossey, L. 1982. *Space, time, and medicine*. Berkeley, Calif.: Shambala.

Doubilet, P.; Begg, C.; Weinstein, M.; Braun, P.; and McNeil, B.J. 1985. Probabilistic sensitivity analysis using Monte Carlo simulation. *Medical Decision Making* 5:157-177.

Durand, B. 1989. Children needing acute and chronic care. Paper presented at the scientific session of the annual meeting of the American Academy of Nursing in Denver, Colo.

Durio, P.; Muzychenko, M.; and Williams, R. 1986. Clinical ladders: Back to the drawing board. *Nursing Management* 17(7):53-54.

Duxbury, M.L.; Henly, G.A.; and Armstrong, G.D. 1982. Measurement of the nurse organizational climate of neonatal intensive care units. *Nursing Research* 31:83-88.

Dvorak, E.M. and Woods, R.P. 1989. *Relationship between certification and practice outcomes*. Chicago: National Certifying Corporation.

Ehrat, K.S. 1985. Liberal education skills in the field of nursing. Ph.D. dissertation. University Microfilms International, 8514906.

Eisenberg, L. 1987. Preventive pediatrics: The promise and the peril. *Pediatrics* 80:415-422.

Enthoven, A. and Kronic, R. 1989. A consumer-choice health plan for the 1990s, parts 1 and 2. *New England Journal of Medicine* 320:29-101.

Epting, R.J.; Haddy, R.I.; and Schaler, M.E. 1987. Nonemergency room use in patients with and without primary care physicians. *Journal of Family Practice* 24:389-392.

Establishing a Mechanism for Deriving Competency Statements for the Two Categories of Nursing Practice. *The American Nurse*, 15 September 1978.

Ethridge, P. and Rusch, S.C. 1989. The professional nurse/case manager in changing organizational structures. In *Series on nursing administration*, vol. 2,
ed.M. Johnson. Redwood City, Calif.: Addison-Wesley.

Everly, G.S. and Falcione, R.L. 1976. Perceived dimensions of job satisfaction for
staff registered nurses. *Nursing Research* 25:346-348.

Fagin, C.M. 1982. Nursing's pivotal role in American health care. In *Nursing in the
1980s*, eds. L. Aiken and S. Gortner, pp. 459-476. Philadelphia: J.B. Lippincott.

Fagin, C.M. and Jacobsen, B.S. 1985. Cost-effectiveness analysis in nursing
research. In *Annual review of nursing research*, vol. 3, eds. H. H. Werley and
J. J. Fitzpatrick, pp. 215-238. New York: Springer.

Farley, P.J. 1985. Who are the underinsured? *Milbank Memorial Fund Quarterly*
63:476-503.

Feetham, S.L. 1986. Hospitals and home care: Inseparable in the '80s. *Pediatric
Nursing* 12:383-386.

Felton, G. 1975. Increasing the quality of nursing care by introducing the concept of
primary nursing: A model project. *Nursing Research* 24:27-32.

———. 1990. Perspectives of the American Association of Colleges of Nursing. In
Current issues and perspectives on differentiated practice, ed. American Organization of Nurse Executives, pp. 70-75. Chicago: American Hospital Association.

Ferguson, M. 1987. *The Aquarian conspiracy: Personal and social transformation in our
time*, rev. ed. Los Angeles: J. P. Tarcher.

Fetter, M.; Feetham, S.; D'Apolito, K.; Chaze, B.A.; Fink, A.; Frink, B.B.; Hougart,
M.; and Rushton, C. 1989. Randomized clinical trials: Issues for researchers.
Nursing Research 38:117-120.

Finley, J.; Young, D.; and Morris, L. 1985. Reimbursement and technology assessment. In *Assessing medical technologies*, ed. Institute of Medicine, pp. 211-227.
Washington, D.C.: National Academy Press.

Fitzpatrick, J.C., ed. *The writings of George Washington from the original manuscript
sources*, vol. III. Washington, D.C.

Fitzpatrick, M.L. 1972. The National Organization for Public Health Nursing, 1912-
1952: Development of a practice field. Ph.D. dissertation. Teachers College,
Columbia University, New York, N.Y.

———. 1975. *The National Organization for Public Health Nursing: Development of a practice field*. New York: National League for Nursing.

Ford, W.C.; Hunt, G.; et al., eds. *Journals of the Continental Congress*, vol. II.
Washington, D.C.

Fox, R.C. 1986. Medicine, science, and technology. In *Applications of social science to
clinical medicine and health policy*, ed. L. Aiken and D. Mechanic, pp. 13-30. New
Brunswick, N.J.: Rutgers University Press.

Frederickson, K. 1990. Interim report on the results of the pilot unit: Theory-based
and professional nursing practice. Montefiore Medical Center, New York, N.Y.

Frederickson, K.; Strauman, T.; Jackson, B.; and Strauman, J. Forthcoming. Physiological status, symptom distress, and sickness impact: Testing hypotheses derived from the Roy Adaptation Model.

Freeman, H.E.; Blendon, R.J.; Aiken, L.H; et al. 1987. Americans report on their access to health care. *Health Affairs* 6:6-8.

French, O.E. 1988. Clinical ladders for nurses: Expect a resurgence of interest but there will be changes. *Nursing Management* 19(2):52-55.

Freund, D.A. and Hurley, R.E. 1987. Managed care in Medicaid: Selected issues in program origins, design, and research. *Annual Review of Public Health* 8:137-163.

Freund, D.A.; Hurley, R.E.; and Taylor, D.E. 1989. Gatekeeping the emergency department: Impact of a Medicaid primary care case management program. *Health Care Management Review* 14:63-71.

Frink, B. 1985. *Technology assessment in nursing*. Philadelphia: University of Pennsylvania.

Froebe, D.; Deets, C.; and Knox, S. 1983. What motivates nurses to join and remain with an organization? *Nursing Leadership* 6:22-33.

Fuszard, B.; Slocum, K.I.; and Wiggers, D.E. 1990. Rural nurses: Surviving the nurse shortage. *Journal of Nursing Administration* 20(5):41-46.

Garrison, L. and Wilensky, G. 1986. Cost containment and incentives for technology. *Health Affairs* 5:46-58.

Gilbert, P. 1989. Executive vice president's report. *Duval County Medical Society* (September):9.

Ginsberg, E. 1949. *The Ginsberg report: A program for the nursing profession.* New York: Macmillan.

Giovanetti, P. 1980. A comparison of team and primary nursing care systems. *Nursing Dimensions* 7:96-100.

_____. 1986. Evaluation of primary nursing. In *Annual review of nursing research*, vol. 4, eds. H.H. Werley, J.J. Fitzpatrick, and R.L. Taunton, pp. 127-151. New York: Springer.

Glaser, W.A. 1986. Payment systems and their effects. In *Applications of social science to clinical medicine and health policy*, eds. L. Aiken and D. Mechanic, pp. 481-499. New Brunswick, N.J.: Rutgers University Press.

Glass, A.J. and Bernucci, R.J., eds. 1966. *Medical department United States Army: Neuropsychiatry in World War II*, vol. 1. Washington, D.C.: U.S. Government Printing Office.

Godfrey, M.A. 1978. Job satisfaction — Or should that be dissatisfaction? How nurses feel about nursing, part 1. *Nursing78* 8(4):89-102.

Goldmark, J. 1923. *Goldmark report: Nursing and nursing education in the United States.* New York: Macmillan.

Goldsmith, J. 1989. A radical prescription for hospitals. *Harvard Business Review* (May-June):104-111.

Goodman, C. 1985. Appendix A: Profiles of 20 technological assessment programs. In *Assessing medical technologies*, ed. Institute of Medicine, pp. 255-260. Washington, D.C.: National Academy Press.

Habenstreit, B. 1986. Health care patterns of nonurgent patients in an inner-city emergency room. *New York State Journal of Medicine* 86:517-521.

Haller, K.B. 1989. Methods to identify patient outcomes dependent on nursing actions. Chicago: National Certifying Corporation.

Harman, W.W. 1977. The coming transformation. *The Futurist* (April).

Hartz, A.J.; Krakauer, H.; Kuhn, E.M.; Young, M.; Jacobsen, S.J.; Gay, G.; Muenz, L.; Katzoff, M.; Bailey, R.C.; and Rimm, A.A. 1989. Hospital characteristics and mortality rates. *New England Journal of Medicine* 321(25):1720-1725.

Haussmann, R.K.D.; Hegyvary, S.T.; and Newman, J.F. 1976. *Monitoring quality of nursing care*, part II. Washington, D.C.: Department of Health, Education, and Welfare.

_____.1977. *Monitoring quality of nursing care*. Hyattsville, Md.: Department of Health, Education, and Welfare.

Hawken, P.L. 1990. Perspectives of the National League for Nursing. In *Current issues and perspectives on differentiated practice*, ed. American Organization of Nurse Executives. Chicago: American Hospital Association.

Hays, A.M. 1968. Nursing behaviors of warrant officer nurses, United States Army Medical Service; as described by warrant officer nurses and their immediate supervisors. Master's dissertation. School of Nursing, The Catholic University of America, Washington, D.C.

Health Insurance Association of America. 1989. *Source book of health insurance data*. Washington, D.C.: Health Insurance Association of America.

Health Insurance Premiums to Soar in '89. *The Wall Street Journal*, 25 October 1988.

Heaton, L.D. Memorandum to Col. Mildred Irene Clark.U.S. Army Center of Military History Archives, Folder 97. Washington, D.C.: Army Nurse Corps.

Hegyvary, S.T. 1991. Issues in outcomes research. *Journal of Nursing Quality Assurance* 5(2):1-6.

Hegyvary, S.T. and Haussman, R.K.D. 1976. The relationship of nursing process and patient outcomes. *Journal of Nursing Administration* 6:18-21.

Henderson, V. 1978. *The nature of nursing: Remarks from the Yale University School of Nursing colloquium*. Videotape no. 3722. New Haven, Conn.: Yale University School of Nursing.

_____.1985. The essence of nursing in high technology. *Nursing Administration Quarterly* 9:1-9.

Hesterly, S. and Sebilia, A.J. 1986. Recognizing clinical excellence. *Journal of Nursing Administration* 16(12):34-38.

Himmelstein, D.U.; Woolhandler, S.; and the Writing Committee of the Working Group on Program Design. 1989. A national health program for the United States: A physician's proposal. *New England Journal of Medicine* 320:102-108.

Hinshaw, A. and Atwood, J. 1982. A patient satisfaction instrument: Precision by replication. *Nursing Research* 31:170-175.

Hinshaw, A.S.; Smeltzer, C.H.; and Atwood, J.R. 1987. Innovative retention strategies for nursing staff. *Journal of Nursing Administration* 17(6):8-16.

Hogan, D.B. 1979. *A study in the philosophy and practice of professional regulation.* Cambridge, Mass.: Ballinger Publishing Co.

Hohlen, M. et al. 1990. Access to office-based physicians under capitation reimbursement and Medicaid case management: Findings from the Children's Medicaid Program. *Medical Care* 28:59-68.

Horn, B.J. and Swain, M.A. 1977. *Development of criterion measures of nursing care.* Hyattsville, Md.: Department of Health, Education, and Welfare.

Hudson Institute. 1987. *Workforce 2000: Work and workers for the 21st century.* Indianapolis: Hudson Institute.

Hudson, T. 1990. Use of health professionals poses payment, authority conflicts. *Hospitals* 5 (October):48.

Hughes, D.; Johnson, K.; Rosenbaum, S.; and Liu, J. 1989. *The health of America's children: Maternal and child health data book.* Washington, D.C.: The Children's Defense Fund.

Hurley, R.E.; Freund, D.; and Taylor, D. 1989. Gatekeeping in emergency departments: Impact of a Medicaid primary care case management program. *Health Care Management Review* 14:63-71.

Hutchinson, M.; Himes, T.; and Davis, L. 1987. Preventing multiple body tube mix-ups. *Nursing* 87:17,57.

Identification and Titling of Establishment of Two Categories of Nursing Practice. *The American Nurse*, 15 September 1978.

Inglehart, J.K. 1982. Federal policies and the poor. *New England Journal of Medicine* 307:836-840.

_____.1985. Medical care of the poor: a growing problem. *New England Journal of Medicine* 313:59-63.

_____ 1987. Health policy report: Problems facing the nursing profession. *New England Journal of Medicine* 317:646-651.

Institute of Medicine. 1983. *Nursing and nursing education: Public policies and private actions.* Washington, D.C.: National Academy Press.

_____.1985a. *Assessing medical technologies.* Washington, D.C.: National Academy Press.

_____.1985b. *Preventing low birthweight: Summary.* Washington, D.C.: National Academy Press.

_____.1988. *Prenatal care: Reaching mothers, reaching infants,* ed. Sarah Brown. Washington, D.C.: National Academy Press.

Inzer, F. and Aspinall, M.J. 1981. Evaluating patient outcomes. *Nursing Outlook* 29:178-181.

Jackson, B.; Strauman, J.; Frederickson, K.; and Strauman, T. In press. Long-term biopsychosocial effects of Interleukin-2 therapy. *Oncology Nursing Forum.*

Jacox, A.; Pillar, B.; and Redman, B. 1990. A classification of nursing technology. *Nursing Outlook* 38(2):81-85.

Jalowiec, A. 1989. Measuring nursing process and practice outcomes. Chicago: National Certifying Corporation.

Jalowiec, A.; Powers, M.J.; and Reichelt, P. 1984. Nurse practitioner and physician care compared for nonurgent emergency room patients. *Nurse Practitioner* 2:39-52.

———.1985. *Levels of practice: Renegotiation of a different level.* Philadelphia: Hospital of the University of Pennsylvania Division of Nursing.

Jamieson, M. and Campbell, J. 1987. The St. Anthony Park Block Nurse Program. *American Journal of Public Health* 77(9): 1227-1228.

Jamieson, M. and Martinson, I. 1983. Block nursing: Neighbors caring for neighbors. *Nursing Outlook* 31(5): 270-273.

Jansen, D.E. 1979. The Henry Street settlement: A response to the needs of the sick poor, 1893-1913. Ph.D. dissertation. Teachers College, Columbia University, New York, N.Y.

Jennett, B. 1986. *High technology medicine: benefits and burdens.* Oxford: Oxford University Press.

Joel, L.A. 1990. Perspectives of the American Nurses Association. In *Current issues and perspectives on differentiated practice,* ed. American Organization of Nurse Executives. Chicago: American Hospital Association.

Johnson, D.E. 1959. The nature of the science of nursing. *Nursing Outlook* 7(4):291-294.

Johnson, J.H. 1988. Differences in the performances of baccalaureate, associate degree, and diploma nurses: A meta-analysis. *Research in Nursing and Health* 11:183-197.

Jones, K. 1975. Study documents effect of primary nursing on renal transplant patients. *Hospitals* 49:85-89.

Kaspar, J. 1986. Health status and utilization: Differences by Medicaid coverage and income. *Health Care Financing Review* 7(4):1-17.

Kenner, C. 1989. Measuring neonatal assessment. Chicago: National Certifying Corporation.

Kent, N.A. and Warner, J.S. An analysis of nursing staff propensities to leave hospital units and medical nursing. University of Rochester School of Nursing, Rochester, N.Y.

Kentucky Board of Nursing. 1990. *Commonwealth of Kentucky Board of Nursing annual report, 1989-90.* Louisville, Ky.: Kentucky Board of Nursing.

Kiely, M.L. and Meister, S.B. 1987. *Literature on prenatal screening for neural tube defects: concordance with standards of technology assessment.* Boston: Harvard University Press.

Kimball, M.C. 1990. Nation's health bill to rise 10.4 percent, U.S. says. *Healthweek* 4(1):1, 52.

Knaus, W.A. and Nash, D.B. 1988. Predicting and evaluating patient outcomes. *Annals of Internal Medicine* 109:521-522.

Kneedler, J.; Collins, S.E.; Gattas, M.A.; and Lavery, S.A. 1987. Competency-based career ladders. *Nursing Management* 18(7):77-78.

Koch, A. 1988. Financing health services. In *Introduction to health services*, 3d ed., eds. S.J. Williams and P.R. Torrens. New York: John Wiley & Sons.

Koerner, J. 1990. The relevance of differentiated practice in today's environment. In *Current issues and perspectives on differentiated practice*, ed. American Organization of Nurse Executives. Chicago: American Hospital Association.

Koerner, J.; Bunkers, L.; Nelson, D., and Santema, K. 1988. Implementing differentiated practice: The Sioux Valley Hospital experience. *Journal of Nursing Administration* 18(6):13-22.

Kramer, M. 1990. The magnet hospitals: Excellence revisited. *Journal of Nursing Administration* 20(9):35-44.

Kramer, M.F. 1989. *Research on the organizational structure, governance, and management influence on resources for quality patient care delivery.* Washington, D.C.: National Center for Nursing Research.

Kramer, M. and Schmalenberg, C. 1988. Magnet hospitals: Institutions of excellence, parts I and II. *Journal of Nursing Administration* 18:1-19.

Lancaster, F.W. 1990. Science and politics. *National Forum: The Phi Kappa Phi Journal* 74(4):2-4.

Lang, N. 1990. Policy and politics of patient outcomes. Paper presented at the Nursing Research Conference at Johns Hopkins University, Baltimore, Md.

Lang, N.M. and Marek, K.D. 1990. The classification of patient outcomes. *Journal of Professional Nursing* 6(3):158-163.

Larson, E. 1985. Infection control issues in critical care: An update. *Heart and Lung* 14:149-155.

Larson, E. and Sherer, B. 1983. The nurse-computer interface: Effectiveness of computerized arrhythmia monitoring. *Dimensions of Cardiac Care Nursing* 2:174-179.

Lawler, E.E., III. 1990. *Strategic pay.* San Francisco: Jossey-Bass.

Lawrence, P. and Lorsch, J. 1967. *Organization and environment: Managing differentiation and integration.* Boston: Harvard University Press.

Lee, E. 1942. *History of the school of nursing of the Presbyterian Hospital School of Nursing, 1892-1942.* New York: G. P. Putnam's Sons.

Lewis, H. 1984. Part-time nursing: How much of a career? *RN* 34-37.

Light, D.W. 1986. Surplus versus cost containment: the changing context for health providers. In *Applications of social science to clinical medicine and health policy*, eds. L. Aiken and D. Mechanic, pp. 519-542. New Brunswick, N.J.: Rutgers University Press.

Linacre, J.M. 1989. The Rasch measurement of robust estimators by means of independent rank orderings. Paper presented at the meeting of the Midwest Objective Measurement Seminar, Chicago.

Lindeman, C. 1989. Keynote address. In *Nursing and technology: Moving into the 21st century*, ed. Department of Health and Human Services, pp. 41-53. Washington, D.C.: U.S. Government Printing Office.

London, P. 1964. *The modes and morals of psychotherapy.* New York: Holt, Rinehart, & Winston.

Lowery, B.J. and Jacobsen, B.S. 1984. On the consequences of overturning turnover: A study of performance and turnover. *Nursing Research* 33:363-367.

Luft, H.S. 1986. Economic incentives and constraints in clinical practice. In *Applications of social science to clinical medicine and health policy*, eds. L. Aiken and D. Mechanic, pp. 500-518. New Brunswick, N.J.: Rutgers University Press.

Lysaught, J.P. 1970. *An abstract for action.* New York: McGraw-Hill.

———.1973. *From abstract into action.* New York: McGraw-Hill.

Machiavelli. 1513. *The Prince*, XV.

Malloch, K.M.; Milton, D.A.; and Jobes, M.O. 1990. A model for differentiated practice. *Journal of Nursing Administration* 20(2):20-26.

Manual of the Medical Department. 1900. Washington, D.C.: U.S. Government Printing Office.

Maraldo, P.J. 1989. The nursing solution. *Health Management Quarterly* 11(4):18-19.

Marek, K. 1988. Classification of outcome measures in nursing practice. In *Classification systems for describing nursing practice*, pp. 37-42. Kansas City, Mo.: American Nurses Association.

Marston. D. 1987. Does categorical teacher certification benefit the mildly handicapped child? *Exceptional Children* 53:423-431.

Martinez, N.H.; Schreiber, M.L.; and Hartman, G.W. In press. Pediatric nurse practitioners: Primary care providers and case managers for chronically ill children at home. *Journal of Pediatric Health Care*.

Martinson, I.; Jamieson, M.; O'Grady, B.; and Sime, M. 1985. The Block Nurse Program. *Journal of Community Health Nursing* 2(1):21-29.

Massachusetts General Hospital. 1921. Memorial and historical volume, together with the proceedings of the centennial of the opening of the hospital, p. 125.

Mattera, M. 1987. Nursing income: Experience begins to pay off. *RN* 50(11):34-40.

Maxwell, A.C. 1918. What Presbyterian Hospital (New York) nurses are doing. *American Journal of Nursing* 18:727-728.

McCloskey, J.C. 1974. Influence of rewards and incentives on staff nurse turnover rate. *Nursing Research* 23:239-247.

———.1983. Nursing education and job effectiveness. *Nursing Research* 32(2):53-58.

_____.In press. Autonomy and social integration: Two requirements for job contentment. *Image: Journal of Nursing Scholarship.*

McCloskey, J.C. and McCain, B.E. 1987. Satisfaction, commitment, and professionalism of newly-employed nurses. *Image* 19:20-24.

_____.1988a. Nurse performance: Strengths and weaknesses. *Nursing Research* 37(5):308-313.

_____.1988b. Variables related to nurse performance. *Image: Journal of Nursing Scholarship* 20(4):203-208.

McClure, M.L. 1976. Entry into professional practice: The New York proposal. *Journal of Nursing Administration* 6(5):12-17.

McClure, M.L.; Poulin, M.A.; Sovie, M.D.; and Wandelt, M.A. 1983. *Magnet hospitals: Attraction and retention of professional nurses.* Kansas City, Mo.: American Academy of Nursing.

McCormack, M.H. 1984. *What they don't teach you at Harvard Business School.* New York: Bantam Books.

McGhan, W.F.; Stimmel, G.L.; Gilman, T.M.; and Segal, J.L. 1982. Pharmacists as drug prescribers. *Evaluation and the Health Professions* 5:115-129.

McGrath, S. 1990. The cost-effectiveness of nurse practitioners. *Nurse Practitioner* 40-42.

McKibbin, R.C. 1990. *The nursing shortage and the 1990s: Realities and remedies.* Kansas City, Mo.: American Nurses Association.

McKinlay, J.B. 1979. A case for refocusing upstream: The political economy of illness. In *Patients, Physicians, and Illness*, 3d ed., ed. E.F. Jaco, pp. 9-25. New York: Free Press.

McNeil, B.J.; Keeler, E.; and Adelstein, S.J. 1975. Primer on certain elements of medical decision making. *New England Journal of Medicine* 293:211-215.

McNeil, B.J. and Parker, S. 1984. Decision analysis for public health: Principles and illustrations. *Annual Review of Public Health* 5:135.

Meister, S.B. 1989. Family health policy: A perspective on its development and trends for the future. In *Proceedings of the national conference on family nursing*, ed. L.G. Krentz, pp. 65-76. Portland, Oreg.: Oregon Health Services University

_____.1991. Children's hospitals REACH out: Content of care and impact in two pilot programs. Final report to The Robert Wood Johnson Foundation.

Meleis, A.I. 1985. *Theoretical nursing: Development and progress.* Philadelphia: J.B. Lippincott

Milio, N. 1970. *9226 Kercheval: The storefront that did not burn.* Ann Arbor, Mich.: University of Michigan Press.

_____.ed. 1983. *Primary care and the public's health.* Lexington, Mass.: Lexington Books.

443

_____.1984. Nursing research and the study of health policy. In *Annual review of nursing research*, eds. H.H. Werley and J.J. Fitzpatrick, pp. 291-306. New York: Springer.

_____.1986. Telematics in the future of health care delivery: Implications for nursing. *Journal of Professional Nursing* 2(1):39-50.

_____.1989. Developing nursing leadership in health policy. *Journal of Professional Nursing* 6:315-321.

_____.1990. The press and policymaking: Clues for creating a health-promoting climate. *International Quarterly of Community Health Education* 10(4):329-346.

Miller, C.A. 1988. Achieving a proper fit between health services and needs. In *Cost, quality, and access in health care*, eds. F.A. Sloan, J.F. Blumstein, and J.M Perrin. San Francisco: Jossey-Bass.

Mitchell, P.H.; Armstrong, S.; Simpson, T. F.; and Lentz, M. 1989. American Association of Critical Care Nurses demonstration project: Profile of excellence in critical care nursing. *Heart and Lung* 18:219-237.

Montag, M.L. 1980. Looking back: An associate degree education in perspective. *Nursing Outlook* 28(4):248-250.

Moos, R.H. 1986. Work environment scale manual, 2nd ed. Palo Alto, Calif.: Consulting Psychologists Press.

Moritz, P.; Hinshaw, A.S.; and Heinrich, J. 1989. Nursing resources and the delivery of patient care. *Journal of Nursing Administration* 19(5):12-17.

Morlock, L. 1990. Dialogue: A case for case management. *Focus on Mental Health Services Research* 3(1):1-2.

Mottaz, C.J. 1988. Work satisfaction among hospital nurses. *Hospital and Health Services Administration* 33(1):57-74.

Mullins, W.S. and Parks, R.J. 1974. *Medical training in World War II*. Washington, D.C.: Office of the Surgeon General.

Mundinger, M. 1985. Health service funding cuts and the declining health of the poor. *New England Journal of Medicine* 1:44-47.

Murphy, M. 1989. Nursing service-delivery systems. In *Nursing's vital signs: Shaping the profession for the 1990s*. Battle Creek, Mich.: W.K. Kellogg Foundation.

Murphy, M. and DeBack, V. 1990. Myths and realities. In *Current issues and perspectives on differentiated practice*, ed. American Organization of Nurse Executives. Chicago: American Hospital Association.

Murphy, R.M. and McNeil, D. 1986. Rural and urban hospital closures: A comparison. *Health Affairs* 5(1).

Mury, E.A., ed. Report of chief nurse, Army Nurse Corps mobilization unit at Ellis Island, New York Harbor. National Archives RG112. Washington, D.C.

Naisbett, J. 1984. *Megatrends*. New York: Warner Books.

National Archives. 1949. *Diary Army Nurse Corps*. National Archives RG112. Washington, D.C.

444

National Center for Health Services Research. 1985. *NCHSR extramural research*. Washington, D.C.: U.S. Government Printing Office.

———.1986. *NCHSR offers grants for research on health care technology assessment*. Washington, D.C.: U.S. Government Printing Office.

National Center for Health Statistics. 1985. *Health: United States, 1984*. Hyattsville, Md.: Department of Health and Human Services.

National Commission on Nursing. 1983. *Summary report and recommendations*. Chicago: The Hospital Research and Education Trust.

National Commission on Nursing Implementation Project. 1986. *Nursing programs now and in the future*. Milwaukee: National Commission on Nursing Implementation Project.

———.1989. *Nursing practice patterns (differentiated practice)*. Milwaukee: National Commission on Nursing Implementation Project.

National Commission to Prevent Infant Mortality Report. *Seattle Times,* 1 March 1990.

National Committee for the Improvement of Nursing Services. 1950. *Nursing schools at the mid-century*. New York: Osmond Johnson, Inc.

National Guidelines Aim to Bring Out Teachers' Best. *Chicago Tribune*, 18 July 1989.

National League for Nursing. 1918. Report of the National Organization for Public Health Nursing executive secretary. NOPHN archives, microfilm no. 11. New York: National League for Nursing.

———.1987. *Competencies of the associate degree nurse*. New York: National League for Nursing.

———.1989. *Characteristics of baccalaureate education*. New York: National League for Nursing.

National League of Nursing Education. 1917. *Standard curriculum for schools of nursing*. Baltimore, Md.: Waverly Press.

——— 1927. *A curriculum for schools of nursing*. National League of Nursing Education.

Naylor, M.D. 1990. *Nursing education and the shortage*. Chicago: American Hospital Association and American Nurses Association.

New Jersey State Nurses Association. 1967. Blueprint for nursing education initiated. *New Jersey Nurse* (May-June):3.

———.1968. Nursing education in transition: A plan for action in New Jersey. *New Jersey Nurse* (January-February):3.

———.1978. Position on nursing education and entry levels into practice. *New Jersey Nurse* (November-December):12.

———.1979. Task force for educational mobility. *New Jersey Nurse* (November-December):3.

_____. 1982. Resolution on educational preparation for practice. *New Jersey Nurse* (November-December):10.

New Salary Wars Promise Solid Gains This Year: Hospitals are Bidding Up Start and Shift Rates. *American Journal of Nursing* 88:113-122.

Newman, M.A. 1986. *Health as expanding consciousness*. St. Louis: C. V. Mosby.

New York State Nurses Association. 1985. *New York State Nurses Association Action Plan: Directions for Nursing in Health Care*. Guilderland, N.Y.: New York State Nurses Association.

Nursing Archives. Emerson's plan for health visitors. Ph.D. dissertation. Teachers College, Columbia University, New York, N.Y.

Nursing Restructuring Renews Focus on Patient-Centered Care. *Hospitals,* 20 April 1990.

Nutt, P. 1984. Decision-modeling methods used to design decision support systems for staffing. *Medical Care* 22:1002-1013.

Nutting, M.A. 1923. Thirty years of progress in nursing. *American Journal of Nursing* 23 (September):1027-1030.

Nutting, M.A. and Dock, L.L. 1907. *A history of nursing*. New York: G.P. Putnam's Sons.

Oberg, C.N. and Polich, C.L. 1988. Medicaid: Entering the third decade. *Health Affairs* 7(4):83-96.

Office of the Surgeon General. 1911. *Annual report of the surgeon general*. Washington, D.C.: U.S. Government Printing Office.

_____. 1920a. *Annual report of the surgeon general*. Washington, D.C.: U.S. Government Printing Office.

_____. 1920b. *Relative rank for members of the Army Nurse Corps*. OTSG circular letter no. 114, RG112. Washington, D.C.: National Archives.

_____. 1923. *Annual report of the surgeon general*. Washington, D.C.: U.S. Government Printing Office.

_____. 1945. Memorandum from Col. Florence A. Blanchfield, Superintendent Army Nurse Corps, to the Chief Professional Administration Service. National Archives RG112. Washington, D.C.: Office of The Surgeon General.

Onek, J.N. 1988. Forestalling adverse consequences of competition. In *Cost, quality, and access in health care*, eds. F.A. Sloan, J.F. Blumstein, and J.M. Perrin, pp. 158-170. San Francisco: Jossey-Bass.

Orem, D.E. 1985. *Nursing: concepts of practice*. New York: McGraw-Hill.

_____. 1990. *Nursing: concepts of practice*. St. Louis: C.V. Mosby Co.

Panel Issues New Warning on Infant Mortality Rate. *Seattle Times*, 1 March 1990.

Parse, R.R. 1981. *Man-living-health: A theory of nursing*. New York: John Wiley & Sons.

_____.1987. *Nursing science: Major paradigms, theories, and critiques.* Philadelphia: W.B. Saunders.

_____.1990. Health: A personal commitment. *Nursing Science Quarterly* 3:136-140.

Parsons, T., ed. 1880. *Memoir of Emily Elizabeth Parsons.* Boston: Little, Brown and Co.

Peplau, H.E. 1956. Historical development of psychiatric nursing: A preliminary statement of some facts and trends. Paper presented at the Working Conference on Graduate Education in Psychiatric Nursing, Williamsburg, Va.

_____.1967. Psychiatric nursing. In *Comprehensive textbook of psychiatry,* eds. A.U. Freedman and H.I. Kaplan. Baltimore, Md.: Williams & Wilkins.

Perez-Woods, R. 1990. Use of a social action research framework to determine the content validity of the NCC certification examinations. In review.

Pettengill, M.M., ed. 1987. *Final report — Associate degree nursing: Facilitating competency development.* Indianapolis: Midwest Alliance in Nursing.

Pettengill, M.M. and Stull, M.K., eds. 1987. *Nurses in agreement: Controlling our future.* Indianapolis: Midwest Alliance in Nursing.

Pierce, P.M. and Freedman, S.A. 1983. The REACH project: An innovative health delivery model for medically-dependent children. *Children's Health Care* 12:86-89.

Pierce, P.M.; Freedman, S.A.; Frauman, A.C.; and DeBusk, F.I. 1985. Reducing costs with a community outreach program. *Pediatric Nursing* 11:361-364.

Pierce, P.M. and Weiss, D.E. 1983. REACH: Monitoring home-based nursing support. *Nursing Management* 17:33-36.

Pillar, B.; Jacox, A.; and Redman, B. 1990. Technology, its assessment, and nursing. *Nursing Outlook* 38:16-19.

Pirsig, R.M. 1974. *Zen and the art of motorcycle maintenance.* New York: William Morrow & Co.

Prescott, P. 1986. Use of nurses from supplemental services: Implications for hospitals. *Nursing Administration Quarterly* 11(1):81-88.

Preziosi, P. 1989. Developing a national health plan: Why now? Why nurses? *Public Policy Bulletin* (Fall).

Primm, P.L. 1986. Entry into practice: Competency statements for BSNs and ADNs. *Nursing Outlook* (May-June):135-137.

_____.1987. Differentiated practice for ADN- and BSN-prepared nurses. *Journal of Professional Nursing* 3:218-225.

_____.1990a. Approaches and strategies. In *Current issues and perspectives on differentiated practice,* ed. American Organization of Nurse Executives, pp. 17-134. Chicago: American Hospital Association.

_____.1990b. Decision-making complexity and accountability scales. Unpublished observations.

Pugliese, G.; Larson, E.; Foote, S.; Jackson, M.M.; and Hierholzer, W.J. 1986. Certification: Philosophy, goals, and methods, with application to the discipline of infection control practice. *American Journal of Infection Control* 14:11-19.

Ramsey, P.G.; Carline, J.D.; Inui, T.S.; Larson, E.B.; LoGerfo, J.P.; and Wenrich, M.D. 1989. Predictive validity of certification by the American Board of Internal Medicine. *Annals of Internal Medicine* 110:719-726.

Ramsey, S. 1927. Remarks on legislation for benefit of army nurse. In *The medical department of the United States Army in the World War*, ed. J.C. Stimson. Washington, D.C.: U.S. Government Printing Office.

Relman, A.S. 1989. Universal health insurance: Its time has come. *New England Journal of Medicine* 320:117-118.

Rexrode, J.S. 1978. Expectations and perceptions for the role of primary care nurse practitioner within the army health care system. Ph.D. dissertation. The Catholic University of America, Washington, D.C.

Rich, R.F. 1990. Policy-making for science and technology. *National Forum: The Phi Kappa Phi Journal* 74(4):16-19.

Richmond, J.B. and Kotelchuck, M.L. 1983. Political influences: Rethinking national health policy. In *Handbook on health professions education*. San Francisco: Jossey-Bass.

Riehl-Sisca, J., ed. 1985. *The science and art of self-care*. Norwalk, Conn.: Appleton-Century-Crofts.

Riis, P. 1988. Ethical aspects of medical technology. In *The economics of medical technology*, eds. F.F. Rutten and S.J. Reiser. New York: Springer-Verlag New York, Inc.

Rinke, L.T. 1987. *Outcome measures in home care*, vol. I. New York: National League for Nursing.

RN Vacancies Hit 12.66% in 1989. 1990. *American Journal of Nursing* 90(11):11.

Roberts, D.E. and Hudson, H.H. 1964. *How to study patient progress*. Washington, D.C.: Department of Health, Education, and Welfare.

Roe, W.I. 1985. Medical technology under PPS: An uncertain future. *Hospitals* 59:892.

Roemer, R.E. 1981. Vocationalism in higher education: Explanations from social theory. *Review of Higher Education* 4:23-46.

Rogers, M. 1989. Keynote speech. First Annual Differentiated Practice Recognition Seminar, Maryvale Samaritan Medical Center, Phoenix, Ariz.

Rossi, A.C., ed. 1973. *The feminist papers: From Adams to de Beauvoir*. New York: Columbia University Press.

Rossi, P.H. and Freeman, H.W. 1989. *Evaluation: A systematic approach*. Newbury Park, Calif.: Sage Publications.

Rotkovich, R. 1986. ICON: A model of nursing practice for the future. *Nursing Management* 17(3):54-56.

Roy, C. 1988. An explication of the philosophical assumptions of the Roy Adaptation Model. *Nursing Science Quarterly* 1(1):26-34.

_____. 1990. Dialogue on a theoretical issue: Strengthening the Roy Adaptation Model through conceptual clarification response. *Nursing Science Quarterly* 3(2):64-66.

Roy, C. and Andrews, H. 1991. *The Roy Adaptation Model: the definitive statement.* Norwalk, Conn.: Appleton & Lange.

Rules and Directions for the Better Regulation of the Military Hospital of the United States. Manuscript Collections, Library of Congress. 78(22):177-182. Washington, D.C.

Russel, M. V. and Williams, E. 1976. *Practice effectiveness of army nurse clinicians.* Ft. Sam Houston, Tex : United States Army, Academy of Health Sciences, Health Case Studies Division.

Sanford, R.C. 1987. Clinical ladders: Do they serve their purpose? *Journal of Nursing Administration* 17(5):34-37.

Schlotfeldt, R.M. 1988. Structuring nursing knowledge: A priority for creating nursing's future. *Nursing Science Quarterly* 1(1):335-338.

Schmal, J.A. 1966. *Experiment in change: An interdisciplinary approach to the integration of psychiatric content in baccalaureate nursing education.* New York: Macmillan.

Schoen, D. and Schoen, R. 1985. A life table analysis of the labor force participation of U.S. nurses, 1949 to 1984. *Research in Nursing and Health* 8:105-116.

Schorr, L.B. and Schorr, D. 1988. *Within our reach.* New York: Doubleday.

Schraeder, B.D. 1989. Measuring nursing management of technology in the NICU. Chicago: National Certifying Corporation.

Schrieber, G.J. and Pouillier, J.P. 1987. Recent trends in international health spending. *Health Affairs* 6(3): 105-112.

Schwab, S. and Pierce, P.M. 1986. Assessment of clinical nursing practice in a rural decentralized case-management system. *Public Health Nursing* 3:111-119.

Secretary's Commission on Nursing, U.S. Department of Health and Human Services. 1988. *Final report.* Washington, D.C.: U.S. Government Printing Office.

Selby, T. 1983. Block Nurse Program provides home care for older residents. *The American Nurse* (Nov./Dec.).

Senate Special Committee on Aging. 1985. *Americans at risk: The case of the medically uninsured.* Washington, D.C.: U.S. Government Printing Office.

Seybolt, J.W. 1979. *Identifying problems in the motivation, performance, and retention of nursing staff.* New York: National League for Nursing.

Seybolt, J.W.; Pavett, C.; and Walker, D.D. 1978. Turnover among nurses: It can be managed. *Journal of Nursing Administration* 8(9):4-9.

Shields, E.A., ed. 1981. *Highlights in the history of the Army Nurse Corps.* Washington, D.C.: U.S. Government Printing Office.

Shukla, R. 1981. Structure vs. people in primary nursing. *Nursing Research* 30:236-241.

Silva, N. and Aderholdt, B. 1989. Computerizing assessment of workload and productivity. *Nursing Management* 20:49-55.

Simpson, K. 1985. Job satisfaction or dissatisfaction reported by registered nurses. *Nursing Administration Quarterly* 9(3):64-73.

Slavitt, D.; Stamps, P.; Piedmont, E.; and Haase, A.M. 1979. Measuring nurses' job satisfaction. *Hospital and Health Services Administration* 24(3):62-76.

Sloan, F.A.; Blumstein, J.F.; and Perrin, J.M. 1988. Finding solutions to problems of access, quality assurance, and cost containment. In *Cost, quality, and access in health care*, eds. F.A. Sloan, J.F. Blumstein, and J.M. Perrin, pp. 1-20. San Francisco: Jossey-Bass.

Smeltzer, C.H. 1990. Consider this: Innovative pay package. *Journal of Nursing Administration* 20(7/8):6-7.

Snizek, W.E. 1972. Hall's professionalism scale: An empirical reassessment. *American Sociological Review* 37:109-114.

South Dakota Board of Nursing. 1988. *South Dakota statewide project for nursing and nursing education: Final report*. Sioux Falls, S.D.: South Dakota Board of Nursing.

Sovie, M.D. 1985. Managing nursing resources in a constrained economic environment. *Nursing Economic$*: 85-94.

Starr, P. 1982. *The social transformation of American medicine*. New York: Basic Books.

Statewide Project Steering Committee. 1988. *Final report of statement project for nursing and nursing education*. Sioux Falls, S.D.

Steering Committee on Future Health Scenarios. 1987. *Anticipating and assessing health care technology*, vol. 1. Dordrecht, Netherlands: Martinus Nijhoff Publishers.

Stimson, J.C. 1927. The Army Nurse Corps. In *The medical department of the United States Army in the World War*, vol. 8, part two. Washington, D.C.: U.S. Government Printing Office.

Strauman, J.; Frederickson, K.; and Jackson, B. 1987. Preliminary report of the biopsychosocial effects of Interleukin-2 cancer therapy. *Journal of New York State Nurses Association* 18:50-60.

Strickland, O.L. 1989. Theoretical models used to measure nursing practice. Chicago: National Certifying Corporation.

Strickland, O.L. and Waltz, C.F. 1988. *Measurement of nursing outcomes*. New York: Springer.

Study Sees RNs Still Gripped by Pay Compression. 1990. *American Journal of Nursing* 90(3):93, 112.

Swanson-Kauffman, K. 1986. Caring in the instance of unexpected early pregnancy loss. *Topics in Clinical Nursing* 8:37-46.

Swets, J.; Pickett, R.; Whitehead, S.; Getty, D.; Schnur, J.; Swets, J.B.; and Freeman, B. 1979. Assessment of diagnostic technologies. *Science* 205:753-759.

Tanner, C.A. 1987. Teaching clinical judgment. *Annual Review of Nursing Research* 5:153-173.

Taylor, E.J. 1926. Psychiatry and the nurse: Discussion for a paper by Arthur H. Ruggles, M.D. *American Journal of Nursing* 26:631.

Temkin-Greener, H. 1986. Medicaid families under managed care: Anticipate behavior. *Medical Care* 24:721-732.

Thwing, M.D. 1919. Discontinuance of the attendant service in Cleveland. *Public Health Nurses Quarterly* 11 (April):243-260.

Tobey, J.A. 1939. *Public health law.* New York: The Commonwealth Fund.

Tonges, M.C. 1989a. Redesigning hospital nursing practice: The professionally advanced care team (ProACT) model, part 1. *Journal of Nursing Administration* 19(7):31-38.

_____. 1989b. Redesigning hospital nursing practice: The professionally advanced care team (ProACT) model, part 2. *Journal of Nursing Administation* 19(9):19-28.

_____. 1990. ProACT: The professionally advanced care team model. In *Patient care delivery models,* eds. G.G. Mayer, M.J. Madden, and E. Lawrenz, pp. 13-35. Rockville, Md.: Aspen.

Toynbee, A. 1972. *A study of history.* New York: Oxford University Press.

Travers, S.T. 1972. Army nursing: Contemporary practice program. Paper presented at Chief Nurses' Conference, April 25-28.

United Hospital Fund. *Confronting the nursing shortage.* New York: United Hospital Fund.

U.S. Bureau of the Census. 1989. *Statistical abstract of the United States: 1988,* 109th ed., table 40. Washington, D.C.: U.S. Government Printing Office.

U.S. Department of Health and Human Services. 1989. *Nursing and technology: Moving into the 21st century.* Washington, D.C.: U.S. Government Printing Office.

Vagts, A. 1959. *A history of militarism: Civilian and military,* rev. ed. New York: Meridian Books.

Wald, L.D. 1906. The Henry Street (the nurses) settlement. *Charities and the Commons* 16 (April 7):36-37.

Wallis, N.E. 1987. Competence assessment in optometric specialty certification: The missing element. *Journal of the American Optometric Association* 58:948-953.

Wandelt, M.; Pierce, P.; and Widdowsen, R. 1981. Why nurses leave nursing and what can be done about it. *American Journal of Nursing* 81:72-77.

Warren, L. 1987. NSNCO meeting report. *American Association of Diabetes Educators News* 13:1.

Waters, Y. 1909. *Visiting nursing in the United States.* Philadelphia: William F. Fell Co.

Webster's Ninth New Collegiate Dictionary. 1991. Springfield, Mass.: Merriam-Webster.

Weinstein, M. and Fineberg, H. 1980. *Clinical decision making*. Philadelphia: W.B. Saunders.

Weisman, C.S.; Alexander, C.S.; and Chase, G.A. 1980. Job satisfaction among hospital nurses: A longitudinal study. *Health Services Research* 15:341-364.

_____.1981. Determinants of hospital staff nurse turnover. *Medical Care* 19:431-443.

Weiss, D.J.; Dawis, R.V.; England, G.W.; and Lofquist, L.H. 1979. *Manual for the Minnesota satisfaction questionnaire*. Minneapolis: University of Minnesota.

Werley, H. and Zorn, C. 1988. The nursing minimum data set: Benefits and implications. In *Perspectives in Nursing: 1987-1989*, pp. 105-114. New York: National League for Nursing.

Werley, H.H. and Lang, N., eds. 1988. The consensually derived nursing minimum data set: Elements and definitions. In *Identification of the nursing minimum data set*, pp. 105-114. New York: Springer.

Western Interstate Commission for Higher Education. 1985. *The preparation and utilization of new nursing graduates*. Boulder, Colo.: Western Interstate Commission for Higher Education.

Wilbur, R.S. 1979. Mandatory continuing medical education and recertification: Who needs them? *Journal of Occupational Medicine* 21:631-634.

Williams, K.R. 1981. Major trends in public health nursing, 1902-1925: The transition from specialized to generalized practice. Ph.D. dissertation. Teachers College, Columbia University, New York, N.Y.

Wilson-Barnett, J. 1981. Care evaluation: Sizing up the scores. *Nursing Mirror* 8(26):31-33.

Winslow, C.E.A. 1923. *Evaluation and significance of the modern public health campaign*. New Haven: Yale University Press.

Witzel, P.A. and Sovie, M.D. 1987. *Council of teaching hospitals: 1986 nursing care hours study*. University of Rochester School of Nursing, Rochester, N.Y.

Woods, R. 1990. Manuscript in preparation.

Zander, K. 1985. Second generation primary nursing. *Journal of Nursing Administration* 15:18-24.